Mechanisms of Pain

Pain is a serious health problem. This book presents an intensive review of the anatomy, physiology, and pharmacology of the systems that mediate nociceptive processing. The authors cover areas that include anatomy, central and peripheral nerve processing, tissue and nerve injury states, as well as preclinical and clinical models of pain. *Mechanisms of Pain* also covers important clinical concepts, with specific emphasis on mechanisms of action. Written by world-renowned global faculty, this book covers important areas of science required to understand pain medicine. Important topics covered include post–tissue and nerve injury pain states of primary afferents and the spinal cord. The authors also cover mechanisms of action of clinically relevant analgesics (opiates and non-opiates), psychological aspects of pain, pathophysiology of migraines, as well as the genetics of pain. This comprehensive book is to guide undergraduates, graduates, and clinicians in the field of pain medicine on important concepts related to the science and practice of pain.

Mechanisms of Pain

Edited by
Krishnan V. Chakravarthy
and Alaa Abd-Elsayed

CRC Press
Taylor & Francis Group
Boca Raton London New York

CRC Press is an imprint of the
Taylor & Francis Group, an **informa** business

Designed cover image: © Shutterstock

First edition published 2025
by CRC Press
2385 NW Executive Center Drive, Suite 320, Boca Raton FL 33431

and by CRC Press
4 Park Square, Milton Park, Abingdon, Oxon, OX14 4RN

CRC Press is an imprint of Taylor & Francis Group, LLC

ISBN: 978-0-367-53317-5 (hbk)
ISBN: 978-0-367-55614-3 (pbk)
ISBN: 978-1-003-09430-2 (ebk)

DOI: 10.1201/9781003094302

Typeset in Times
by Apex CoVantage, LLC

Contents

About the Editors

Dr. Krishnan V. Chakravarthy, MD, PhD, is an interventional pain and spine physician. He is the president and co-founder of Solaris Research Institute (SRI). Currently, he is also a partner at Innovative Pain Treatment Solutions and Surgery Center in Temecula, CA. He is also the founder of the Empower You Chronic Pain Foundation, focusing on patient access, advocacy, and knowledge. Dr. Chakravarthy is an affiliate professor in the Department of Anesthesiology and an affiliate professor in the Department of Nanoengineering at UCSD Health and VA San Diego Healthcare. Dr. Chakravarthy instructs medical students, residents, and fellows at UC San Diego School of Medicine, in addition to running his own institute and clinical work at the VA hospital. His research interests include incorporating new technology into advancing pain care. His research work has been featured in national and international venues and has been published in top journals, including *Anesthesiology*, *Proceedings of the National Academy of Sciences of the United States of America*, and *Pain*. He has, to date, lectured in over 400 regional, national, and international venues and has more than a hundred published works. Expertscape's PubMed-based algorithms placed Dr. Chakravarthy in the top 0.1% of scholars writing about pain management over the past ten years, defining him as a "world expert." He has won numerous national and international awards for his clinical and research work, most notably including the American Society of Pain and Neuroscience Young Innovator Award. He is considered an international thought leader in the pain space and serves on the advisory board of several major companies as well as the editorial board of several national and international journals. He has been involved in pioneering several first clinical cases in the United States and has been a founding faculty member of "restorative neurostimulation" and "closed-loop" stimulation. An entrepreneur, Dr. Chakravarthy is the founder of several biotechnology start-up companies. He has served as chair on several committees and in executive officer positions in organizations such as the International Neuromodulation Society, Pacific Spine and Pain Society, and American Society of Pain and Neuroscience. Currently, he is the president of the American Society of Pain and Neuroscience.

Dr. Alaa Abd-Elsayed, MD serves as the medical director of UW Health Pain Services, the medical director of UW Health Pain Clinic, and the division chief of chronic pain management and an associate professor of anesthesiology at the University of Wisconsin, Madison, Wisconsin, USA. He has published more than 350 peer-reviewed manuscripts, edited more than 30 books, authored dozens of book chapters, and serves on the editorial board of several prestigious journals, including *Pain Physician*, *Pain Practice*, *Journal of Pain Research*, *Neuromodulation*, *Pain and Therapy*, *Advances in Therapy*, and *Interventional Pain Medicine*. In addition, Dr. Abd-Elsayed serves as the editor-in-chief for *Pain Medicine Case Reports*. Dr. Abd-Elsayed serves on the board of directors of the American Society of Interventional Pain Physicians (ASIPP), the North American Neuromodulation Society (NANS), and the council of advisors of the American Society of Pain and Neuroscience.

Contributors

Abd-Elsayed, Alaa
University of Wisconsin School of Medicine and Public Health
Madison, Wisconsin

Abdallah, Rany T.
APICO Pain Management Bear
Bear, Delaware

Broachwala, Mustafa
University of California–San Diego
San Diego, California

Case, Laura
Department of Anesthesiology
University of California–San Diego
San Diego, California

Caylor, Jacob
Pain Specialists of America
Cedar Park, Texas

Chen, Jeffrey L.
University of California–San Diego Medical Center
San Diego, California

Cui, Christina
Department of Anesthesiology, Center for Pain Medicine
University of California–San Diego School of Medicine
San Diego, California

Ezell, Jacob
Department of Pain Management
Cleveland Clinic, Mayfield Heights
Mayfield Heights, Ohio

Furnish, Timothy
Department of Anesthesiology
University of California–San Diego Health
San Diego, California

Grate, Jeremy C.
Anesthesiology and Perioperative Medicine
Mayo Clinic, Rochester
Rochester, Minnesota

Green, Maja
Solaris Research Institute Inc., Clayton
Melbourne, Australia

Hassan, Amna
Mayo Clinic, Rochester
Rochester, Minnesota

Hernandez, Brandon A.
University of Wisconsin Health University Hospital
Madison, Wisconsin

Kalia, Hemant
CRISP (Center for Research and Innovation in Spine and Pain)
Rochester, New York

Lerman, Imanuel
Department of Anesthesiology, Center for Pain Medicine
University of California–San Diego School of Medicine
San Diego, California
Department of Radiology
VA San Diego Healthcare System
San Diego, California
Department of Electrical and Computer Engineering
University of California–San Diego
San Diego, California
VA Center of Excellence for Stress and Mental Health
VA San Diego Healthcare System
San Diego, California

Moheimani, Roya
Coast Spine Sports Medicine
Orange County and Santa Ana, California

Moskatel, Leon S.
Department of Neurology, Division of Headache
Stanford University
Palo Alto, California

Nazemian, Vida
Solaris Research Institute Inc., Clayton
Melbourne, Australia

Nelson, Eric
Western University of Health Sciences
Pomona, California

Reddy, Rajiv
Department of Anesthesiology, Center for Pain Medicine
University of California–San Diego School of Medicine
San Diego, California

Reyes, Zabrina
Tulane University School of Medicine
New Orleans, Louisiana

Rutledge, Thomas
VA San Diego Healthcare System and Department of Psychiatry
University of California–San Diego
San Diego, California

Schuster, Nathaniel M.
Department of Anesthesiology
University of California–San Diego Health
San Diego, California

Sheen, Soun
University of Massachusetts Chan Medical School
Worcester, Massachusetts

Shubayev, Veronica I.
Department of Anesthesiology
University of California–San Diego
VA San Diego Healthcare System
San Diego, California

Suh, Hyungseok
Department of Anesthesiology
Kyung Hee University
Seoul, South Korea

Towne, Brooke
Pacific Pain Consultants Encinitas
Encinitas, California

Tram, Jennifer
David Geffen School of Medicine
University of California–Los Angeles
VA Greater Los Angeles Healthcare System
Los Angeles, California

Villatoro-Lopez, Jasmin
University of Delaware
Newark, Delaware

Woolley, Christopher A
Interventional Pain Management
Sierra Neurosurgery Group
Reno, Nevada

Yin, Sopyda
Department of Anesthesiology, Center for Pain Medicine
University of California–San Diego School of Medicine,
San Diego, California

Zeidan, Fadel
Department of Anesthesiology
University of California–San Diego
San Diego, California

Zhang, Grace
Department of Physical Medicine and Rehabilitation
University of California–Los Angeles
VA Greater Los Angeles Healthcare System
Los Angeles, California

Zheng, Danielle
University of California–San Diego
San Diego, California

1 Pain
Introductory and Key Concepts in the Basis of Pain

Jennifer Tram, Grace Zhang, and Roya Moheimani

1.1 INTRODUCTION

Pain is a very complex experience that includes both sensory-discriminative and affective-motivational components that influence how patients respond to and remember pain. Our understanding of pain physiology continues to develop with research in pharmacology, nanotechnology, immunology, biochemistry, and genetics, such as prior research into the behaviors of *Paramecia* and *Tritonia*. This chapter discusses microorganism models of pain, pain terminology, neuroplasticity, and the sensory-discriminative and affective-motivational aspects of pain.

1.2 EVOLUTIONARY BASIS OF PAIN: FUNDAMENTAL DARWINISM

The scientific community's understanding of pain physiology continues to develop with emerging research in pharmacology, nanotechnology, immunology, biochemistry, and genetics.

What is currently known is that positive biological pressure toward attractants and, conversely, resistance against averse states are natural tenets of fundamental Darwinism. Pain behavior can be traced back to two evolutionary imperatives—obtaining nutrients and avoiding harm, which are universally expressed in the biology of all organisms (Walters and Williams 2019).

One example illustrating the evolutionary development of response to pain is the *Paramecia*'s response to chemical environmental cues. Elevated extracellular levels of glutamate, released by the bacteria, algae, and yeast, on which the *Paramecia* feed, activate receptor-mediated signal transduction to move this single-celled eukaryote forward. Conversely, inosine monophosphate (IMP), which displaces glutamate from its binding site, produces an inhibitory effect. It is believed that these extracellular cues allow the *Paramecium* to respond to stimuli that may be perceived as attractants or threats.

Simply put, the elevation of glutamate concentrations, linked to high concentrations of bacteria, will signal the organism to respond and forage. Specifically, glutamate plays a role in the chemosensory transduction pathway by lowering extracellular K^+ levels and increasing intracellular cAMP, a cyclic nucleotide second messenger

DOI: 10.1201/9781003094302-1

facilitating depolarization and enhancing ciliary beating. This subsequently leads to the repolarization of voltage-dependent K^+ channels and increases ciliary beating to rapidly move the organism forward (Yang et al. 1997). Conversely, high levels of IMP will alert the organism to sense toxic conditions and depolarize its cell membrane, thus setting off repulsion behaviors in ciliary beat and movement patterns (Van Houten, Yang, and Bergeron 2000). Interestingly, while other attractants may also hyperpolarize the cell membrane, glutamate alone specifically triggers the second messenger response of cAMP. Studies investigating this particular attractant are therefore instrumental, and it has been shown that glutamate also plays a role in mammalian and human responses to the pleasant "umami" taste attractant (Yang et al. 1997).

Several animal studies examining motor responses to sensory inputs further support the presence of pain-like behavior in nonconscious organisms. Investigation of the startle response in *Tritonia diomedea* shows that the mollusk will initiate an escape swim upon an aversive stimulus to one of its peripheral nerves (Frost et al. 2015). Likely an evolutionary response to the organism's natural predator, the sea star, *Pycnopodia helianthoides*, the *Tritonia* activates an escape swim circuit through a synaptic pathway comprised of command neurons and excitatory interneurons. Dorsal swim interneurons receive sensory input from afferent neurons, triggering rapid firing of interneurons and subsequent motor activation of a series of ventral and dorsal body flexion movements to escape (Katz and Frost 1995). Interestingly, the response is attenuated if only a weak stimulus is present, illustrating the mollusk's ability to subsequently tailor its all-or-none reflex (Frost et al. 2003). This is a phenomenon known as prepulse inhibition.

1.3 APPROACH-AVOIDANCE BEHAVIOR

The study of both *Paramecia* and *Tritonia* provides insight into the development of neural systems as a response to evolutionary pressures. The central pattern generator (CPG) in *Tritonia*, in particular, drives the mollusk's approach-avoidance behavior to mechanical and chemical afferent inputs (Katz and Frost 1995). Mechanoreceptive and chemoreceptive S-neurons translate signals across synaptic firing pathways to interneurons that activate the CPG and initiate motor response (Katz and Frost 1995). The regulation of this swim circuit pathway is dependent on the strength of stimulation; a single S-neuron alone does not activate the response. Similarly, mechanical stimulation alone does not activate the escape swim circuit. Prepulse inhibition will recruit inhibitory interneurons to prevent inhibition of motor patterns in the setting of a weak stimulus (Frost et al. 2003). On the other hand, a strong stimulus will trigger a cascade of excitatory interneurons to activate the CPG and, ultimately, contribute to a positive feedback loop. In short, different stimuli will either activate an "approach" or "avoid" response, exemplifying a functional polarity in neuronal behavior.

Investigation of *Tritonia*'s swimming behavior provides a simplified model of neural plasticity, which can contribute to the understanding of more complex neural circuitry involved in human pain. Human pain is linked to emotion, particularly anxiety and fear, which can trigger an avoidance response (Becker et al. 2018). Over time, this lends to the alteration of brain circuitry to connect pain with more of an emotional, rather than nociceptive, response (Becker et al. 2018). These learned maladaptive behaviors can often be exhibited in chronic pain patients and are important to address during motivational interviewing.

1.4 EVOLUTIONARY ADVANTAGES OF ACUTE PAIN SENSATION

Although unpleasant, acute pain is essential for life and survival and encourages avoidance of harmful stimuli. Case reports of individuals with congenital insensitivity to pain illustrate the necessity of sensorimotor responses to noxious stimuli (Nagasako, Oaklander, and Dworkin, 2003). These individuals were noted to die early in childhood as they were unable to sense pain (classified as a form of neuropathy) or generate an aversive response (Nagasako, Oaklander, and Dworkin 2003). A similar example of bodily damage incurred from insensitivity to pain includes the development of Charcot joints (Armstrong and Herr 2021). Altered pain and proprioceptive responses result in a destructive joint, a consequence of repetitive microtrauma to the weight-bearing joint.

1.5 NOCICEPTION

The nociceptive pathway is a neural feedback response enabling an organism to escape threatening stimuli. Winning him a Nobel Prize in 1932, C. S, Sherrington's discovery of the nociceptive flexion reflex pointed to the existence of a spinal reflex loop involving nociceptors. Similar to the quick, reflexive drawback one would experience when touching a hot stove, Sherrington's study demonstrated the presence of a flexion–withdrawal reflex away from high electrical stimulation to animal limbs (Skljarevski and Ramadan 2002). Years later, this nociceptive reflex would be studied in humans as the nociceptive flexion reflex (NFR). Similar to Sherrington's study, a polysynaptic withdrawal reflex could be elicited in all limbs with transcutaneous electrical stimulation of nerves. Decreased NFR thresholds are thought to be a contributor to the perception of acute pain. Repetitive stimulation of the sural nerve creates a temporal summation effect, leading to increased NFR and pain. This mechanism is thought to play a role in the pain central sensitization phenomenon (Skljarevski and Ramadan 2002).

In acute pain, peripheral nerve endings sense a stimulus and signal the release of pro-inflammatory cytokines, leading to widespread neuroinflammation when the stimulus is prolonged. An example of this is the conformational change that occurs in Vanilloid receptor channels in nociceptive neurons. Detection of a stimulus leads to the influx of calcium and subsequent depolarization, leading to the recruitment of pro-inflammatory cytokines, such as substance P and neurokinin A (Armstrong and Herr 2021). When these nociceptors are overly sensitive, a phenomenon known as allodynia may be observed. This describes the sensation of pain to typically non-painful stimuli, which is likely the result of oversensitive nociceptors responding to sub-noxious stimuli (Armstrong and Herr 2021).

Finally, it is important to note that pain itself brings about an emotional experience. As such, pain is inexplicably linked to consciousness, verbalization, and feeling. Without these cognitive and social aspects of pain, the processing of sensorimotor response to stimuli alone is merely termed *nociception*. Understanding the ability of emotion to modulate the pain experience is crucial in pain psychology. Not uncommonly, catastrophizing thoughts and anxiety lead to avoidant behavior in patients who are unable to adjust to pain (Lumley et al. 2011). This can be mapped out to the medial pain system, involving the anterior cingulate cortex, amygdala, and medial prefrontal cortex (Lumley et al. 2011). On the other hand, it is important to also encourage patients to refrain from suppressing feelings related to pain, as the presence of adaptive emotion is beneficial and protective (Lumley et al. 2011).

1.6 DEFINING PAIN

In 1979, the International Association for the Study of Pain (IASP) formally defined *pain* as "an unpleasant sensory and emotional experience associated with actual or potential tissue damage, or described in terms of such damage" (Raja et al. 2020). In response to concerns that this definition did not adequately address the psychological or ethical component of pain, the definition was later revised to "an unpleasant sensory and emotional experience associated with, or resembling that associated with actual or potential tissue damage" (Raja et al. 2020). The removal of the phrase "described in terms" also stemmed from concerns that the definition excluded individuals such as young children or people with intellectual disabilities who were unable to effectively verbalize or communicate their pain.

At its core, pain is an unpleasant experience that is often tied to emotional distress but does not necessarily need to be associated with actual or potential tissue damage. The presence of a noxious stimulus, and the resultant activation of the nociceptive pathway, does not always confer pain. Notably, the IASP definition of *pain* does not mention a stimulus and focuses instead on the emotional, unpleasant experience of pain.

Pain is a subjective and emotional experience influenced by biological, psychological, and social factors that are learned over a lifetime (Cohen, Quintner, and van Rysewyk 2018). It can vary greatly in terms of characterization, localization, severity, and duration between patients. Therefore, a patient's complaint of pain should be respected, as should the effects it has on their social and mental well-being.

The Cartesian model of pain proposed by Rene Descartes suggests that there is a fixed relationship between a stimulus and the degree of the response. It relies on the presence of a stimulus for the production and perception of pain along nociceptive pathways (Melzack and Katz 2013). In recent years, however, the popularity of the Cartesian model has lessened in favor of the biopsychosocial or neuromatrix model, which recognizes the psychological aspect of pain. The neuromatrix model implies that pain sensation and experience are primarily generated in the brain, as opposed to nociceptive pathways in local tissue or the peripheral nervous system. Therefore, according to this model, pain can occur even in the absence of a physical stimulus or tissue damage (Melzack 2001). This model is especially relevant when characterizing chronic pain conditions such as phantom limb pain or nonspecific pain that does not have an easily identifiable source (Melzack 1990).

The response to pain can be verbal, physiological, or behavioral. Table 1.1 provides examples of how the pain response can be separated into verbal, physiological, or behavioral responses.

TABLE 1.1
Examples of Types of Responses to Pain

Type of Response	Examples
Verbal	• "My pain is consistently a 6 out of 10." • "The sunburn on my shoulder hurts." • "I feel a burning pain on the side of my cheek."
Physiological	• Tachycardia • Tachypnea • Mydriasis • Diaphoresis • Piloerection
Behavioral	• Association of stimulus with pain • Avoidance of painful stimulus • Guarding

Verbal response to pain can be elicited by asking patients to rank their pain on a scale of 1 to 10, typically with 0 representing no pain and 10 representing the worst pain imaginable. Examples of quantifiable physiological responses include changes in blood pressure, heart rate, or respiratory rate (Cho and Hong 2021). Behavioral response to pain can vary from a quick reflex away from the painful stimulus to deliberate avoidance of the painful stimulus in the future. *Escape latency* is generally defined as the time taken for the individual to physically withdraw from the painful stimulus. Physiological and behavioral responses have been most useful in inferring pain in animal models.

1.7 PAIN TERMINOLOGY

The IASP has defined *allodynia* as "pain due to a stimulus that does not normally provoke pain." Allodynia implies the role of plasticity in pain encoding and reduction in the threshold for pain. Sometimes, *allodynia* is differentiated from *sensitization* in that allodynia occurs only in individuals who can verbally express pain, although the two are commonly used interchangeably.

There are two types of allodynia based on mechanism: dynamic mechanical allodynia and static mechanical allodynia. Dynamic allodynia is mediated by the physical movement of a usually non-noxious stimulus across hair follicles or Pacinian corpuscles in the skin (Buonocore et al. 2016). The mechanism behind dynamic allodynia has not been fully elucidated. Activation of A-beta mechanoreceptors, sensitization of peripheral nociceptive receptors, or changes in nociceptive processing within the central nervous system may all contribute to the pathogenesis of allodynia (Buonocore et al. 2016). Postherpetic neuralgia is a classic example of dynamic allodynia. Static mechanical allodynia is evoked by sustained stimulation of slowly adapting mechanical nociceptors (Landerholm and Hansson 2011). Static allodynia can be induced via the application of von Frey monofilaments to the skin.

Quantitative sensory testing with von Frey monofilaments or tuning forks can be used to differentiate between the two types.

Hyperalgesia is an increased response to a stimulus that is normally painful. It is not necessarily associated with a change in the pain threshold but, rather, is usually associated with an increase in the suprathreshold response.

Hyperalgesia can be further characterized based on location; hyperalgesia that occurs at the injury site is termed *primary hyperalgesia*, while hyperalgesia that occurs in undamaged tissue outside of the injury site is referred to as *secondary hyperalgesia* (Treede et al. 1992). This distinction was first clarified by the Hardy, Wolff, and Goodell experiments in the 1940s. In this study, pain sensation was induced through the application of a heat radiation lamp to local skin. The researchers noted that the threshold for mechanical and thermal nociception was reduced in the immediate injury site, whereas only the mechanical threshold was reduced in tissue adjacent to the injury site (Hardy, Wolff, and Goodell 1947). Therefore, primary hyperalgesia is likely mediated by changes in the peripheral and central nervous system, while secondary hyperalgesia is likely caused by changes in the central nervous system. This central sensitization causes an increased response to a nociceptive stimulus that previously evoked a less-intense response.

Hyperesthesia is a more general term that implies increased sensitivity to a stimulus and encompasses both hyperalgesia and allodynia. In 1994, IASP defined *hyperpathia* as "a painful syndrome characterized by an abnormally painful reaction to a stimulus, especially a repetitive stimulus, as well as an increased threshold." It involves a persistent stimulus that causes an intense pain response (Helme, Finnerup, and Jensen 2018). Hyperpathia is less commonly reported in the literature and is usually associated with neuropathic pain. *Analgesia* is an absence of pain or nociception, which can be preceded by *hypoalgesia*, which is a reduced pain response to a usually painful stimulus. Hypoalgesia is associated with a rightward shift in the stimulus–response curve. Hypoalgesia and analgesia can be achieved with various pharmacological agents, such as seen with the opioid family.

1.8 THE COMPLEX PAIN STATE

The experience and perception of pain are inherently complex. Melzack and Casey have proposed two distinct components of pain: the sensory-discriminative and the affective-motivational aspects. The sensory-discriminative part of pain focuses on its characterization, including location, intensity, duration, and quality (Novembre, Zanon, and Silani 2015). The affective-motivational component involves higher-order functions, such as memory, emotion, and suffering, and explains how anticipation of future pain can contribute to the pain experience and psychological distress (Auvray, Myin, and Spence 2010). For example, animal models have demonstrated anticipatory pain responses through significantly increased activity of nociceptive neurons at temperatures immediately below the level at which tissue injury and pain would occur (Auvray, Myin, and Spence 2010). In some cases, this anticipatory pain may be even more debilitating or distressing than the pain induced by the stimulus itself. The primary somatosensory cortex is implicated in sensory-discriminative pain, while the anterior insula and cingulate cortex are responsible for affective-motivational pain (Novembre, Zanon, and Silani 2015).

1.9 CONCLUSION

Animal studies in *Paramecia* and *Tritonia* have demonstrated the presence of pain-like and approach-avoidance behavior in simple-cell organisms. There are several evolutionary benefits of acute pain, specifically, the avoidance of painful or detrimental environmental stimuli. The International Association for the Study of Pain has defined *pain* as "an unpleasant sensory and emotional experience associated with, or resembling that associated with, actual or potential tissue damage." Of note, pain requires consciousness and verbalization, as the processing of sensorimotor responses to noxious stimuli alone is *nociception*. The Cartesian model explains pain as a fixed relationship between peripheral stimulus and response, while the neuromatrix model recognizes the role of the central nervous system in the generation of pain. Pain processing also involves some degree of neuroplasticity, as demonstrated by the development of hyperalgesia, allodynia, and hyperpathia. Finally, *pain* is a highly complex experience that includes sensory-discriminative and affective-motivational components that influence how patients respond to and remember pain.

REFERENCES

Armstrong, S. A., and M. J. Herr. 2021. "Physiology, Nociception." StatPearls Publishing accessed May 9. https://www.ncbi.nlm.nih.gov/books/NBK551562/.

Auvray, M., E. Myin, and C. Spence. 2010. "The Sensory-Discriminative and Affective-Motivational Aspects of Pain." *Neurosci Biobehav Rev* 34 (2):214–23. doi: 10.1016/j.neubiorev.2008.07.008.

Becker, S., E. Navratilova, F. Nees, and S. Van Damme. 2018. "Emotional and Motivational Pain Processing: Current State of Knowledge and Perspectives in Translational Research." *Pain Res Manag* 2018:5457870. doi: 10.1155/2018/5457870.

Buonocore, M., L. Demartini, A. M. Aloisi, and C. Bonezzi. 2016. "Dynamic Mechanical Allodynia—One Clinical Sign, Several Mechanisms: Five Illustrative Cases." *Pain Pract* 16 (3): E48–55. doi: 10.1111/papr.12416.

Cho, Y., and G. S. Hong. 2021. "Behavioral and Physiological Pain Responses in Brain-Injured Patients Who Are Unable to Communicate in the Intensive Care Unit." *Pain Manag Nurs* 22 (1):80–85. doi: 10.1016/j.pmn.2020.08.006.

Cohen, M., J. Quintner, and S. van Rysewyk. 2018. "Reconsidering the International Association for the Study of Pain Definition of Pain." *Pain Rep* 3 (2): e634. doi: 10.1097/PR9.0000000000000634.

Frost, W. N., T. A. Hoppe, J. Wang, and L.-M. Tian. 2015. "Swim Initiation Neurons in Tritonia Diomedea1." *American Zoologist* 41 (4):952–961. doi: 10.1093/icb/41.4.952.

Frost, W. N., L. M. Tian, T. A. Hoppe, D. L. Mongeluzi, and J. Wang. 2003. "A Cellular Mechanism for Prepulse Inhibition." *Neuron* 40 (5):991–1001. doi: 10.1016/s0896–6273(03)00731–1.

Hardy, J. D., H. G. Wolff, and H. Goodell. 1947. "Studies on Pain: Discrimination of Differences in Intensity of a Pain Stimulus as a Basis of a Scale of Pain Intensity." *J Clin Invest* 26 (6):1152–8. doi: 10.1172/JCI101907.

Helme, R. D., N. B. Finnerup, and T. S. Jensen. 2018. "Hyperpathia: 'to Be or Not to Be: That Is the Question'." *Pain* 159 (6):1005–9. doi: 10.1097/j.pain.0000000000001149.

Katz, P. S., and W. N. Frost. 1995. "Intrinsic Neuromodulation in the Tritonia Swim Cpg: The Serotonergic Dorsal Swim Interneurons Act Presynaptically to Enhance Transmitter Release from Interneuron C2." *J Neurosci* 15 (9):6035–45.

Landerholm, A. H., and P. T. Hansson. 2011. "The Perception Threshold Counterpart to Dynamic and Static Mechanical Allodynia Assessed Using von Frey Filaments in Peripheral Neuropathic Pain Patients." *Scand J Pain* 2 (1):9–16. doi: 10.1016/j.sjpain.2010.08.001.

Lumley, M. A., J. L. Cohen, G. S. Borszcz, A. Cano, A. M. Radcliffe, L. S. Porter, H. Schubiner, and F. J. Keefe. 2011. "Pain and Emotion: A Biopsychosocial Review of Recent Research." *J Clin Psychol* 67 (9):942–68. doi: 10.1002/jclp.20816.

Melzack, R. 1990. "Phantom Limbs and The Concept of A Neuromatrix." *Trends Neurosci* 13 (3):88–92. doi: 10.1016/0166–2236(90)90179-e.

Melzack, R. 2001. "Pain and The Neuromatrix in The Brain." *J Dent Educ* 65 (12):1378–82.

Melzack, R., and J. Katz. 2013. "Pain." *Wiley Interdiscip Rev Cogn Sci* 4 (1):1–15. doi: 10.1002/wcs.1201.

Nagasako, E. M., A. L. Oaklander, and R. H. Dworkin. 2003. "Congenital Insensitivity to Pain: An Update." *Pain* 101 (3):213–9. doi: 10.1016/S0304-3959(02)00482-7.

Novembre, G., M. Zanon, and G. Silani. 2015. "Empathy for Social Exclusion Involves the Sensory-Discriminative Component of Pain: A Within-Subject fMRI Study." *Soc Cogn Affect Neurosci* 10 (2):153–64. doi: 10.1093/scan/nsu038.

Raja, S. N., D. B. Carr, M. Cohen, N. B. Finnerup, H. Flor, S. Gibson, F. J. Keefe, J. S. Mogil, M. Ringkamp, K. A. Sluka, X. J. Song, B. Stevens, M. D. Sullivan, P. R. Tutelman, T. Ushida, and K. Vader. 2020. "The Revised International Association for the Study of Pain Definition of Pain: Concepts, Challenges, and Compromises." *Pain* 161 (9):1976–82. doi: 10.1097/j.pain.0000000000001939.

Skljarevski, V., and N. M. Ramadan. 2002. "The Nociceptive Flexion Reflex in Humans—Review Article." *Pain* 96 (1–2):3–8. doi: 10.1016/s0304–3959(02)00018–0.

Treede, R. D., R. A. Meyer, S. N. Raja, and J. N. Campbell. 1992. "Peripheral and Central Mechanisms of Cutaneous Hyperalgesia." *Prog Neurobiol* 38 (4):397–421. doi: 10.1016/0301–0082(92)90027-c.

Van Houten, J. L., W. Q. Yang, and A. Bergeron. 2000. "Chemosensory Signal Transduction in Paramecium." *J Nutr* 130 (4S Suppl):946S–9S. doi: 10.1093/jn/130.4.946S.

Walters, E. T., and A. C. C. Williams. 2019. "Evolution of Mechanisms and Behaviour Important for Pain." *Philos Trans R Soc Lond B Biol Sci* 374 (1785):20190275. doi: 10.1098/rstb.2019.0275.

Yang, W. Q., C. Braun, H. Plattner, J. Purvee, and J. L. Van Houten. 1997. "Cyclic Nucleotides in Glutamate Chemosensory Signal Transduction of Paramecium." *J Cell Sci* 110 (Pt 20):2567–72.

2 Organization of the Nervous System

Gross Anatomy

Brandon A. Hernandez, Jeremy C. Grate, and Alaa Abd-Elsayed

2.1 INTRODUCTION

This chapter will review the anatomy of the central and peripheral nervous system. There is a series of key terms to understand before diving deeper into the gross anatomy of the nervous system.

White matter. Myelinated axons. Surrounds the gray matter within the spinal cord. Found throughout the periphery and composes the majority of tissue within the cerebral hemispheres, cerebellum, and brain stem.

Gray matter. Nerve cell bodies, ganglia, dendrites, synapses, and unmyelinated axons. Forms an "H" shape within the spinal cord and can be found throughout the periphery and the surface of cerebral hemispheres.

Ganglion. A cluster of neuronal axons. Typically found within the PNS near major sites of innervation.

Nerve fiber. Typically refers to a cluster of nerve axons that serve a common function. It may reference a bundle of axons that serve different functions but travel within the same fascia.

2.1.1 Central Nervous System

2.1.1.1 Overview

The central nervous system can be thought of as the center of executive control within the nervous system. The CNS is home to the brain and the spinal cord, which serve as the crucial centers of nervous interaction and are necessary for much of the perception and interpretation of sense and thought.

2.1.1.2 Gross Anatomy

The CNS can be divided into cranial and vertebral components. The cranial portion of the CNS consists of the cerebrum, cerebellum, and brain stem, while the vertebral component consists of the spinal cord. There are two cranial nerves (cranial nerves I and II) that are commonly considered to be part of the central nervous system.[1]

DOI: 10.1201/9781003094302-2

2.1.1.3 Cranial CNS

2.1.1.3.1 Meninges

The brain is covered by three layers of meninges: the dura mater, arachnoid mater, and pia mater. The *dura mater* is the outermost meningeal layer that lines the periosteum of the skull.[1] The *arachnoid mater* is the middle meningeal layer and is composed of a loose and vascular network of tissue throughout the brain. The *pia mater* is the innermost meningeal layer, which closely adheres to the gyri and sulci of the brain.[1]

2.1.1.3.2 Lobes, Fissures, and Gyri of the Cerebral Cortex

The *cerebral cortex* refers to the outermost layer of the cerebrum. The lobes of the cerebral cortex are named based on the cranial bones, which they underlie and are separated by fissures or sulci. The frontal and parietal lobes are divided by the central fissure. The precentral gyrus, a component of the frontal lobe, is found anterior to the central fissure, while the postcentral gyrus, a component of the parietal lobe, is found posterior to the fissure. The temporal lobes are separated from the frontal and parietal lobes by the lateral fissure of Sylvius. The parietal and temporal lobes are further separated from the occipital lobe via the parieto-occipital fissure. Finally, the two cerebral hemispheres (left and right) are separated by the central longitudinal fissure.[1] The two cerebral hemispheres are joined together via the corpus callosum, which is a large bundle of nerve fibers and is typically considered to be a part of the brain stem.[2]

2.1.1.3.3 Limbic System

The limbic system lies just deep to the cerebral cortex and is primarily superficial to the corpus callosum. The system begins centrally but wraps laterally within both hemispheres, terminating at the amygdala and hippocampus, which form the largest portions of the system. The limbic system contains cortical and subcortical components. The cortical components are the cingulate cortex and the parahippocampal gyri. Some portions of the insula and prefrontal cortex are also considered part of the limbic system. The subcortical components of the limbic system are the hippocampus, amygdala, and hypothalamus.[2]

2.1.1.4 Brain Stem

Deep in the cerebral cortex lies the brain stem. The brain stem is further subdivided into the midbrain, pons, and medulla. The *midbrain* is continuous with the pons and medulla but forms the upper 1.5 cm of the brain stem.[2] The *pons* lies between the midbrain and the medulla and bulges anteriorly, forming the next 2.5 cm of the brain stem. The medulla is the most inferior portion of the brain stem and lies just anterior to the bulk of the cerebellum, composing the inferior 2.5 cm of the brain stem.[2]

2.1.1.4.1 Ventricles

Cerebrospinal fluid circulates throughout the brain and spinal cord via a system of ducts and chambers referred to as ventricles. [1] There are four ventricles contained within the brain. The lateral ventricles are the most superior and can be found on the medial aspects of the cerebral hemispheres. The foramen of Munro connects the lateral ventricles to the third ventricle, which is further connected to the fourth ventricle via the aqueduct of Sylvius. The fourth ventricle lies within the pons and further drains into the median and lateral apertures.[1] The central canal also extends from the fourth ventricle and carries CSF to the caudal medulla and spinal cord.[2]

2.1.1.4.2 Cerebellum

The cerebellum is approximately 1/10 of the size of the cerebrum and lies posterior to the brain stem and fourth ventricle within the posterior cranial fossa.[3] The cerebellum is rostrally separated from the cerebrum via the tentorium cerebelli, which is an extension of the dura mater. The cerebellum is superficially lined by an outer layer of gray matter that surrounds a body of white matter called the arbor vitae.[3] The *arbor vitae* further surrounds three pairs of cerebellar nuclei, which, listed medial to lateral, are referred to as the fastigial, interposed, and dentate nuclei.[3] The cerebellum is divided into three lobes via two transverse fissures, the primary and posterolateral fissures. The primary fissure separates the cerebellum into anterior and posterior lobes, while the posterolateral fissure divides the cerebellum into posterior and flocculonodular nodes.[3]

The cerebellum is attached to the brain stem via three pairs of peduncles: the inferior, middle, and superior peduncle. The middle peduncle is the largest of the three.[3]

2.1.1.4.3 Cranial Nerves I and II

Cranial nerve I, the olfactory nerve, conveys information about smell from the nasal cavity to the brain. The nerve CN1 is composed of white matter and is not surrounded by Schwann cells.[4] The axons of the olfactory nerve travel from the anterior cranial fossa through the cribriform plate and extend to the mucosa of the nasal cavity.[5] The olfactory bulb marks the termination point of the olfactory tract within the anterior cranial fossa, while the axons that travel to the nasal mucosa are often referred to as the olfactory nerves.[4] Cranial nerve II, the optic nerve, originates from the posterior pole of the ocular globe. It is important to understand that there are two bilateral optic nerves, one for each eye.[4] The optic nerve is divided into four segments: intraocular, intraorbital, intracanalicular, and prechiasmatic segments. The intraorbital is the longest segment of the optic nerve, followed by the prechiasmatic, then intracanalicular. The intraocular segment of the optic nerve is the shortest segment by far, measuring 1 mm long on average. Each optic nerve extends from the optic chiasm, where nasal fibers of the nerve cross. From here, the fibers of the nerve continue to extend posteriorly as two separate, bilateral optic tracts.[4] These optic tracts travel along the cerebral peduncles and synapse at the lateral geniculate nuclei. Additional nerve fibers that relay optic information extend from the lateral geniculate body, terminating at the primary visual cortex, which resides in the occipital lobe.[5]

2.1.2 Spinal Cord CNS

In an adult, the spinal cord originates from the top first cervical vertebra (C1) and terminates at the bottom edge of the first lumbar vertebra (L1).[1] The spinal column, cord, and nerves can be divided into cervical and thoracic sections. The general structure of the spinal cord remains consistent throughout each section in that vertebral bodies house the central cord, carrying myelinated and unmyelinated nerve axons, bodies, and nuclei, while pairs of spinal nerves extend from junctions between the vertebrae. The cervical portion is the most superior and is composed of 7 vertebral bodies and 8 pairs of spinal nerves extending from the central cord. The thoracic portion begins just inferior to the cervical portion (below the 7th cervical vertebrae) and is composed of 12 vertebrae and 12 pairs of spinal nerves. The 11th and 12th thoracic vertebrae typically mark the first point at which the spinal cord fibers begin to transition from a solid columnar cord into a more tapered appearance. The tapering that begins at the distal portion of the thoracic spinal cord is referred to as the conus medullaris. While the bony spine will continue to form lumbar, sacral, and coccygeal vertebrae, the nervous tissue composing the spinal cord terminates approximately at the first lumbar vertebrae.[1] It is relevant to note that the lumbar vertebrae have independent vertebral bodies, while the sacral and coccygeal vertebrae are fused. There are additional spinal nerve pairs: 5 lumbar, 5 sacral, and 1 coccygeal. These additional spinal nerve pairs extend distally to form the cauda equina.[1]

The spinal cord itself can be separated between outer white matter and inner gray matter. The gray matter forms an "H" shape within the center of the cord and is composed of neuron cell bodies, axons, and dendrites. The white matter surrounds this central gray matter, filling out the remainder of the columnar spinal cord, and is composed primarily of nerve fiber tracts. The same meninges discussed previously cover the spinal cord.[1]

2.1.3 Peripheral Nervous System

2.1.3.1 Overview

While the CNS is composed of the brain, brain stem, and spinal cord, the peripheral nervous system is composed of everything outside of this. It is made up of peripheral nerves, cranial nerves, spinal nerves, and their roots and branches.

2.1.3.2 Gross Anatomy

2.1.3.2.1 Spinal Nerves

There are 31 pairs of spinal nerves; 8 cervical, 12 thoracic, 5 lumbar, 5 sacral, and 1 coccygeal. Spinal nerves play an intermediary role between the CNS and the periphery. Each spinal nerve is made up of nerve fibers that extend from the dorsal and ventral roots of the spinal cord.[6] Within the intervertebral foramina is where the root fibers join together to form a spinal nerve to exit the vertebral canal. This holds for each nerve, except the C1 spinal nerve; this nerve exits the vertebral column in between the atlas and the occiput.[6] The spinal cord does not travel the entire length of the vertebral column. Due to this, more cranially located spinal nerves exit the spinal cord horizontally before entering the periphery, while the more caudally located spinal nerves have to travel more inferiorly within the spinal column before exiting; these are referred to as the cauda equina. Spinal nerves C1 to C7 exit the vertebral column above the vertebrae they are associated with. Spinal nerve C8 exits between C7 and T1, and each subsequent spinal nerve below this exits caudally concerning their vertebrae.[6]

Once the spinal nerve exits the vertebral column, it divides into a dorsal ramus and a ventral ramus, with the dorsal ramus usually being grossly smaller in size. The dorsal ramus branches innervate paraspinal muscles along with dermatomes in relation to the vertebral level. The much larger ventral ramus sends fibers to all major neural plexuses to provide sensorimotor innervation.[6]

The 12 spinal nerves originating from the thoracic spine make up the thoracic nerves. A *plexus* is a network of nerves or vessels.[7] Once the spinal nerve branches into the dorsal and ventral rami, the ventral rami of different levels of the spinal column come together to form the cervical plexus, the brachial plexus, and the lumbosacral plexus, which is made up of the lumbar and sacral plexuses. The cervical plexus is composed of the anterior rami of spinal nerves C1 to C5. The Brachial plexus consists of the ventral roots of C5–C8, with contribution from spinal nerve T1.[7] The lumbar and sacral plexuses overlap, and that is why it is called the lumbosacral plexus; however, they exist as two separate bundles anatomically. The lumbar plexus consists of branches from anterior roots of spinal nerves L1–L4 and sits superior to the pelvic rim while also going through the psoas muscle. Housed in the pelvic girdle, the major branches of the sacral plexus come from below the pelvic rim.[7]

2.1.3.2.2 Cranial Nerves

There are 12 cranial nerves, and technically, nerves I (olfactory nerve) and II (optic nerve) originate from the cerebellum, so they are a part of the CNS. The PNS contains the cranial nerves that originate from the brain stem, nerves III (oculomotor), IV (trochlear), V (trigeminal), VI (abducens), VII (facial), VIII (vestibulocochlear), IX (glossopharyngeal), X (vagus), XI (accessory), and XII (hypoglossal).[4]

Cranial nerve III (oculomotor) has somatic motor fibers that originate from the nuclear complex of the midbrain and parasympathetic fibers that arise from the Edinger–Westphal nucleus dorsal to the oculomotor nuclear complex.[4] The nerve runs superior to the posterior cerebral artery and inferior to the superior cerebellar artery, ultimately traveling through the superior orbital fissure to reach the orbit.[6]

Cranial nerve IV (trochlear) originates from the posterior brain stem and, similar to the oculomotor nerve, runs between the superior cerebellar artery and posterior cerebral artery, entering the orbit via the superior orbital fissure.[4, 6]

Cranial nerve V (trigeminal) is the largest cranial nerve and presents with three branches. The nerve itself originates from the midbrain and runs anteriorly from here, branching into V1, V2, and V3 divisions.[6] The ophthalmic (V1) division runs through the superior orbital fissure into the orbit. The maxillary (V2) division runs through the foramen rotundum, travels across the pterygopalatine fossa, and enters the orbit via the inferior orbital fissure. The maxillary division ultimately terminates at the face after traveling through the infraorbital foramen. The mandibular (V3) division travels through the foramen ovale to exit the skull and divides into additional branches.[4] Two key branches are the lingual and inferior alveolar branches. The lingual nerve of V3 travels inferior to the tongue. The inferior alveolar nerve of V3 travels through the mandibular foramen into the mandible.[4, 6]

Cranial nerve VI (abducens) originates from the abducens nucleus beneath the pons and enters the orbit via the superior orbital fissure.[4,6]

Cranial nerve VII (facial) consists of a proper and intermediate nerve complex.[6] The proper nerve contains motor fibers and originates from the pons, traveling through the temporal bone, passing through the facial canal, ultimately giving off three segments: labyrinthine, tympanic, and mastoid. The nerve exits the skull via the stylomastoid foramen and passes through the parotid gland. The chorda tympani segment of the nerve emerges from the mastoid portion of the nerve. The intermediate nerve contains sensory and parasympathetic motor fibers and originates from the superior salivatory nucleus and tracts anteriorly via the greater petrosal segment of the nerve.[6]

Cranial nerve VIII (vestibulocochlear) is composed of two separate nerves, the cochlear and the vestibular nerves, and originates from the brain stem. Both nerves travel across the internal acoustic meatus with the facial nerve and terminate at the cochlea, saccule, utricle, and semicircular canals.[4]

Cranial nerve IX (glossopharyngeal) originates from the lateral medulla and exits the skull via the jugular foramen. From here, the nerve branches into a lingual branch, which terminates in the posterior sublingual space and continues posteriorly to form pharyngeal, sinus, stylopharyngeus, and tympanic branches.[4, 6]

Cranial nerve X (vagus) originates from the lateral medulla and exits the skull via the jugular foramen, between the glossopharyngeal and accessory nerves.[6] The vagus nerve forms a superior ganglion within the jugular foramen and an inferior ganglion below the jugular foramen. It travels posteriorly in a vertical fashion into the upper mediastinum, branching here into the recurrent laryngeal nerve.[4] The nerve continues to dive posteriorly in a vertical fashion, entering the abdominal cavity through the esophageal hiatus.[6]

Cranial nerve XI (accessory) has cranial roots originating from the lateral cerebellomedullary cistern and spinal roots originating from the cervical spinal cord and travels superiorly via the foramen magnum.[4, 8] The roots then join and travel through the jugular foramen, posterior to the glossopharyngeal and vagus nerves. The nerve terminates at the trapezius and sternocleidomastoid muscles.[6, 8]

Cranial nerve XII (hypoglossal) originates from the medulla oblongata and exits the skull via the hypoglossal canal. From here, it runs medial to the glossopharyngeal, vagus, and accessory nerves and deep to the digastric muscle.[4] It ultimately innervates the extrinsic and intrinsic muscles of the tongue.[8]

2.1.3.2.3 Peripheral Nerves

Peripheral nerves may originate from spinal nerve roots, dorsal and ventral rami, and nerve plexuses or may be found independently throughout the body.[9] These nerves often have their branches, ultimately innervating all tissue and organs that are not already innervated by the central nervous system. Peripheral nerves contain a mix of myelinated and unmyelinated fibers, as well as somatic and autonomic fibers. The nerves themselves are arranged in fascicles, which contain individual nerve fibers. Each fascicle is surrounded by the perineurium, which contains layers of perineurial cells and collagen. Peripheral nerve fascicles are embedded in connective tissue, termed the epifascicular epineurium. The outer layers of this structure of connective tissue condense to form the nerve sheath. The organization of peripheral nerve fascicles can be incredibly variable; however, from a gross perspective, it is important to simply understand that a peripheral nerve may vary in diameter throughout its course throughout the body. Peripheral nerves can ultimately be seen as originating as larger, fascicular bundles of fibers encapsulated in connective tissue that ultimately branch into smaller and smaller nerve fibers, allowing the peripheral nerves to innervate the vast body area that they do.[9]

Two primary divisions of the autonomic nervous system (ANS) are evident within the peripheral nerves: sympathetic and parasympathetic divisions of the ANS. Autonomic neuronal bodies originate from the gray matter of the lateral horn of the spinal cord.[6] From the thoracic and lumbar regions of the spinal cord (T1–L2), sympathetic nerve axons and somatomotor axons exit the spinal cord via the ventral root. Sympathetic fibers originating from the spinal cord tend to terminate abruptly at the prevertebral ganglia located just outside of the spinal cord. Parasympathetic nerve fibers originate from the cranial and sacral regions of the spinal cord. These fibers are much longer than their sympathetic counterparts, which typically allows them to travel to the visceral ganglia or target tissue before terminating.[6]

REFERENCES

1. Schnell, Sally, and Mary Ellen Maher de Leon. "Anatomy of the central nervous system." *Seminars in Oncology Nursing*. Vol. 14. No. 1. WB Saunders, 1998.
2. Vanderah, Todd, and Douglas J. Gould. *Nolte's The Human Brain E-Book: An Introduction to its Functional Anatomy*. Elsevier Health Sciences, 2020.
3. Roostaei, Tina, et al. "The human cerebellum: a review of physiologic neuroanatomy." *Neurologic Clinics* 32.4 (2014): 859–869.
4. Romano, Nicola, Margherita Federici, and Antonio Castaldi. "Imaging of cranial nerves: a pictorial overview." *Insights into Imaging* 10.1 (2019): 1–21.
5. Naidich, T. P., M. Castillo, S. Cha, and J. Smirniotopoulos. *Imaging of the Brain*. Elsevier, 2013.

6. Kaiser, Joshua T., and Julian G. Lugo-Pico. "Neuroanatomy, spinal nerves." *StatPearls [Internet]* (2019).
7. van Alfen, N., and M. J. Malessy. "Diagnosis of brachial and lumbosacral plexus lesions." *Handbook of Clinical Neurology* 115 (2013): 293–310.
8. Sheth, S, and B. F. Branstetter 4th, and E. J. Escott. "Appearance of normal cranial nerves on steady-state free precession MR images." *Radiographics* 29.4 (2009): 1045–1055
9. Stewart, John D. "Peripheral nerve fascicles: anatomy and clinical relevance." *Muscle & Nerve* 28.5 (2003): 525–541.

3 Neurophysiology of Pain—Peripheral

Brandon A. Hernandez, Jeremy C. Grate, and Alaa Abd-Elsayed

3.1 INTRODUCTION

Pain is, unfortunately, an experience common to everyday life for all humans. The experience, however, is unique to everyone. The emotional and/or physical response that one has to a pain signal is what differentiates pain from the closely related term *nociception*. This unpleasant response defines *perception*, which is the final step of pain processing. The International Association for the Study of Pain revised its definition of *pain* in 2020 for the first time in 31 years. It is now defined as "[a]n unpleasant sensory and emotional experience associated with, or resembling that associated with actual or potential tissue damage." To understand what pain and pathological states of pain are, we first need to distinguish *pain* and *nociception*. It is then necessary to understand the anatomy and physiology of the nervous system. A commonly used method of dividing the nervous system is into the central nervous system and the peripheral nervous system. Here, we will describe the fundamentals of the peripheral nervous system, followed by how the peripheral nervous system is used to signal nociception, ending with certain pathologic states of pain.

3.2 DEFINITIONS: PAIN AND NOCICEPTION

The IASP has developed consensus definitions of important vocabulary innate to the understanding of pain. Key definitions are highlighted here, while a complete reference can be found on the IASP website.

> Nociception: The neural process of encoding noxious stimuli.
>
> (IASP)

> Nociception functions as an important alarm system alerting the individual to potential and actual tissue damage.
>
> (Sneddon)

> Pain: An unpleasant sensory and emotional experience associated with, or resembling that associated with, actual or potential tissue damage.
>
> (IASP)

DOI: 10.1201/9781003094302-3

The body's response to nociception may be automatic (as in sympathetic stimulation, with elevated heart rate and blood pressure) or behavioral (motor withdrawal reflexes). The sensation of pain is not necessarily implied by these responses.

Six keynotes and etymology are provided by the IASP:

- "Pain is always a personal experience that is influenced to varying degrees by biological, psychological, and social factors." (IASP)
- "Pain and nociception are different phenomena. Pain cannot be inferred solely from activity in sensory neurons." (IASP)
- "Through their life experiences, individuals learn the concept of pain." (IASP)
- "A person's report of an experience as pain should be respected." (IASP)
- "Although pain usually serves an adaptive role, it may have adverse effects on function and social and psychological well-being." (IASP)
- "Verbal description is only one of several behaviors to express pain; inability to communicate does not negate the possibility that a human or a nonhuman animal experiences pain." (IASP)

3.2.1 Peripheral Nervous System

3.2.1.1 Pain Signaling Pathway

In contrast to the definition of *pain*, *nociception* is the encoding and processing of noxious stimuli without any regard to the perception of these stimuli. This includes the transduction, transmission, and modulation of a pain stimulus initiated at the periphery and traveling to the central nervous system. These components of the pain processing pathway will be broken down into individual steps. Generally, nociception involves a process of neuronal signaling from the periphery to the central nervous system, either the spinal cord or the brain. This process starts with the activation of nociceptors in the tissues which suffer damage. This can be either thermal, mechanical, or chemical stress. For these noxious signals to become sensed, they need to be converted to neuronal signals, a process termed *transduction*. After the transduction of the signal, the neural passing of information centrally is called transmission. This subjective awareness of these pain signals is termed perception. Lastly, *modulation* is the modification of these nociceptive neuronal signals at any point along this pathway. Modulation typically refers to methods of decreasing the transmission of neural signals of nociception. The entire process of nociception, from transduction to perception, takes place throughout the entire nervous system, both peripheral and central.

3.2.2 Anatomy of the Peripheral Nervous System

3.2.2.1 Fibers

To best understand the transmission of nociceptive signals, certain anatomy becomes important to understand and appreciate. First, different types of nerve fibers transmit pain signals. To help explain the differences in how different types of tissue stimulation and damage elicit different perceptive experiences, we will explore these different types of nerve fibers.

First, peripheral nerve fibers come in many forms (A_α, A_β, A_δ, and C fibers). They are free nerve endings that respond to thermal, mechanical, and chemical stimuli, but typically only at damaging or aversive thresholds. A fibers are myelinated, whereas C fibers are not myelinated. Recall that *myelin* is an insulating sheath around nerve fibers produced by Schwann cells in the peripheral nervous system. This insulating sheath increases the speed at which impulses are conducted along the nerve fibers. Therefore, all types of A fibers will transmit signals faster than C fibers. A_α is the fastest-conducting and is responsible for proprioception; therefore, we will ignore these to discuss nociception. A_β fibers are the next fastest (conducting at 35–90 m/s) and are used to conduct signals from mechanoreceptors. These are what transmit signals from touch and pressure from the skin. A_δ is the slowest of the A fibers (conduct at 5–40 m/s) and transmits touch and thermal (cold and heat) signals from the skin. C fibers are unmyelinated and are the slowest-conducting (0.5–2 m/s) and transmit mechanical, thermal, and chemical signals (Sneddon).

Notice that both A fibers and C fibers transmit mechanical and thermal signals. A_δ and C fibers are the major pain-conducting fibers. It has been described that Aδ fibers are the signals of "first pain" due to myelination and the rapid conduction velocity. C fibers are responsible for "second pain," the longer-term, pressing, or dull pain perceived (Beissner). First pain is typically thought of as the immediate, instant pain sensation felt when experiencing a stimulus, such as touching a hot stove. The second pain is the lingering, burning pain that remains after touching the hot stove.

3.2.2.2 First-Order, Second-Order, Third-Order Neurons

First-order neurons are termed as such because they are the first neurons to carry signals from a stimulus in the periphery toward the CNS. These first-order neurons carry signals from the periphery to the spinal cord, synapsing with second-order neurons in the dorsal horn of the spinal cord. Second-order neurons carry signals to the thalamus along ascending pathways in the spinal cord, ultimately synapsing with third-order neurons. These third-order neurons carry signals from the thalamus to the primary sensory cortex of the brain, where higher-level processing and perception can occur (Aguggia).

3.2.2.3 Inflammatory Mediators

Certain inflammatory mediators exist in the periphery and are released for a variety of reactionary reasons. Such insults include surgical incision or other tissue injury. Inflammatory mediators activate peripheral nociceptors, act to sensitize functional nociceptors, and activate dormant nociceptors. The process of sensitization of peripheral nociceptors is important because they decrease the threshold for activation, increase the discharge rate with activation, and increase the rate of spontaneous discharge (Carr). These mediators include peptides, neurotransmitters, lipids, and neurotrophins, such as bradykinin, serotonin, prostaglandins, and nerve growth factor, respectively.

3.2.2.4 Neurotransmitters Involved in Pain

A variety of neurotransmitters are involved in modulating pain signals. These can be both excitatory and inhibitory and typically are from descending signals acting upon neuronal synapses. Excitatory neurotransmitters include, but are not limited to, glutamate, aspartate, vasoactive intestinal peptide, cholecystokinin, gastrin-releasing peptide, angiotensin, and substance P. Inhibitory neurotransmitters include, but are not limited to, enkephalins, endorphins, and somatostatin. Nociceptors can also release neurotransmitters, which also contribute to the inflammatory response, including substance P, which is released from the peripheral terminal (Besson).

3.3 TRANSDUCTION

All senses are perceived by humans in the brain in the form of neuronal signals. For the body to ultimately perceive pain from a noxious stimulus, the stimulus must first be converted to a neural signal. This process of transforming the stimulus into a neural signal is termed *transduction.* To initiate this process, nociceptors must be activated. *Nociceptors* are neurons that transmit a noxious stimulus from peripheral tissue to the spinal cord—that is, they are primary afferent neurons with free nerve endings in our skin, muscles, and viscera that sense noxious stimuli. The part of this nociceptor neuron that receives the input from a stimulus is termed the nociceptor transducer. This transducer is found on the membrane of the peripheral terminals of nociceptors (Osterweis).

The cell bodies of these neurons reside in the dorsal root ganglion of the spinal cord or the trigeminal ganglion of the face. Each primary afferent neuron is a pseudounipolar neuron that has a peripheral axon that travels to the periphery to receive information, and a central axon that transmits the information to the CNS (Bausbaum). A single afferent neuron with all its receptor endings makes up a sensory unit. The area in which these receptor endings reside makes up a receptive field and can overlap with other surrounding receptive fields. The degree of overlap and receptor density is what determines our ability to localize a painful stimulus (Pradeep).

Transducers respond to three types of stimuli: mechanical, thermal, and chemical. Different transducers are required to respond to each of these types of stimuli; however, each transducer shares a common chemical signaling pathway once activated. A noxious stimulus, whether thermal, mechanical, or chemical, leads to specific ion channels and G protein–linked receptors being activated, which either open or close, allowing for current to flow, generating an inward sodium or other cation current creating generator potentials, ultimately depolarizing the neuron. Once these generator potentials reach a threshold potential, voltage-gated sodium channels allow further sodium influx, and the signal propagates down the neuronal axon as an action potential. The frequency and duration of actional potentials from a nerve are influenced by the intensity and duration of the stimulus on the transducer (Gold). A common family of receptors that respond to noxious stimuli by causing generator potentials sufficient to cause an action potential are the transient receptor potential channels (TRP channels).

Transient receptor potential channels (TRP) are non-selective cation channels that respond to multiple stimuli and include TRPV 1, 2, and 3 receptors, which sense noxious heat, and TRPM8, which senses noxious cold (Stucky). A few other nociceptors that have been discovered are acid-sensing ion channels (ASICs), which sense hydrogen ions; P2X receptors, which sense ATP released during tissue damage; and Piezo receptors, which respond to mechanical stimuli (Woolf, Volkers).

3.4 TRANSMISSION

Once a noxious stimulus, be it mechanical, thermal, or chemical, is transduced to neuronal signals by transducers, the signal needs to be carried from the periphery to the central nervous system. The transfer of a pain signal by action potentials and by synaptic signaling along a peripheral nerve toward the spinal cord and ascending upward to the thalamus defines *transmission*. First, the first-order neurons (primary afferent fibers: A_β, A_δ, and C) carry the signal of the action potentials from the peripheral nerves to the central nervous system; specifically, they enter the spinal cord through Lissauer's (posterolateral) tract and terminate in the dorsal horn of the spinal cord. The cell bodies of these nociceptors exist in the dorsal root ganglion (Basbaum). When this action potential from the first-order neuron reaches the dorsal horn of the spinal cord, it synapses on a second-order neuron that will carry the signal from the spinal cord to the brain.

If the first-order neuron's action potentials are sufficiently frequent in arriving at the dorsal horn, neurotransmitters are released into the synapse in the dorsal horn of the spinal cord. Excitatory neurotransmitters (pain propagating) released in this synapse include glutamate, aspartate, vasoactive intestinal polypeptide, cholecystokinin, gastrin-releasing peptide, angiotensin, and substance P. Glutamate is the fastest of these. However, the other neuropeptides are more sustained via G protein–coupled receptors (Woolf). Inhibitory neurotransmitters responsible for the modulation and dampening of pain signals include enkephalins, endorphins, and somatostatin (Ganong). It is here in the synapse of the dorsal horn that both local modulation and descending modulation occur, permitting either amplification or reduction in the signal that is passed up the spinal cord to the brain.

Upon receiving a signal from the synapse in the dorsal horn of the spinal cord, second-order pain transmission neurons are activated and transmit the signal to the brain. Second-order neurons first decussate or cross from one side of the spinal cord to the opposite side via the anterior commissure in the same level of the spinal cord that the first-order neuron entered. The axons of the second-order neurons then subsequently travel up to the brain via various tracts in the spinal cord. Nociceptive information is typically found and carried in axons that travel along the spinothalamic tract, located in the anterolateral spinal cord. This pathway terminates in the ventroposterolateral (VPL) thalamus. Other nociceptive information has been found to travel in other tracts: spinoreticular tract (SRT), spinomesencephalic tract (SMT), spinocervical tract, and post-synaptic dorsal columns (Willis).

3.5 PERCEPTION

Perception of pain is the subjective awareness of pain. This process occurs as a nociceptive signal is processed in various centers of the brain. Generally, signals transmitted from the thalamus to higher centers that produce cortical responses ultimately generate the perception of pain. Certain areas of the brain are consistently activated by pain and are referred to as primary centers. There are also secondary or ancillary centers, where activation is variable among subjects (Pichurko).

3.6 MODULATION

Modulation is the alteration of the intensity of a noxious stimulus as it travels up the ascending pathway. Rubbing our head immediately after we bump it into an object to help alleviate the pain we experience is an example of a simple type of pain modulation explained by the "gate control theory." In 1965, Wall and Melzack proposed that by stimulating Aβ fibers near the site of injury, the transmission of concurrent nociceptive inputs is inhibited (Melzack). This idea postulates that there is a "gate" in the spinal cord that either permits the nociceptive signal to proceed or the signal is blocked. Since then, other mechanisms of modulation have been elucidated. Interneurons in the dorsal root ganglion and dorsal horn release endogenous opioid peptides, such as enkephalin and dynorphin, which reduce sensory transmission (Ganong). One notable descending inhibitory pathway originates in the locus coeruleus, which inhibits primary afferent terminals via norepinephrine-induced activation of α2 receptors (Llorca-Torralba). Other brain regions that can produce descending inhibition of pain processing include the sensory cortex, thalamus, hypothalamus, midbrain, pons, and medulla (Gebhart).

3.6.1 Pathologic States of Pain

The pain that one experiences when they grab a hot pan or step on a sharp nail can be described as physiologic pain. Physiologic pain is essential for survival as it elicits reflex withdrawal and avoidance of painful stimuli to protect us from further harm. When the nervous system becomes altered, pain may no longer be protective and may persist long after the initial noxious stimulus has resolved, leading to the development of pathologic pain.

3.7 WINDUP

Under normal circumstances, stimulation of peripheral nociceptors results in a proportional response in the dorsal horn. This response may become altered and increase disproportionally when a stimulus is repeated above a certain frequency. Mendell and Wall described this altered response to repeated stimuli in 1965 (Mendell). They found that brief C fiber stimulation led to neurons firing at a rate proportional to the amplitude of the input; however, repetitive C fiber stimulation at a frequency >0.5 and <10 Hz resulted in a nonlinear increase in the response of the dorsal horn neuron (Mendell, Mannion). This disproportionate increase in response to each successive input is termed *windup*. This results behaviorally in increased pain sensation to the same noxious stimulus (Mannion).

3.8 HYPERALGESIA/ALLODYNIA

As tissues are injured, the sensitivity of the nociceptive afferent fibers may increase to further ensure adequate tissue protection. The two conditions of this hypersensitivity that are known are hyperalgesia and allodynia. *Hyperalgesia* is a heightened pain response to a known noxious stimulus, whereas *allodynia* is a pain response to a normally non-painful stimulus (Aguggia, Sandkuhler). These two processes may occur due to peripheral and central sensitization. *Peripheral sensitization* is the result of nociceptive afferent fibers having a lower stimulation threshold secondary to the local release of chemicals at the site of tissue injury. Examples of these chemicals are potassium, bradykinin, substance P, histamine, serotonin, and prostaglandins, which can either activate or sensitize nociceptors (Ganong, Latremoliere). *Central sensitization* is often not uniformly defined but, in general, refers to changes in the processing of noxious stimuli in the central nervous system, leading to pain hypersensitivity (Latremoliere). Dysfunction within the nervous system at either the peripheral or central level may cause hyperalgesia and/or allodynia that persists after the resolution of the noxious stimulus, leading to the development of pathologic pain (Sandkuhler).

3.9 NEUROPATHIC PAIN

Neuropathic pain is defined by the IASP as "pain caused by a lesion or disease of the somatosensory nervous system." Either the peripheral or central nervous system can be affected, leading to peripheral, central, or mixed neuropathic pain. As opposed to nociceptive pain, neuropathic pain does not appear to have any protective function. It differs from other forms of chronic pain in that it no longer has an intact pain pathway. Nerve injury leading to neuropathic pain may be caused by trauma, toxin-induced injury, or a disease, such as diabetes. As the nerve is damaged, it may lead to spontaneous firing, along with alterations in the conduction and neurotransmitter properties of the nerve. The clinical manifestations across all forms of neuropathic pain are similar and include signs of hypersensitivity and hyposensitivity (Baron). These can include burning, tingling, numbness, "pins and needles" sensations, hyperalgesia, and allodynia. The pathophysiology is complex, but research has shown that increased expression and gain of function mutations in ion channels, along with upregulation of receptor proteins, are a few of the mechanisms involved (Baron). Diagnosing neuropathic pain as an entity distinct from nociceptive pain is very important to ensure proper treatment is initiated.

REFERENCES

Aguggia, M. "Neurophysiology of Pain." *Neurological Sciences*, vol. 24, no. S2, 2003, doi:10.1007/s100720300042.

Baliki, Marwan N., and A. Vania Apkarian. "Nociception, Pain, Negative Moods, and Behavior Selection." *Neuron*, vol. 87, no. 3, 2015, pp. 474–491, doi:10.1016/j.neuron.2015.06.005.

Baron, Ralf, et al. "Neuropathic Pain: Diagnosis, Pathophysiological Mechanisms, and Treatment." *The Lancet Neurology*, vol. 9, no. 8, 2010, pp. 807–819, doi:10.1016/s1474-4422(10)70143-5.

Basbaum, Allan I., et al. "Cellular and Molecular Mechanisms of Pain." *Cell*, vol. 139, no. 2, 2009, pp. 267–284, doi: 10.1016/j.cell.2009.09.028.

Beissner, Florian, et al. "Quick Discrimination of Adelta and C Fiber Mediated Pain Based on Three Verbal Descriptors." *PLoS ONE*, vol. 5, no. 9, 2010, doi:10.1371/journal.pone.0012944.

Besson, J. M. "The Neurobiology of Pain." *The Lancet*, vol. 353, no. 9164, 1999, pp. 1610–1615, doi:10.1016/s0140-6736(99)01313-6.

Carr, Daniel B, and Leonidas C Goudas. "Acute Pain." *The Lancet*, vol. 353, no. 9169, 1999, pp. 2051–2058, doi:10.1016/s0140-6736(99)03313-9.

Dinakar, Pradeep, and Alexandra Marion Stillman. "Pathogenesis of Pain." *Seminars in Pediatric Neurology*, vol. 23, no. 3, 2016, pp. 201–208, doi:10.1016/j.spen.2016.10.003.

Doleys, Daniel M. *Pain: Dynamics and Complexities*. Oxford University Press, 2014.

Ganong, William F., et al., "Somatosensory Neurotransmission: Touch, Pain, & Temperature." *Review of Medical Physiology*, McGraw-Hill Medical, 2015.

Gebhart, G. F. "Descending Modulation of Pain." *Neuroscience & Biobehavioral Reviews*, vol. 27, no. 8, 2004, pp. 729–737, doi:10.1016/j.neubiorev.2003.11.008.

Gold, Michael S. "Molecular Biology of Sensory Transduction." *Wall and Melzack's Textbook of Pain*, Elsevier, Saunders, 2013, pp. 31–47.

"IASP Terminology." *IASP*, 14 Dec. 2018, www.iasp-pain.org/Education/Content.aspx?ItemNumber=1698.

Koltzenburg, Martin. "Neural Mechanisms of Cutaneous Nociceptive Pain." *The Clinical Journal of Pain*, vol. 16, no. Supplement, 2000, doi:10.1097/00002508-200009001-00004.

Latremoliere, Alban, and Clifford J. Woolf. "Central Sensitization: A Generator of Pain Hypersensitivity by Central Neural Plasticity." *The Journal of Pain*, vol. 10, no. 9, 2009, pp. 895–926, doi:10.1016/j.jpain.2009.06.012.

Llorca-Torralba, Meritxell, et al. "Noradrenergic Locus Coeruleus Pathways in Pain Modulation." *Neuroscience*, vol. 338, 2016, pp. 93–113, doi:10.1016/j.neuroscience.2016.05.057.

Loeser, John D, and Ronald Melzack. "Pain: An Overview." *The Lancet*, vol. 353, no. 9164, 1999, pp. 1607–1609, doi:10.1016/s0140–6736(99)01311–2.

Mannion, Richard J., and Clifford J. Woolf. "Pain Mechanisms and Management: A Central Perspective." *The Clinical Journal of Pain*, vol. 16, no. Supplement, 2000, doi:10.1097/00002508-200009001-00006.

Melzack, R., and P. D. Wall. "Pain Mechanisms: A New Theory." *Science*, vol. 150, no. 3699, 1965, pp. 971–978, doi:10.1126/science.150.3699.971.

Mendell, Lorne M., and Patrick D. Wall. "Responses of Single Dorsal Cord Cells to Peripheral Cutaneous Unmyelinated Fibres." *Nature*, vol. 206, no. 4979, 1965, pp. 97–99, doi:10.1038/206097a0.

Osterweis, Marian et al. "The Anatomy and Physiology of Pain." *Pain and Disability: Clinical, Behavioral, and Public Policy Perspectives*, National Academy Press, 1988, pp. 123–145.

Pichurko, Adrian, and Richard E. Harris. "Neurobiology of Acute and Chronic Pain." *Oxford Textbook of Neuroscience and Anaesthesiology*, Oxford University Press, 2019, pp. 111–119.

Sandkühler, Jürgen. "Models and Mechanisms of Hyperalgesia and Allodynia." *Physiological Reviews*, vol. 89, no. 2, 2009, pp. 707–758, doi:10.1152/physrev.00025.2008.

Sneddon, Lynne U. "Comparative Physiology of Nociception and Pain." *Physiology*, vol. 33, no. 1, 2018, pp. 63–73, doi:10.1152/physiol.00022.2017.

Stucky, Cheryl L., et al. "Roles of Transient Receptor Potential Channels in Pain." *Brain Research Reviews*, vol. 60, no. 1, 2009, pp. 2–23, doi:10.1016/j.brainresrev.2008.12.018.

Volkers, Linda, et al. "Piezo Channels: from Structure to Function." *Pflügers Archiv—European Journal of Physiology*, vol. 467, no. 1, 2014, pp. 95–99, doi:10.1007/s00424-014-1578-z.

Willis, W. D. "Nociceptive Pathways: Anatomy and Physiology of Nociceptive Ascending Pathways." *Philosophical Transactions of the Royal Society of London. B, Biological Sciences*, vol. 308, no. 1136, 1985, pp. 253–268, doi:10.1098/rstb.1985.0025.

Woolf, Clifford J. "Pain: Moving from Symptom Control toward Mechanism-Specific Pharmacologic Management." *Annals of Internal Medicine*, vol. 140, no. 6, 2004, p. 441, doi:10.7326/0003-4819-140-8-200404200-00010.

Woolf, Clifford J., and Qiufu Ma. "Nociceptors—Noxious Stimulus Detectors." *Neuron*, vol. 55, no. 3, 2007, pp. 353–364, doi: 10.1016/j.neuron.2007.07.016.

4 DRG/Peripheral Nerve
Multicellular Modality and Coding

Hyungseok Suh and Veronica I. Shubayev

4.1 INTRODUCTION

The International Association for the Study of Pain (IASP) defines *pain* as "an unpleasant sensory and emotional experience associated with, or resembling that associated with, actual or potential tissue damage" (Raja 2020). As such, sensory capability for actual or potential tissue damage is a key component of pain. The peripheral nervous system (PNS) is what grants an individual this sensory capability, with the dorsal root ganglia (DRG) and peripheral nerves comprising the core structures of the PNS. To adequately understand pain, one must first develop a solid understanding of the anatomy, morphology, physiology, and support structures associated with the dorsal root ganglia and peripheral nerves. This chapter aims to provide readers with a succinct, rational, and focused approach to building their comprehension of these concepts so that they may more optimally address the complex phenomenon of pain and relieve suffering in their patients.

4.2 ANATOMY OF MAJOR STRUCTURES IN PRIMARY AFFERENT NEURON

4.2.1 Structure of the Peripheral Nerve

The nerve can be divided into three concentric groupings of fibrous membranes: the epineurium, perineurium, and endoneurium. The *epineurium*, or nerve sheath, is the outermost membrane that surrounds the entire nerve. The *perineurium* is the next smaller grouping membrane, which surrounds bundles of axons called nerve fascicles. The cells of the perineurium have tight junctions and help create a specially protected environment around nerve fibers. Lastly, at the smallest level, the *endoneurium* is the membrane that surrounds each myelin sheath that surrounds axons. Cross sections of these structures at increasing levels of magnification are seen in Figure 4.1.

4.2.2 Primary Afferent Neuron

The cell bodies of primary sensory neurons are located in the DRG and attached to two axons: the dorsal root in the central nervous system (central terminal) and the spinal nerve in the peripheral nervous system (distal terminal; Figure 4.2). The DRG cell body extends

 DOI: 10.1201/9781003094302-4

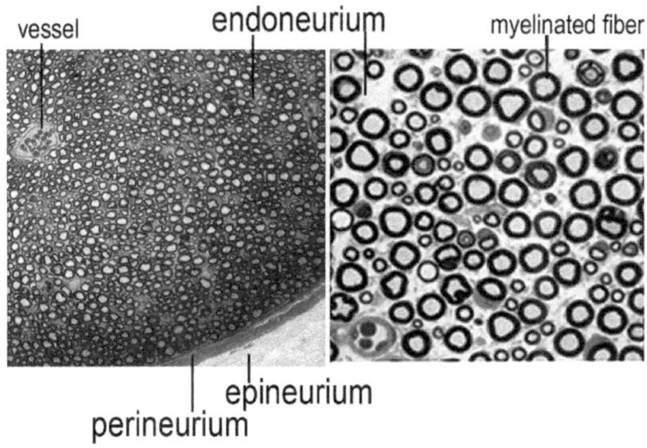

FIGURE 4.1 The peripheral nerve: the epineurium, perineurium, and endoneurium.

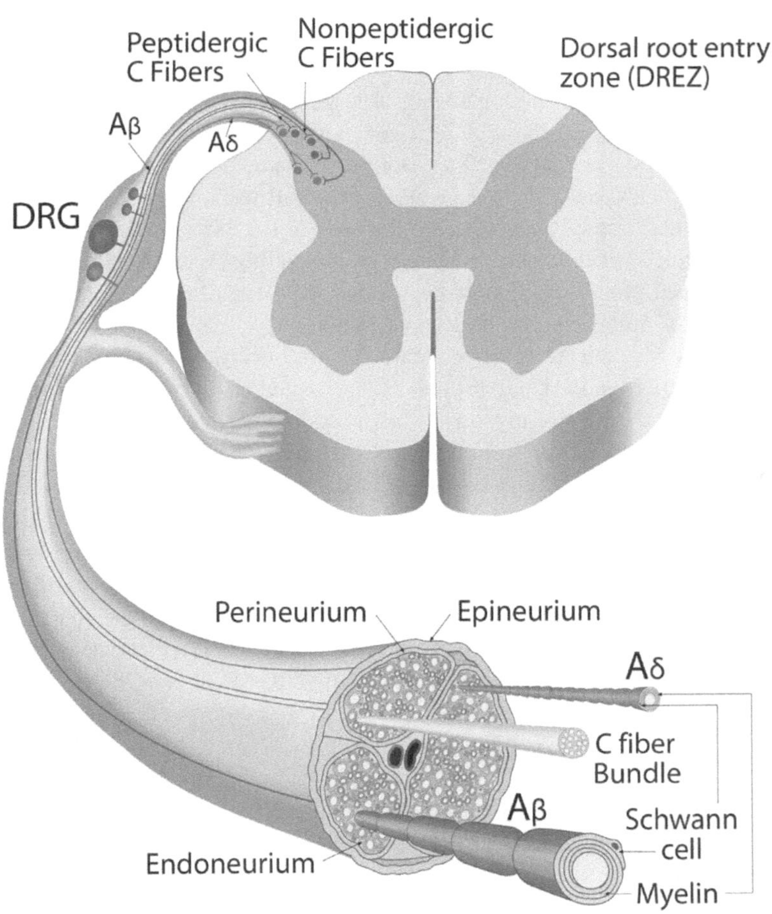

FIGURE 4.2 Primary afferent neurons.

bidirectionally to two axons via a bifurcated short-necked structure called the glomerulus, which is the reason that the primary afferent neuron is classified as pseudounipolar. Of note, the glomerulus and axons are extensions of the cell body and thus comprise a continuous channel of neuronal cytoplasm. Due to this continuous nature, action potentials traveling in the axons can also traverse into and depolarize the cell body.

From an embryological perspective, the DRG arises from the neural crest and sends sprouts, which become axons centrally into its somite, spinal cord, and peripherally to a target of sensory innervation. The DRG cell body then buds off from these axons by a glomerulus. This glomerulus is the route by which products synthesized in the cell body are transported to the central and peripheral terminals.

Due to the key role of primary afferent neurons in sensory/pain transmission from the periphery to the central nervous system, it has been recognized for decades as a key structure for the treatment of chronic pain. Thus, established therapies, including anesthesia, ganglionectomy, dorsal root entry zone (DREZ) lesioning, radiofrequency ablation/stimulation, and steroid injection, and the development of novel analgesic therapeutics aim to target primary afferent neurons (Esposito 2019).

4.2.2.1 Myelinated *vs.* Unmyelinated Fibers

Myelin is the lipid-rich insulating sheath of large-diameter (>1 μm) axons. The process of myelination ensures a rapid, efficient, saltatory nerve conduction of the mammalian nervous systems (Salzer 2015). Both myelinated and unmyelinated fibers are surrounded by Schwann cells, the primary glial cell responsible for myelination in the peripheral nervous system; however, the ratio of the axon to Schwann cell and to myelination effects differ. In myelinated fibers, including A-afferent fibers (as well as motor fiber), each axon is myelinated by a Schwann cell at a 1:1 ratio. Slow-conducting C fibers transmit impulses via the Remak bundle. Myelinating Schwann cells wrap their membranes around the A afferent axon in concentric layers to form a multilamellar myelin sheath. Myelin sheath propels voltage-gated sodium (Na^+) channels (Navs) to concentrate in the gaps of myelin, called nodes of Ranvier, so that currents underlying the action potential hop from one node to another, a phenomenon known as saltatory nerve conduction. Myelin damage causing ectopic insertion of Navs along the A afferent axon is believed to contribute to neuropathic pain, pain caused by injury or disease of the somatosensory nervous system (Devor 2009), discussed in what follows.

Contrasting this, in unmyelinated (C afferent) primary afferents, multiple axons are grouped within a single Schwann cell into Remak bundles. Schwann cells associated with C fibers are nonmyelinating. Figure 4.3 shows the differences in size and Schwann cell ratio between myelinated and unmyelinated fibers.

4.2.3 Types of DRG: A vs. B

Cell bodies of DRG can be divided into two main groups based on their size and histological staining qualities. Large-type A cells are connected to large, thickly myelinated A beta fibers and some thinly myelinated A delta fibers. Small-type B cells are connected to C fibers and some smaller A delta fibers. Selective immunohistochemical staining is used extensively to classify DRG cells. The most common neurotransmitter, glutamate, is present in cells of all sizes. In contrast, peptides are expressed in

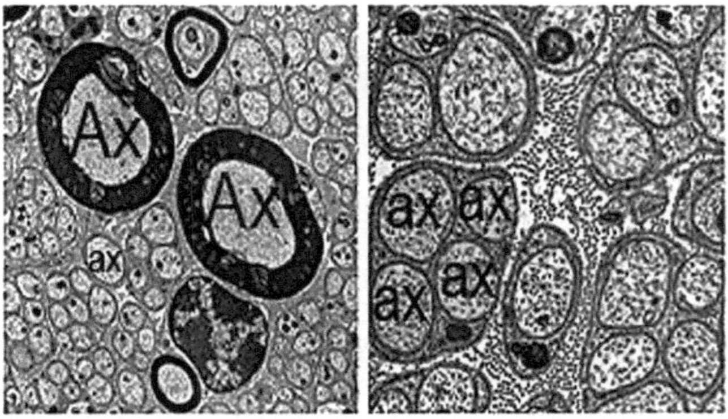

FIGURE 4.3 Myelinated and unmyelinated fibers.

TABLE 4.1
Classification of DRG Neurons by Surface Markers, Characteristics, and Neuropeptides

Marker	Characteristic	Sensory Cell Type
Parvalbumin	Calcium-binding protein found in subsets of sensory neurons, inhibitory interneurons, and motor neurons	Proprioceptors and Ap fibers
CGRP	Neuronal peptide transmitter	Peptidergic C fibers, subpopulation of AS fibers
Substance P	Neuronal peptide transmitter	Peptidergic C fibers
TRPV1	Capsaicin receptor which transduces high-intensity thermal and low-PH signals	Peptidergic C fibers
NF200	Found on large-cell (type A) proprioceptors	Myelinated AS fibers, Ap fibers, and non-peptidergic C fibers
IB4	Surface lectin found on subpopulation of small (type B) dark cells and not present on large (type A) cells	

a more selective fashion, with calcitonin gene–related peptide (CGRP), vasopressin, and oxytocin each histologically labeling more than 30% of the total DRG population, while substance P labels between 10 and 30% of DRG neurons. Frequently, peptides may be co-localized, with almost all substance P cells containing CGRP; however, many CGRP neurons may not contain substance P. Table 4.1 details the general classification of DRG neurons by surface markers, characteristics, and neuropeptides.

4.3 NERVE ENDINGS, RECEPTORS, AND TRANSDUCTION

4.3.1 Free Nerve Endings and Specialized Nerve Ending

In the periphery, various types of stimuli are sensed by the nervous system through free nerve endings and specialized nerve endings. Free nerve endings are utilized by small unmyelinated fibers (C fibers), which are activated by polymodal stimulation (e.g., thermal, mechanical, chemical). In the skin, free nerve endings are located at the junction of the dermis and the epidermis. Figure 4.4 demonstrates examples of nerve endings of the skin. Each free ending has several types of channels and receptors (both inhibitory and excitatory). Specialized nerve endings are utilized by large-diameter myelinated fibers (Aβ and Aδ), which are activated by stimulation specific to each specialized nerve ending (e.g., light touch, pressure, vibration, non-extreme temperature, hair movement). When a nerve ending is activated, it initiates a depolarization event (generator potential), which allows the inflow of cations (+ ions, mostly Na^+ and, to a lesser degree, Ca^{2+}), which makes the membrane resting potential (about −80 to −60 mV) more positive. If the sum of total generator potentials elicited for a specific region is large enough, it will initiate an action potential that will be propagated throughout the axon and DRG cell body.

4.3.2 Silent Nociceptors

Silent nociceptors are mechanically insensitive. They are found on many small afferents innervating the skin and joint viscera and normally have exceedingly high

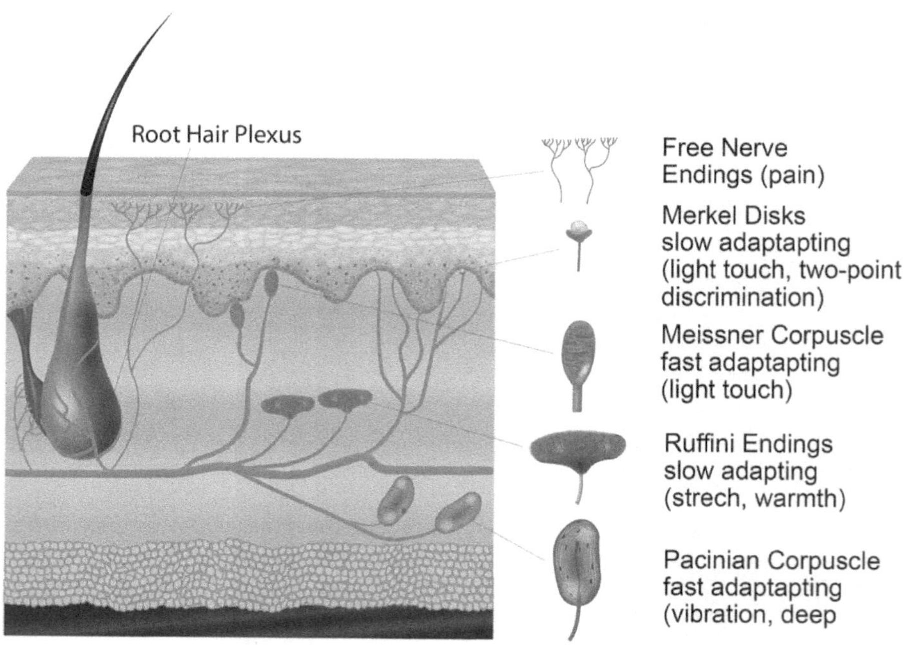

FIGURE 4.4 Nerve endings of the skin.

activation thresholds. However, after exposure to inflammatory chemicals (e.g., bradykinin, serotonin, histamine, prostaglandin E2, and low PH) created by local tissue injury, they can show a profound sensitization. This mechanism is thought to be important, especially in arthritic pain.

4.4 PROPAGATION OF THE ACTION POTENTIAL/ SIGNAL TRANSMISSION

4.4.1 Conduction of Action Potential

As discussed earlier, a generator potential of sufficient size will result in an action potential. This entails the axonal membrane becoming transiently permeable to Na^+, and the internal potential of the neuron becomes increasingly positive. Once the internal potential is increased from its baseline (−80 to −60 mV) to approximately −55 mV, an auto-depolarization phenomenon occurs until the cell's potential is about +10 to +20 mV. At this point, the Na^+ channels close, and immediate repolarization occurs via K^+ channels being transiently opened and K^+ being pumped out of the cell, thus returning the cell to its normal baseline of −80 to −60 mV). This is followed by a brief refractory period in which the Na^+ channels are inactivated.

4.4.2 Function of Afferent Fibers

A peripheral nerve consists of bundles of nerve cells (neurons) and their fibers (axons). Several classifications of peripheral nerve fibers have been made based on their specific features, such as myelination, diameter, or conduction velocity. By the presence of their myelination, nerve fibers are classified as A, B (myelinated), and C (nonmyelinated). Especially in the A group, fibers can be divided into four subgroups, α, β, γ, and δ (in size order) (Terzis and Smith 1990; Barrett and Ganong 2012). Generally, the larger fibers, such as Aα or Aβ, take part in proprioception or touch, whereas the smaller fibers, like Aδ or C, play in autonomic functions as well as pain or temperature. However, they can show relatively different sensitivity to several clinical factors, such as local anesthetics, hypoxia, or pressure (Barrett and Ganong 2012; Varga and Mravec 2015).

Regarding the normal pathway of pain sensation, which generally consists of transduction, transmission, and modulation of electrical signals of neurons after the presence of noxious stimuli, Aδ and C fibers are mainly nociceptive in function. Aδ fibers are the smallest myelinated nerves, which have a relatively fast conduction velocity (~30 m/s). They are responsive to a brief pricking type of pain. C fibers are nonmyelinated, polymodal nerves and have a relatively slow conduction velocity (~2 m/s). They are responsive to dull, poorly localized sensations as well as activated by thermal, mechanical, or chemical stimuli (Yam et al. 2018).

Neuropathic pain, which follows nerve injury or nerve impairment, is distinguished from general pain conditions, which are so-called nociceptive. It originates from the nervous system directly by definition, and also, an abnormal peripheral/central sensitization process can be observed in its manifestation. It has been widely accepted that the neuroma formed after nerve injury may generate spontaneous electrical activity or show ectopic sensitivity to other, non-nociceptive stimuli. Damaged nerve fibers due to stretching, compression, or transection may alter the process in the initiation or propagation of the action potentials and cause a spontaneous or hyper-excitability on the affected site. In addition to the abnormal electrical activities, the sensitization process after nerve injury can occur at the protein (i.e., voltage-gated Na^+ channel) or dorsal root of the spinal cord through increased release of excitatory neurotransmitters and enhanced efficacy at the neuronal synapse (Fukuoka et al. 2001; Basbaum 1999; Campbell and Meyer 2006).

4.4.3 Differences between Fiber Types in Susceptibility to Drugs and Metabolic Changes

Each fiber type demonstrates different susceptibilities to drugs and metabolic changes. C fibers are the most susceptible to local anesthetics and the least susceptible to block by pressure or hypoxia. Thus, lower concentrations of lidocaine can block C fibers selectively compared to A fibers. In cases in which there is ectopic activity (spontaneous firing) in C fibers, it is blocked at lower concentrations of plasma lidocaine than normal stimulus-driven action potentials. A fibers, on the other hand, are more sensitive to pressure block and hypoxia than C fibers. Through knowledge of these principles, we can better clinically deduce the mechanisms for different types of pain and how they are mediated/perpetuated.

4.5 NONNEURONAL CELLS OF THE PERIPHERAL NERVOUS SYSTEM

4.5.1 Glial Cells

Glial cells support peripheral nerve axons in their function. Schwann cells (SCs) and satellite glial cells (SGCs) are unique glia of the PNS. After PNS injury, communication between axons and glial cells is key to neuronal survival and successful regeneration. Various inflammatory cytokines, chemokines, proteinoids, neurotrophins, kinins, ATP, and other mediators are released by neurons, glial, and immune cells, leading to neuroinflammation. This neuroinflammatory process has been shown to play a critical role in the physiologic change after nerve injury and the development of neuropathic pain (Myers et al. 2006).

4.5.1.1 Schwann Cells

SCs are major neuroglial cells of the PNS which dynamically communicate with peripheral nerve axons (Lavdas and Matsas 2009). SCs comprise approximately 90% of all endoneurial cells and serve the extremely important function of structural, trophic, and metabolic support in the peripheral nerves. The two main types of SCs, *myelinated* and *unmyelinated*, are derived from the SC precursor cell originating from the neural crest. The processes of SC differentiation, survival, and proliferation are regulated by the neuregulin-1/Erb and other receptors (Lavdas and Matsas 2009). In later embryonic nerves, SC precursors converted to immature SCs, which envelope the axons and form the axon/SC family. The single axon segregation from the axon/SC families becomes individually ensheathed by an SC (*myelination*) (Kristján R. Jessen, Mirsky, and Lloyd 2015).

For myelination, SCs wrap around and subsequently circumnavigate the axon. The compaction of SC cytoplasm occurs and results in the formation of compact myelin. The extracellular space can be reduced to 2 nm, and the extracellular matrix forms the basal lamina, which separates SC from the axon (Court, Wrabetz, and Feltri 2006). In the PNS, the axonal ensheathment occurs by active spiral progression of the inner layer of the myelin, finally producing the myelin sheath, a short segment of lipid-rich, nonconductive, modified plasma membrane. Myelin sheath can be divided into two domains: peripheral myelin protein (P0, PMP-22), which is a compact myelin that can stabilize the myelin structure, and myelin basic protein (MBP), which is a non-compact myelin that links the adjacent cytoplasmic surfaces, contributing to the interaction between neuron and SC in the peripheral nerves (Lavdas and Matsas 2009).

After peripheral nerve injury, or as part of Wallerian degeneration, SCs respond by the reversal of differentiation and its reprogramming. Genes for myelination are rapidly downregulated, and immature SC-characterizing molecules are upregulated (Jessen and Mirsky, 2008). The reprogramming of the axon/SC complex includes the upregulation of neurotrophic factors that promote axonal elongation and the activation of immune response, including tumor necrosis factor α (TNFα), interleukin-1α (Il-1α). The immune response is required to promote SC repair, the formation of regeneration tracks to guide axon growth, and the activation of SC autophagy for myelin breakdown (Jessen and Mirsky 2016). In the sequential event of Wallerian degeneration after peripheral nerve injury, the matrix metalloproteinase (MMP) cytokine network contributes to neuroinflammation and the development of neuropathic pain (Hong et al. 2017; Myers et al. 2006).

4.5.1.2 Satellite Cells

SGCs are small, flat perineuronal cells that line the circumference of neurons in the PNS ganglia, including DRGs. SGCs originate from the neural crest. In the early stages of embryonic development, one SGC is connected to multiple neurons, and as development proceeds, each neuron is enveloped by numerous SGCs. SGCs express a high number of proteins or surface molecules, but the glutamine synthetase and glial fibrillary acidic protein (GFAP) are commonly used for their identification (Milosavljević et al. 2021; Pannese 1969; Hanani 2005).

Along with the unique characteristic morphology of surrounding neurons, SGCs can slow down the diffusion of substances from extracellular space or uptake by transporters from the neurons (i.e., glutamate transporter). SGCs communicate with each other via gap junctions, which perform functional coupling (Hanani 2005). Through the NO–cGMP pathway, SGCs communicate with the neuron in the regulation of neuroprotective functions (Thippeswamy et al. 2005).

After peripheral nerve injury, DRGs have a critical role in the transmission and processing of external sensory stimuli during pathological pain (Jang and Garraway 2024). Glutamate is the most abundant nociceptive neurotransmitter in the PNS contributing to peripheral inflammation and neuropathic pain (Woolf and Salter, 2000). In response to peripheral nerve injury, SGCs proliferate (Gehrmann, Monaco, and Kreutzberg 1991) and contribute to ectopic neuronal discharge through the release of inflammatory cytokines, such as TNFα, IL-1β, or IL-6, and other mediators (Lee et al. 2004; Zanella et al. 2008).

4.5.2 Macrophages

Macrophages both control inflammation and promote nerve repair after injury. In many tissues, including the PNS, tissue-resident macrophages are present under homeostatic conditions. In addition, hematogenous macrophages infiltrate into tissues in response to injury (Griffin, George, and Ho 1993). Macrophage infiltration can be observed at the distal nerve segment within three days post-injury and peaks at seven days post-injury (Liu et al. 2019). Chemokine C-C motif ligand 2 (CCL2) and other major chemokines attract macrophages to distal axons and DRG neurons expressing its C-C chemokine receptor type 2 (CCR2) and other relevant receptors (Zigmond and Echevarria 2019).

Both M1 and M2 macrophage phenotypes, considered, respectively, as pro- and anti-inflammatory, infiltrate the damaged nerve. M1 macrophages produce pro-inflammatory TNFα, IL-1β, or IL-6 and are known to be involved in phagocytosis during the early phase of Wallerian degeneration or nerve injury. In contrast, M2 macrophages producing anti-inflammatory IL-10 or TNFβ are believed to be important for nerve regeneration. Local M1–M2 and M2–M1 polarization also occurs at the site of injury throughout nerve regeneration (Rios et al. 2021). During nerve repair, macrophages can facilitate local angiogenesis, axon regeneration and activate the migration and proliferation of SCs (Liu et al. 2019).

Although not fully understood, macrophage infiltration and macrophage-associated demyelination contribute to the pathogenesis of peripheral inflammatory neuropathies, such as Guillain–Barré syndrome. In the case of diabetic polyneuropathy, a long-term complication of diabetes, persistent hyperglycemia can contribute to macrophage infiltration and cause neuroinflammation by the glycosylation of myelin product or stimulate the production of inflammatory cytokines (Msheik et al. 2022).

4.5.3 Vasculature

The blood supply to PNS, known as *vasa nervorum*, consists of two major components: an extrinsic circulation, which has arterioles and venules in the epineurium, and an intrinsic plexus of capillaries in the endoneurium. The two circulations are connected with transperineurial anastomosis of penetrating capillaries (Myers 1991). The extrinsic circulation, which originates from regional systemic vascular flow, can be sympathetically innervated and affected by the mechanical or metabolic environment. The intrinsic circulation is not innervated and does not respond to mechanical or metabolic environments. Between the extrinsic and intrinsic vasa nervorum, multiple penetrating branches interconnect and form a microcirculation network. The peri/endoneurial capillaries are tightly connected and strongly interactive with the peri/endoneurium in the formation of the blood–nerve barrier (Gugala et al. 2018).

This blood–nerve barrier, similar to the blood–brain barrier, displays high transendothelial electrical resistance, low permeability to solutes, and low transendothelial water flow (Prahm, Heinzel, and Kolbenschlag 2022). It is worth noting that DRGs are devoid of the conventional blood–nerve and/or blood–brain barriers.

During the regeneration process after nerve injury, which is one of the unique features of PNS, SCs and macrophages play a critical role in neovascularization. Also, the newly formed blood vessels can induce or lead SC entry into the site of injury and provide axonal regrowth (Cattin et al. 2015).

4.6 AXONAL TRANSPORT

The DRG cell body synthesizes various materials and substances important for normal neuronal functioning, and these are transported anterogradely in an energy-dependent process to the central and peripheral axon terminals. Likewise, SCs produce structural and trophic factors to the neuronal cell body via retrograde axonal transport of proteins and mRNA. Axonally transported materials are traditionally grouped into one of five categories (I--V) with different transport velocities. After peripheral nerve injury, axonal transport serves an essential function in transporting protein and mRNA content between neuronal soma and the proximal segment of the nerve injury (Cavalli et al. 2005). Axonal transport is present in myelinated and unmyelinated fibers. Interestingly, the transport rate is particularly sensitive to temperature and slows progressively as temperature declines (0 at 11°C), as well as metabolic energy availability, with rapid deterioration in ischemic conditions. Also of note, the health status of the neuron determines which materials are synthesized: in normal states, the DRG devotes transcription machinery primarily toward making neurotransmitters (for communication between neurons and other organ systems); however, after nerve injury, the DRG adjusts accordingly and shifts its efforts toward the manufacturing of skeletal proteins for regeneration.

4.7 CONCLUSION

As discussed in this chapter, the peripheral nerve and DRG hosting the primary afferent axons and soma, respectively, have intricate and nuanced architecture and histology, with numerous interrelated components pertinent to pain transmission and clinical implications of pain states. Developing a deep insight into the anatomy and physiology of these structures will allow researchers and clinicians to appropriately employ available and develop novel treatment modalities, including pharmacological, interventional, psychological, and nutritional, to relieve chronic pain suffering in patients.

REFERENCES

Barrett, Kim E., and William F. Ganong, eds. 2012. *Ganong's Review of Medical Physiology*. 24. ed. A Lange Medical Book. New York: McGraw-Hill Med.

Basbaum, Allan I. 1999. "Distinct Neurochemical Features of Acute and Persistent Pain." *Proceedings of the National Academy of Sciences* 96 (14): 7739–43. doi: 10.1073/pnas.96.14.7739.

Campbell, James N., and Richard A. Meyer. 2006. "Mechanisms of Neuropathic Pain." *Neuron* 52 (1): 77–92. doi: 10.1016/j.neuron.2006.09.021.

Cattin, Anne-Laure, Jemima J. Burden, Lucie Van Emmenis, Francesca E. Mackenzie, Julian J.A. Hoving, Noelia Garcia Calavia, Yanping Guo, et al. 2015. "Macrophage-Induced Blood Vessels Guide Schwann Cell-Mediated Regeneration of Peripheral Nerves." *Cell* 162 (5): 1127–39. doi: 10.1016/j.cell.2015.07.021.

Cavalli, V., P. Kujala, J. Klumperman, and L. S. Goldstein. 2005. "Sunday Driver Links Axonal Transport to Damage Signaling." *Journal of Cell Biology* 168 (5): 775–87.

Court, Felipe A, Lawrence Wrabetz, and M Laura Feltri. 2006. "Basal Lamina: Schwann Cells Wrap to the Rhythm of Space-Time." *Current Opinion in Neurobiology* 16 (5): 501–7. doi: 10.1016/j.conb.2006.08.005.

Devor, M. 2009. "Ectopic Discharge in Abeta Afferents as A Source of Neuropathic Pain." *Experimental Brain Research* 196 (1): 115–28.

Esposito, M. F., R. Malayil, M. Hanes, and T. Deer. 2019. "Unique Characteristics of the Dorsal Root Ganglion as a Target for Neuromodulation." *Pain Medicine (Malden, Mass.)* 20 (Suppl 1): S23–S30. doi: 10.1093/pm/pnz012.

Fukuoka, Tetsuo, Eiji Kondo, Yi Dai, Norio Hashimoto, and Koichi Noguchi. 2001. "Brain-Derived Neurotrophic Factor Increases in the Uninjured Dorsal Root Ganglion Neurons in Selective Spinal Nerve Ligation Model." *The Journal of Neuroscience* 21 (13): 4891–900. doi: 10.1523/JNEUROSCI.21-13-04891.2001.

Gehrmann, Jochen, Salvatore Monaco, and Georg W. Kreutzberg. 1991. "Spinal Cord Microglial Cells and DRG Satellite Cells Rapidly Respond to Transection of the Rat Sciatic Nerve." *Restorative Neurology and Neuroscience* 2 (4–6): 181–98. doi: 10.3233/RNN-1991-245605.

Griffin, John W., Rachel George, and Tony Ho. 1993. "Macrophage Systems in Peripheral Nerves. A Review:" *Journal of Neuropathology and Experimental Neurology* 52 (6): 553–60. doi: 10.1097/00005072-199311000-00001.

Gugala, Zbigniew, Elizabeth A. Olmsted-Davis, Yuqing Xiong, Eleanor L. Davis, and Alan R. Davis. 2018. "Trauma-Induced Heterotopic Ossification Regulates the Blood-Nerve Barrier." *Frontiers in Neurology* 9 (June): 408. doi: 10.3389/fneur.2018.00408.

Hanani, Menachem. 2005. "Satellite Glial Cells in Sensory Ganglia: From Form to Function." *Brain Research Reviews* 48 (3): 457–76. doi: 10.1016/j.brainresrev.2004.09.001.

Hong, Sanghyun, Albert G. Remacle, Sergei A. Shiryaev, Wonjun Choi, Swathi K. Hullugundi, Jennifer Dolkas, Mila Angert, et al. 2017. "Reciprocal Relationship between Membrane Type 1 Matrix Metalloproteinase and the Algesic Peptides of Myelin Basic Protein Contributes to Chronic Neuropathic Pain." *Brain, Behavior, and Immunity* 60 (February): 282–92. doi: 10.1016/j.bbi.2016.11.003.

Jang, Kyeongran, and Sandra M. Garraway. 2024. "A Review of Dorsal Root Ganglia and Primary Sensory Neuron Plasticity Mediating Inflammatory and Chronic Neuropathic Pain." *Neurobiology of Pain* 15 (January): 100151. doi: 10.1016/j.ynpai.2024.100151.

Jessen, K. R., and R. Mirsky. 2016. "The Repair Schwann Cell and Its Function in Regenerating Nerves." *The Journal of Physiology* 594 (13): 3521–31. doi: 10.1113/JP270874.

Jessen, Kristján R., and Rhona Mirsky. 2008. "Negative Regulation of Myelination: Relevance for Development, Injury, and Demyelinating Disease." *Glia* 56 (14): 1552–65. doi: 10.1002/glia.20761.

Jessen, Kristján R., Rhona Mirsky, and Alison C. Lloyd. 2015. "Schwann Cells: Development and Role in Nerve Repair." *Cold Spring Harbor Perspectives in Biology* 7 (7): a020487. doi: 10.1101/cshperspect. a020487.

Lavdas, A.A., and R. Matsas. 2009. "Schwann Cell Morphology☆." In *Reference Module in Biomedical Sciences*, 475–84. Elsevier. doi: 10.1016/B978-0-12-801238-3.04758-9.

Lee, Hye-Lim, Kyung-Min Lee, Sun-Joo Son, Sung-Hun Hwang, and Hee-Jung Cho. 2004. "Temporal Expression of Cytokines and Their Receptors mRNAs in a Neuropathic Pain Model." *Neuroreport* 15 (18): 2807–11.

Liu, Ping, Jiang Peng, Gong-Hai Han, Xiao Ding, Shuai Wei, Gang Gao, Kun Huang, Feng Chang, and Yu Wang. 2019. "Role of Macrophages in Peripheral Nerve Injury and Repair." *Neural Regeneration Research* 14 (8): 1335. doi: 10.4103/1673–5374.253510.

Milosavljević, A., J. Jančić, A. Mirčić, A. Dožić, J. Boljanović, M. Milisavljević, and M. Ćetković. 2021. "Morphological and Functional Characteristics of Satellite Glial Cells in the Peripheral Nervous System." *Folia Morphologica* 80 (4): 745–55. doi: 10.5603/FM.a2020.0141.

Msheik, Zeina, Mohamed El Massry, Amandine Rovini, Fabrice Billet, and Alexis Desmoulière. 2022. "The Macrophage: A Key Player in the Pathophysiology of Peripheral Neuropathies." *Journal of Neuroinflammation* 19 (1): 97. doi: 10.1186/s12974-022-02454-6.

Myers, R. R. 1991. "Anatomy and Microanatomy of Peripheral Nerve." *Neurosurgery Clinics of North America* 2 (1): 1–20.

Myers, Robert R., W. Marie Campana, and Veronica I. Shubayev. 2006. "The Role of Neuroinflammation in Neuropathic Pain: Mechanisms and Therapeutic Targets." *Drug Discovery Today* 11 (1–2): 8–20. doi: 10.1016/S1359-6446(05)03637–8.

Pannese, Ennio. 1969. "Electron Microscopical Study on the Development of the Satellite Cell Sheath in Spinal Ganglia." *Journal of Comparative Neurology* 135 (4): 381–421. doi: 10.1002/cne.901350403.

Prahm, Cosima, Johannes Heinzel, and Jonas Kolbenschlag. 2022. "Blood Supply and Microcirculation of the Peripheral Nerve." In *Peripheral Nerve Tissue Engineering and Regeneration*, edited by James B. Phillips, David Hercher, and Thomas Hausner, 35–79. Reference Series in Biomedical Engineering. Cham: Springer International Publishing. doi: 10.1007/978-3-030-21052-6_21.

Raja, Srinivasa N., Daniel B. Carr, Miltonc Cohen, Nanna B. Finnerup, Hertaf Flor, Stepheng Gibson, Francis J. Keefe, Jeffrey S. Mogil, Matthiasj Ringkamp, Kathleen A. Sluka, Xue-Junl Song, Bonniem Stevens, Mark D. Sullivan, Perri R. Tutelman, Takahirop Ushida, Kyleq Vader. 2020. "The Revised International Association for the Study of Pain Definition of Pain: Concepts, Challenges, and Compromises." *Pain* 161 (9): 1976–82. doi: 10.1097/j.pain.0000000000001939.

Rios, Rachel, Albina Jablonka-Shariff, Curtis Broberg, and Alison K. Snyder-Warwick. 2021. "Macrophage Roles in Peripheral Nervous System Injury and Pathology: Allies in Neuromuscular Junction Recovery." *Molecular and Cellular Neuroscience* 111 (March): 103590. doi: 10.1016/j.mcn.2021.103590.

Salzer J. L. (2015). "Schwann Cell Myelination." *Cold Spring Harbor Perspectives in Biology* 7 (8): a020529. doi: 10.1101/cshperspect.a020529.

Terzis, Julia K., and Kevin L. Smith. 1990. *The Peripheral Nerve: Structure, Function and Reconstruction*. Norfolk, Va: Hampton Pr. [u.a.].

Thippeswamy, Thimmasettappa, Jennifer S. Mckay, Richard Morris, John Quinn, Liang-Fong Wong, and David Murphy. 2005. "Glial-mediated Neuroprotection: Evidence for the Protective Role of the NO-cGMP Pathway via Neuron–Glial Communication in the Peripheral Nervous System." *Glia* 49 (2): 197–210. doi: 10.1002/glia.20105.

Varga, Ivan, and Boris Mravec. 2015. "Nerve Fiber Types." In *Nerves and Nerve Injuries*, 107–13. Elsevier. doi: 10.1016/B978-0-12-410390-0.00008-1.

Woolf, Clifford J., and Michael W. Salter. 2000. "Neuronal Plasticity: Increasing the Gain in Pain." *Science* 288 (5472): 1765–68. doi: 10.1126/science.288.5472.1765.

Yam, Mun Fei, Yean Chun Loh, Chu Shan Tan, Siti Khadijah Adam, Nizar Abdul Manan, and Rusliza Basir. 2018. "General Pathways of Pain Sensation and the Major

Neurotransmitters Involved in Pain Regulation." *International Journal of Molecular Sciences* 19 (8): 2164. doi: 10.3390/ijms19082164.

Zanella, John M., Eric N. Burright, Keith Hildebrand, Chris Hobot, Mark Cox, Laura Christoferson, and William F. McKay. 2008. "Effect of Etanercept, a Tumor Necrosis Factor-Alpha Inhibitor, on Neuropathic Pain in the Rat Chronic Constriction Injury Model:" *Spine* 33 (3): 227–34. doi: 10.1097/BRS.0b013e318162340a.

Zigmond, Richard E., and Franklin D. Echevarria. 2019. "Macrophage Biology in the Peripheral Nervous System after Injury." *Progress in Neurobiology* 173 (February): 102–21. doi: 10.1016/j.pneurobio.2018.12.001.

5 Peripheral Nerve and Dorsal Root Ganglion (DRG) Pharmacology

Mechanisms, Therapeutic Targets, and Clinical Applications

Maja Green, Vida Nazemian, and Amna Hassan

5.1 INTRODUCTION

The dorsal root ganglion (DRG) occupies a central role in the peripheral nervous system, serving as the site of cell bodies for primary sensory neurons. These neurons are integral to the transmission of sensory information, particularly pain, from the periphery to the central nervous system. The DRG is strategically positioned at the junction where central (dorsal root) and peripheral (spinal nerve) axons converge, creating a continuous neuronal cytoplasm that extends from the periphery to the spinal cord (Figure 5.1). This unique anatomical and physiological configuration makes the DRG a critical hub in pain perception and a key target for therapeutic intervention (1).

At the molecular level, the DRG functions as a dynamic biochemical factory, synthesizing a wide array of neurotransmitters, modulators, receptors, and ion channels that are essential for sensory signal transduction. These molecules are produced in the cell bodies of DRG neurons and transported along axons to various sites, including nerve terminals and synapses, where they play pivotal roles in modulating neuronal excitability and synaptic transmission. The ability of DRG neurons to produce and regulate these molecules is fundamental to their role in pain perception, as well as in the broader context of sensory processing (1, 3). The ion channels expressed by DRG neurons, such as voltage-gated sodium (Na^+), potassium (K^+), and calcium (Ca^{2+}) channels, are particularly significant in the context of pain. These channels regulate the generation and propagation of action potentials along the axons, thereby controlling the release of neurotransmitters and modulators at synaptic terminals. Dysregulation of these ion channels, whether through genetic mutations, injury, or inflammation, can lead to abnormal neuronal excitability, contributing to the development and maintenance of chronic pain states. Understanding the molecular

DOI: 10.1201/9781003094302-5

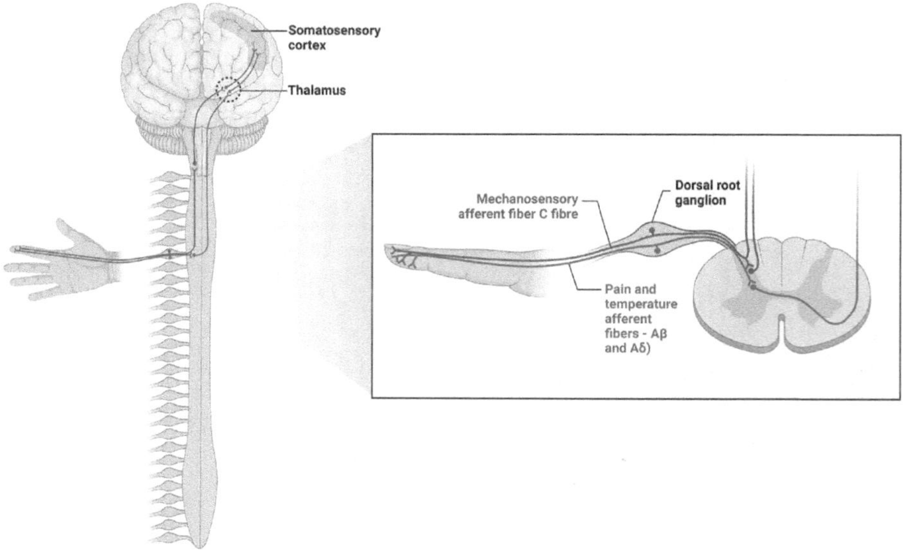

FIGURE 5.1 This figure illustrates the nociceptive pathways involved in pain perception, highlighting the role of different sensory afferent fibers and their connection to the DRG. The mechanosensory afferent C fibers (depicted in red) and the pain and temperature afferent fibers, including Aβ and Aδ fibers (depicted in blue), converge at the DRG before transmitting sensory information to the spinal cord. The nociceptive signals are then relayed to higher brain centers via the spinothalamic tract, ultimately reaching the thalamus and somatosensory cortex, where pain is perceived and processed. The inset provides a close-up of the DRG, showing its central role in integrating and transmitting nociceptive information from peripheral tissues to the central nervous system. This figure emphasizes the anatomical and functional pathways critical for nociception and the perception of pain, underscoring the significance of DRG neurons in the modulation and transmission of pain signals.

Source: (2).

mechanisms governing these ion channels is crucial for identifying new therapeutic targets in pain management (4–6).

In addition to ion channels, DRG neurons produce a variety of neurotransmitters and modulators that influence pain perception. Excitatory neurotransmitters such as glutamate play a key role in amplifying pain signals, while inhibitory neurotransmitters like γ-aminobutyric acid (GABA) help dampen these signals. The balance between excitatory and inhibitory influences is critical for maintaining normal sensory function, and disruptions in this balance are often implicated in chronic pain conditions. Inflammatory mediators, including cytokines and chemokines, further modulate DRG function by sensitizing neurons to noxious stimuli and promoting neuroinflammation, which can exacerbate pain (7–10).

Clinically, the DRG has become an important focus for the development of novel pain therapies. Interventions targeting DRG neurons and their associated pathways, such as neuromodulation techniques and pharmacological agents that modulate ion channel function, offer promising avenues for the treatment of chronic pain. These approaches aim to normalize the aberrant activity of DRG neurons, thereby reducing pain and improving the quality of life for patients (11).

The following sections of this chapter will delve deeper into the molecular and pharmacological mechanisms underlying DRG function, with a particular emphasis on their relevance to pain perception and therapeutic potential. By elucidating the complex interplay of ion channels, neurotransmitters, and intracellular signaling pathways within DRG neurons, this review aims to provide a comprehensive understanding of how these processes contribute to the pathophysiology of pain and how they can be targeted for clinical benefit.

5.2 ION CHANNEL SUBTYPES IN DRG NEURONS: MOLECULAR AND FUNCTIONAL DIVERSITY

The DRG contains the cell bodies of primary sensory neurons, which extend axons to peripheral tissues and the central nervous system (CNS). A key feature of these neurons is their expression of various ion channels, which are crucial for the initiation, propagation, and modulation of action potentials that underlie nociception. Ion channels in DRG neurons are specialized transmembrane proteins that selectively allow the passage of ions, such as sodium (Na^+), potassium (K^+), calcium (Ca^{2+}), and chloride (Cl^-) across the cell membrane. These channels are essential for generating the electrical signals that transmit sensory information, including pain (4, 5, 12). The diversity of ion channel subtypes in DRG neurons reflects the complex and nuanced nature of nociceptive signal processing.

5.2.1 Voltage-Gated Sodium Channels (Nav): Molecular Mechanisms and Clinical Implications in Pain Perception

Voltage-gated sodium channels (Nav) are integral membrane proteins that play a crucial role in the initiation and propagation of action potentials in excitable cells, including neurons of the DRG. These channels are responsible for the rapid influx of sodium ions (Na^+) into the cell upon membrane depolarization, a process that is fundamental to the generation of electrical signals in the nervous system (13). In the context of pain perception, Nav channels are particularly significant, as they are involved in the transmission of nociceptive signals, those that convey information about noxious stimuli that may cause harm.

5.2.2 Structure and Function of Nav Channels

Nav channels are composed of a large α-subunit, which forms the pore through which Na^+ ions pass, and auxiliary β-subunits, which modulate the channel's properties and interactions with other proteins. The α-subunit is organized into four homologous domains (DI–DIV), each containing six transmembrane segments (S1–S6). The S4 segment in each domain acts as the voltage sensor, responding to changes in membrane potential by moving outward, which triggers the opening of the channel. The S5 and S6 segments, along with the intervening pore loop, form the ion-conducting pore of the channel (14, 15).

When the membrane potential of a neuron becomes less negative (depolarizes), the voltage sensors in the Nav channels detect this change and induce a conformational shift that opens the channel, allowing Na^+ ions to flow into the cell. This influx of Na^+ ions further depolarizes the membrane, leading to the propagation of the action potential along the axon. The rapid opening and subsequent inactivation of Nav channels are tightly regulated processes that ensure the precise timing of action potentials, which is essential for proper nervous system function (16).

5.2.3 Nav Subtypes in Pain Perception

There are nine known subtypes of Nav channels, designated Nav1.1 to Nav1.9, each encoded by a distinct gene (5, 14, 15). Among these, Nav1.7, Nav1.8, and Nav1.9 are particularly important in the context of pain perception due to their expression in DRG neurons and their involvement in nociceptive signaling (Table 5.1).

TABLE 5.1
Nav Subtypes and Their Function in Pain Perception

Nav Subtype	Function
Nav1.7	Highly expressed in DRG neurons and is crucial for setting the threshold for action potential initiation. This channel is exquisitely sensitive to small depolarizations, allowing it to amplify weak stimuli and contribute to the fine-tuning of sensory input. Nav1.7's role in pain perception is underscored by genetic studies linking mutations in the SCN9A gene, which encodes Nav1.7, to distinct pain disorders. For instance, gain-of-function mutations in Nav1.7 lead to conditions such as primary erythromelalgia, characterized by severe burning pain, while loss-of-function mutations result in congenital insensitivity to pain, a condition where individuals cannot perceive pain. These clinical findings highlight Nav1.7 as a key player in both the normal and the pathological transmission of pain signals (17).
Nav1.8	Nav1.8 is unique among sodium channels in that it is resistant to tetrodotoxin (TTX), a potent neurotoxin that blocks most other Nav channels. This channel is predominantly expressed in small-diameter, unmyelinated C fibers, which are responsible for transmitting slow, chronic pain signals. Nav1.8 activates at more depolarized membrane potentials compared to other Nav channels and has slower inactivation kinetics. These properties enable Nav1.8 to support sustained, repetitive firing of action potentials, a feature that is particularly important in chronic pain conditions, where continuous nociceptive signaling occurs. The role of Nav1.8 in persistent pain has made it a target for the development of analgesic drugs that can selectively inhibit this channel, thereby reducing chronic pain without affecting other sensory modalities (15).
Nav1.9	Characterized by its low threshold for activation and its ability to generate subthreshold depolarizations. This channel contributes to the overall excitability of DRG neurons by maintaining a depolarized membrane potential, which can enhance the responsiveness of these neurons to other stimuli. Nav1.9 is particularly important in inflammatory pain, where its activity is modulated by inflammatory mediators, such as prostaglandins and bradykinin. These mediators enhance the function of Nav1.9, leading to increased neuronal excitability and pain sensitivity, a process known as peripheral sensitization (15). The involvement of Nav1.9 in the amplification of pain signals makes it a promising target for interventions aimed at reducing pain in inflammatory conditions.

The following table highlights the distinct roles of each Nav subtype in pain perception, highlighting their potential as therapeutic targets for managing different types of pain, including chronic and inflammatory pain conditions.

5.2.4 The Role of Potassium Channels in Neuronal Excitability and Pain Modulation

Potassium channels play a crucial role in maintaining the electrical stability of neurons by regulating the outflow of K^+ ions, which is essential for returning the membrane potential to its resting state after depolarization. These channels are vital in controlling the excitability of neurons and ensuring that action potentials are properly terminated. In the context of pain perception, potassium channels help modulate the activity of neurons within the DRG, where their function can influence both normal and pathological pain states (18–20). Several subtypes of potassium channels are involved in repolarizing the neuronal membrane and modulating neuronal excitability in DRG neurons, as outlined in Table 5.2.

TABLE 5.2
Key Functions of Kv Channel Subtypes in DRG Neurons and Their Roles in Pain Modulation

Kv Subtype	Function
Kv1.1 and Kv1.2	Part of the delayed rectifier family of potassium channels, which is integral in bringing the membrane potential back to its resting state after the propagation of an action potential. These channels are expressed in both large, myelinated A fibers, which transmit rapid, sharp pain, and small, unmyelinated C fibers, which are responsible for slower, chronic pain signals (21). Dysfunctions in Kv1.1 and Kv1.2 channels can lead to hyperexcitability of DRG neurons, a condition often associated with neuropathic pain, where abnormal firing patterns contribute to persistent and sometimes debilitating pain sensations.
Kv7 (KCNQ) channels	The Kv7 family, particularly Kv7.2 and Kv7.3, is essential for maintaining the resting membrane potential and modulating neuronal excitability. These channels produce a slowly activating and non-inactivating current, known as the M-current, which stabilizes the membrane potential and prevents excessive excitability. Mutations in Kv7 channels are associated with various inherited neurological disorders, including epilepsy and specific pain syndromes (21, 22). Due to their pivotal role in controlling neuronal excitability, pharmacological agents that activate Kv7 channels are being explored as potential therapies for pain management, particularly in conditions where reducing neuronal excitability is beneficial.
A-type potassium channels (Kv4.2 and Kv4.3)	A-type potassium channels, such as Kv4.2 and Kv4.3, are characterized by their rapid activation and inactivation kinetics. These channels are crucial for the early phase of repolarization following an action potential, thus helping control the frequency of action potential firing. By limiting the duration of action potentials and the subsequent refractory period, A-type channels prevent excessive neuronal activity and modulate the response to repetitive stimuli. Dysfunctions in these channels can lead to an increased firing rate, contributing to heightened pain perception and conditions such as hyperalgesia, where patients experience exaggerated pain responses to normally non-painful stimuli (19, 23, 24).

Kv1.1 and Kv1.2 channels are crucial for resetting the membrane potential after action potentials, affecting both acute and chronic pain transmission. Kv7 channels maintain the resting membrane potential and prevent excessive excitability, with therapeutic implications in pain management. A-type Kv channels, like Kv4.2 and Kv4.3, control action potential firing frequency and prevent hyperexcitability, with dysfunctions in these channels linked to heightened pain perception and hyperalgesia.

5.2.5 Molecular and Physiological Implications

The activity of potassium channels is tightly regulated by the membrane potential and intracellular signaling pathways. For example, Kv channels are modulated by phosphorylation, which can alter their activity and, consequently, neuronal excitability. Additionally, potassium channel dysfunctions, often due to genetic mutations or pathophysiological conditions, can lead to aberrant pain signaling. In neuropathic pain, for example, a decrease in potassium channel activity can result in prolonged depolarization and an increase in action potential firing, contributing to chronic pain states (19).

5.2.6 Biophysics of Potassium Channel Function

From a biophysical perspective, potassium channels selectively allow K^+ ions to flow out of the neuron, driven by both the concentration gradient and the electrical gradient across the membrane. The structure of these channels, particularly the selectivity filter, ensures that only K^+ ions pass through despite the presence of other cations like Na^+. The gating of these channels, which involves conformational changes in response to voltage changes across the membrane, is a critical aspect of their function. This gating mechanism allows the channels to open rapidly during depolarization and close during repolarization, thus shaping the action potential and influencing the timing and frequency of neuronal firing (25–27).

Potassium channels, particularly the Kv1, Kv7, and A-type channels, are central to the regulation of neuronal excitability and the modulation of pain signals. Their function is essential for maintaining normal sensory processing, and their dysfunction can lead to pathological pain states (26, 28). Understanding these channels' molecular and biophysical properties is crucial for developing targeted therapies aimed at alleviating pain in clinical settings.

5.3 CHLORIDE CHANNEL'S ROLE IN PAIN PERCEPTION AND SIGNALING

Chloride channels are integral to the regulation of neuronal excitability and play a significant role in modulating pain perception. Unlike sodium and calcium channels, which are typically associated with excitatory processes in neurons, chloride channels are primarily involved in inhibitory signaling. This inhibitory action is crucial for maintaining the balance between excitation and inhibition in the nervous system, a balance that is often disrupted in chronic pain states. The primary role of chloride channels in pain perception is mediated through their interaction with neurotransmitter systems, particularly the GABAergic system (29). By controlling the flow of chloride ions across neuronal membranes, these channels influence the membrane potential and, consequently, the likelihood of action potential generation (30). This section will explore the specific chloride channels involved in pain signaling, emphasizing their molecular mechanisms and clinical implications.

Chloride channels (Cl^-) consist of $GABA_A$ receptor channels and KCC2 (K^+–Cl^- cotransporter):

- *$GABA_A$ receptor channels*. The $GABA_A$ receptor is a key player in the modulation of neuronal excitability through chloride ion conductance. When GABA, the primary inhibitory neurotransmitter in the central nervous system, binds to the $GABA_A$ receptor, it triggers the opening of the chloride channel. This allows Cl^- ions to flow into the neuron, resulting in hyperpolarization of the membrane. Hyperpolarization increases the negative charge inside the cell, making it less likely for the neuron to reach the threshold necessary for action potential generation. This inhibitory mechanism is vital for controlling excessive neuronal firing and is particularly important in the context of pain management, where dysregulated neuronal excitability can lead to conditions such as hyperalgesia (increased sensitivity to pain) and allodynia (pain from normally non-painful stimuli). In the context of pain perception, the efficacy of $GABA_A$ receptor–mediated inhibition can be influenced by the intracellular concentration of chloride ions. This concentration is tightly regulated by the activity of various chloride transporters, which either maintain or disrupt the chloride gradient across the neuronal membrane (31–33).
- *KCC2 (K^+–Cl^- cotransporter*. One of the most critical regulators of intracellular chloride levels is the KCC2 cotransporter. KCC2 actively extrudes chloride ions from the neuron, maintaining a low intracellular Cl^- concentration. This low concentration is essential for the hyperpolarizing effect of $GABA_A$ receptor activation. When KCC2 function is optimal, the influx of Cl^- through $GABA_A$ receptors effectively inhibits neuronal firing, thereby dampening pain signals. However, in chronic pain conditions, the expression or function of KCC2 is often compromised. Reduced KCC2 activity leads to an accumulation of intracellular chloride, which can invert the normal hyperpolarizing effect of $GABA_A$ receptor activation. Instead of causing inhibition, the $GABA_A$ receptor may then cause depolarization, effectively reducing the inhibitory control over pain pathways and contributing to heightened pain sensitivity. This phenomenon, known as GABAergic disinhibition, is a significant factor in the pathophysiology of chronic pain, particularly in conditions where pain persists despite the absence of an obvious noxious stimulus (34–39). The dysregulation of KCC2 and the resulting loss of inhibitory control over pain pathways represent a crucial mechanism by which chronic pain develops and is maintained. Consequently, restoring KCC2 function has emerged as a potential therapeutic strategy for treating chronic pain. Pharmacological agents that enhance KCC2 activity or mimic

its function could potentially restore the chloride gradient, re-establish GABAergic inhibition, and thereby reduce pain (40).

5.3.1 Clinical Implications of Chloride Channels

The role of chloride channels, particularly those associated with the $GABA_A$ receptor and KCC2, in pain perception offers promising avenues for therapeutic intervention. Enhancing the function of KCC2 to restore the inhibitory tone in pain pathways is a promising approach to treating chronic pain. Additionally, the modulation of $GABA_A$ receptor activity, either through direct agonists or through the regulation of chloride ion conductance, offers another layer of potential intervention (29). Understanding the intricate balance of chloride ion homeostasis and its impact on neuronal excitability is essential for developing new pain therapies that target these fundamental mechanisms.

5.3.2 Voltage-Gated Calcium Channels (VGCC): Molecular Mechanisms and Therapeutic Targets in Pain Management

Voltage-gated calcium channels (VGCCs) play a critical role in neuronal function by allowing the influx of Ca^{2+} ions into the cell, which serves multiple vital purposes: initiating neurotransmitter release at synaptic terminals, depolarizing the neuronal membrane, and activating intracellular signaling pathways through second messengers.

5.4 FUNCTIONS OF α1 SUBUNITS AND CHANNELS

These channels are composed of a primary α1 subunit, which forms the ion-conducting pore, and several auxiliary subunits, α2δ, β, and ϒ, that modulate channel function, membrane trafficking, and drug sensitivity (41, 42).

5.4.1 α1 Subunits and Channel Types

The α1 subunit is the core component of VGCCs, determining the channel's properties and its classification into one of several types: L, P, N, R, and T (43–46). Each type of channel has distinct physiological roles and patterns of expression (Table 5.3).

The following table is an overview of α1 subunits and the associated channel types in VGCCs. Each channel type plays a distinct role in neuronal function, from regulating synaptic plasticity and neurotransmitter release to modulating pain signals. This table highlights the involvement of these channels in various physiological processes and their implications in neurological disorders and pain management.

In addition to α1 subunits, auxiliary subunits play a critical role in modulating the functional properties of VGCCs, significantly impacting their behavior and interactions with pharmacological agents. The α2δ subunit enhances VGCC expression on the cell surface and modulates channel kinetics and voltage dependence. This subunit is particularly important as it is the target of gabapentin and pregabalin, two widely used analgesics that bind to α2δ, reducing calcium influx and, consequently,

TABLE 5.3
Functions of α1 Subunits and Channels

α1 Subunits and Channel Types	Function
L-type (CaV1.x)	L-type channels are primarily involved in long-lasting calcium currents and are essential for various functions, including muscle contraction and gene expression regulation. In neurons, they contribute to synaptic plasticity and are implicated in the modulation of pain signals (47).
P/Q-type (CaV2.1)	Primarily found in pre-synaptic terminals, where they are crucial for neurotransmitter release. Dysfunctions in P/Q-type channels can lead to neurological disorders, including certain forms of migraine and ataxia, as well as altered pain perception (48).
N-type (CaV2.2)	Involved in neurotransmitter release in the central and peripheral nervous systems. They are key players in the transmission of pain signals. Ziconotide, a synthetic peptide derived from the venom of the marine snail *Conus magus*, selectively inhibits N-type channels, providing potent analgesia for chronic pain conditions (49–51).
R-type (CaV2.3)	These channels are less well understood but are known to contribute to neurotransmitter release in certain neuronal populations and are involved in modulating synaptic activity, particularly in the hippocampus and cerebellum (52, 53).
T-type (CaV3.x)	Characterized by their transient, low-threshold activation. They contribute to the pacemaking activity in neurons and are involved in the generation of rhythmic oscillations in the brain. These channels have been linked to neuropathic pain, epilepsy, and cardiac arrhythmias (54).

decreasing neurotransmitter release and neuronal excitability in pain pathways (55). The β subunit is crucial for VGCC functionality, influencing the channel's gating properties, voltage sensitivity, and trafficking to the plasma membrane, ensuring proper VGCC operation. Although the ϒ subunit is less well understood, it is believed to contribute to fine-tuning VGCC function and stabilizing the channel complex at the membrane, further supporting the precise regulation of calcium influx and its downstream effects in neuronal signaling (56–58).

5.4.2 Pharmacological Implications

VGCCs are key targets for pain management therapies due to their pivotal role in neurotransmitter release and neuronal excitability. The pharmacological modulation of these channels, particularly through drugs targeting specific subunits, like the α2δ (gabapentin, pregabalin) and N-type (ziconotide), offers effective strategies for treating chronic pain conditions (59, 60). These interventions highlight the importance of understanding VGCC subunit composition and their physiological roles, which can lead to the development of more selective and effective pain therapies (Figure 5.2).

On the left, the excitatory synapse details the process of action potential propagation leading to the opening of voltage-gated sodium (Na^+) channels, which is crucial

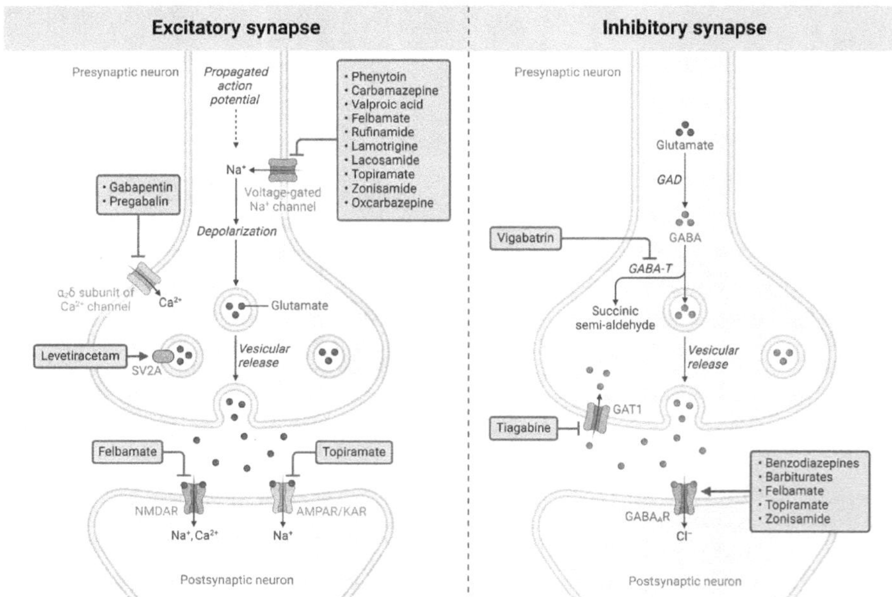

FIGURE 5.2 This figure illustrates the mechanisms of action of various pharmacological agents at excitatory and inhibitory synapses, with a focus on their roles in pain modulation and therapy.

for neuronal depolarization. Calcium (Ca^{2+}) influx through voltage-gated Ca^{2+} channels triggers the release of the neurotransmitter glutamate, a key player in pain signal transmission. Pain therapies like gabapentin and pregabalin target the α2δ subunit of the Ca^{2+} channel, effectively reducing neurotransmitter release and decreasing pain signal propagation. Additionally, drugs such as phenytoin and carbamazepine inhibit voltage-gated Na^+ channels, diminishing neuronal excitability and providing analgesic effects by preventing the initiation of pain signals. Topiramate and felbamate act on post-synaptic receptors, including NMDA and AMPA/Kainate receptors, to dampen excitatory neurotransmission and modulate pain perception.

On the right, the inhibitory synapse illustrates the role of gamma-aminobutyric acid (GABA) in reducing neuronal excitability and modulating pain. Vigabatrin inhibits GABA transaminase (GABA-T), increasing the availability of GABA and enhancing its inhibitory effects, which is critical in the context of pain relief. Tiagabine blocks GAT1, preventing GABA reuptake and prolonging its inhibitory action on post-synaptic neurons. Additionally, benzodiazepines and barbiturates enhance $GABA_A$ receptor function, contributing to their analgesic properties by amplifying inhibitory neurotransmission and reducing pain signals.

5.4.2.1 Neurotransmitters

In the intricate landscape of pain perception, neurotransmitters play a pivotal role in transmitting signals that dictate the experience of pain. The DRG, a critical hub within the peripheral nervous system, is central to this process. The DRG neurons synthesize and release various neurotransmitters that influence nociceptive signaling, thereby modulating the body's response to pain stimuli. Upon depolarization, typically initiated by an action potential, neurotransmitters stored in the axon terminals are released into the synaptic cleft. This release is a finely tuned process involving VGCCs, which allow the influx of calcium ions necessary for neurotransmitter vesicle fusion and exocytosis. The neurotransmitters then interact with receptors on adjacent neurons or other target cells, leading to either excitatory or inhibitory effects on pain transmission (61, 62).

5.4.3 Excitatory Neurotransmitters

Among the excitatory neurotransmitters, glutamate is the most prevalent in the nervous system and is critically involved in pain pathways. Glutamate is synthesized in both the DRG neuron cell bodies and their axon terminals, highlighting its widespread role in pain modulation. The primary receptors for glutamate, NMDA and AMPA, are key players in central sensitization, a process where increased responsiveness of neurons to stimuli contributes to the development and maintenance of chronic pain. This sensitization is often a hallmark of pathological pain states, where normal sensory inputs are perceived as painful.

Another important excitatory neurotransmitter is calcitonin gene–related peptide (CGRP), predominantly produced by the DRG and involved in the transmission of noxious stimuli. CGRP works synergistically with other neurotransmitters, like Substance P, to enhance pain signals and contribute to central sensitization. The interaction of CGRP with its receptors, such as the calcitonin receptor–like receptor (CALCRL), further integrates the central nervous system's control over pain pathways, underscoring its significance in both acute and chronic pain scenarios (63–69).

5.4.4 Inhibitory Neurotransmitters

In contrast, opioid peptides, such as β-endorphins, enkephalins, and dynorphins, serve as the body's natural analgesics by binding to opioid receptors (μ, δ, and κ variants) within the central and peripheral nervous systems. These G protein–coupled receptors, upon activation, inhibit VGCCs and reduce cAMP levels, leading to decreased neurotransmitter release and a reduction in pain signal transmission. The clinical relevance of these pathways is evident in the use of exogenous opioids, like morphine and fentanyl, which exploit these same mechanisms to provide potent pain relief (67, 69, 70).

Cannabinoids also contribute to the modulation of pain through their interaction with CB1 and CB2 receptors, both of which are G protein–coupled receptors similar to opioid receptors. The activation of these receptors by endogenous (e.g., anandamide) or exogenous cannabinoids (e.g., THC and CBD) results in the inhibition of VGCCs, a reduction of cAMP levels, and a subsequent decrease in neurotransmitter release. The presence of CB1 receptors in the DRG highlights their role in modulating pain at the peripheral level, making cannabinoids a therapeutic target for pain management (71–74).

5.4.5 Inflammatory Neurotransmitters

Substance P is a prominent neuropeptide involved in both pain transmission and the inflammatory response. It is particularly notable for its role in neurogenic inflammation, where it mediates interactions between neurons and immune cells, thus modulating the immune response in the context of pain. Substance P's receptors, particularly neurokinin 1 (NK1), are highly expressed in pain pathways, and its co-localization with glutamate in the same axon terminals suggests a dual role in both pain and inflammation. This dual role makes substance P a critical target in efforts to develop treatments for pain conditions that have a significant inflammatory component (75–77).

5.4.6 Mechanisms of Neurotransmitter Release

The release of neurotransmitters is a complex process governed by synaptic vesicle dynamics. Neurotransmitters are stored in vesicles within the axon terminals, and upon depolarization, VGCCs open to allow calcium influx, which triggers the vesicles to fuse with the pre-synaptic membrane. This fusion is mediated by the SNARE complex, enabling the neurotransmitter to be released into the synaptic cleft through exocytosis. This process is tightly regulated, and disruptions can have profound effects on pain signaling (78–81).

Medications like gabapentin, pregabalin, and ziconotide target VGCCs, thereby inhibiting the release of neurotransmitters and reducing the transmission of pain signals. These drugs represent a cornerstone of pharmacological pain management, particularly in conditions characterized by heightened neuronal excitability (81–83) (Figure 5.2). In addition to VGCC-mediated release, neurotransmission can also be modulated by direct inhibition of exocytosis, as seen with *botulinum toxin*. This potent neurotoxin cleaves the SNARE complex, effectively blocking neurotransmitter release and leading to muscle paralysis. Its application in pain management, particularly in conditions like spasticity and chronic migraine, has been linked to its ability to inhibit the release of pain-related neuropeptides, such as CGRP (84–86).

5.4.7 Glutamate Recycling

The recycling of glutamate, the primary excitatory neurotransmitter, is critical for maintaining synaptic homeostasis and preventing excitotoxicity. Glutamate is taken up by astrocytes from the synaptic cleft, converted into glutamine, and then shuttled back to neurons, where it is reconverted to glutamate. Disruptions in this cycle can lead to altered pain perception, with either increased or decreased glutamate levels contributing to pain hypersensitivity or attenuation, respectively (87–89). The implications of this mechanism extend beyond pain, offering insights into the treatment of neurodegenerative diseases, such as Alzheimer's and Huntington's, where glutamate dysregulation plays a key role (90).

5.5 CONCLUSION

DRG serves as a critical nexus in the peripheral nervous system, playing a fundamental role in the transmission of sensory signals, particularly pain, from the periphery to the central nervous system. This chapter has explored the complex interplay of molecular mechanisms within DRG neurons, focusing on ion channels, neurotransmitters, and the processes governing neurotransmitter release, each of which contributes significantly to pain perception and modulation.

Voltage-gated sodium (Nav), potassium (Kv), and calcium (VGCC) channels are vital in regulating the excitability of DRG neurons. Their precise function in initiating and propagating action potentials underscores their importance in nociceptive signaling. Dysfunction or dysregulation of these channels, whether through genetic mutations, injury, or chronic inflammation, can lead to aberrant neuronal activity, contributing to the development and persistence of chronic pain states. This understanding provides a solid foundation for targeting these channels in the development of novel pain therapeutics.

The neurotransmitter systems within the DRG, including excitatory transmitters like glutamate and CGRP and inhibitory transmitters such as opioid peptides and cannabinoids, further modulate pain signaling. These neurotransmitters are critical in the balance between excitation and inhibition, a balance that is often disrupted in chronic pain. The interplay between neurotransmitters and their receptors not only dictates the experience of pain but also offers multiple avenues for therapeutic intervention, particularly in modulating the effects of these neurotransmitters to manage pain more effectively.

Chloride channels, particularly those associated with GABAergic signaling and the KCC2 cotransporter, play a crucial role in maintaining an inhibitory tone within the nervous system. The dysregulation of these channels in chronic pain conditions highlights the importance of restoring inhibitory control as a therapeutic strategy. The potential to enhance GABAergic inhibition through the modulation of chloride channels offers a promising approach to reducing pain sensitivity and improving patient outcomes.

Voltage-gated calcium channels (VGCCs) emerge as key players in neurotransmitter release and neuronal excitability, with their various subtypes contributing to the fine-tuning of pain signaling. The targeting of specific VGCC subunits, such as the $\alpha 2\delta$ subunit, by drugs like gabapentin and pregabalin underscores the clinical relevance of these channels in pain management. The modulation of VGCCs represents a cornerstone in the pharmacological treatment of chronic pain, offering targeted approaches to diminish pain signaling at its source.

Finally, the mechanisms governing neurotransmitter release, including synaptic vesicle dynamics and the role of VGCCs, are critical to understanding how pain signals are transmitted and modulated. Pharmacological agents that inhibit these processes, such as gabapentin, pregabalin, and botulinum toxin, demonstrate the therapeutic potential of targeting neurotransmitter release in pain management.

In conclusion, the DRG and its associated molecular mechanisms offer a rich landscape for understanding the pathophysiology of pain and developing targeted interventions. The integration of molecular insights with clinical applications holds the promise of more effective pain therapies tailored to modulate specific pathways involved in nociception. As our understanding of DRG function deepens, so too will our ability to manage and treat chronic pain, improving the quality of life for patients who suffer from this debilitating condition.

REFERENCES

1. Li S, Brimmers A, van Boekel RLM, Vissers KCP, Coenen MJH. A systematic review of genome-wide association studies for pain, nociception, neuropathy, and pain treatment responses. Pain. 2023;164(9):1891–911.
2. Heijmans L, Mons MR, Joosten EA. A systematic review on descending serotonergic projections and modulation of spinal nociception in chronic neuropathic pain and after spinal cord stimulation. Mol Pain. 2021;17:17448069211043965.
3. Hum B, Christophides A, Jin Z, Elias M, Taneja K, Bergese SD. The validity and applications of the analgesia nociception index: A narrative review. Front Surg. 2023;10:1234246.
4. Zhang J, Yao J, Rong M. Editorial: Role of Ion Channels in Pain. Front Pharmacol. 2022;13:884665.
5. Wang X, Li X. Regulation of pain neurotransmitters and chondrocytes metabolism mediated by voltage-gated ion channels: A narrative review. Heliyon. 2023;9(7): e17989.
6. Matta C, Takacs R, Ducza L, Ebeid RA, CHoi H, Mobasheri A. Ion channels involved in inflammation and pain in osteoarthritis and related musculoskeletal disorders. Am J Physiol Cell Physiol. 2023;325(1):C257–C71.
7. Yam MF, Loh YC, Tan CS, Khadijah Adam S, Abdul MaNan N, Basir R. General Pathways of Pain Sensation and the Major Neurotransmitters Involved in Pain Regulation. Int J Mol Sci. 2018;19(8).
8. Willis WD. Role of neurotransmitters in sensitization of pain responses. Ann N Y Acad Sci. 2001; 933:142–56.
9. Otsuka M, Yanagisawa M. Pain and neurotransmitters. Cell Mol Neurobiol. 1990;10(3):293–302.
10. Ban EG, Brassai A, Vizi ES. The role of the endogenous neurotransmitters associated with neuropathic pain and in the opioid crisis: The innate pain-relieving system. Brain Res Bull. 2020;155:129–36.
11. Podgorski Iii E, Mascaro P, Patin D. Comparison of FDA-approved electrical neuromodulation techniques for focal neuropathic pain: A narrative review of DRG, HF10, and Burst Neuromodulation. Pain Physician. 2021;24(4): E407–E23.
12. Mazzotta G, Sarchielli P, GAggioli A, Gallai V. Study of pressure pain and cellular concentration of neurotransmitters related to nociception in episodic tension-type headache patients. Headache. 1997;37(9):565–71.
13. Goodwin G, McMahon SB. The physiological function of different voltage-gated sodium channels in pain. Nat Rev Neurosci. 2021;22(5):263–74.
14. Schuelert N, McDougall JJ. Involvement of Nav 1.8 sodium ion channels in the transduction of mechanical pain in a rodent model of osteoarthritis. Arthritis Res Ther. 2012;14(1):R5.
15. Coskun C, Ocal I, Gunay I. A Low-Frequency Pulsed Magnetic Field Reduces Neuropathic Pain by Regulating NaV(1.8) and NaV(1.9) Sodium Channels at the Transcriptional Level in Diabetic Rats. Bioelectromagnetics. 2021;42(5):357–70.
16. Mao M, Fan W, Zheng Y, Qi P, Xi M, Yao Y. Upregulation of N-Type Voltage-Gated Calcium Channels Induces Neuropathic Pain in Experimental Autoimmune Neuritis. Evid Based Complement Alternat Med. 2022;2022:8547095.

17. Eagles DA, Chow CY, King GF. Fifteen years of Na(V) 1.7 channels as an analgesic target: Why has excellent in vitro pharmacology not translated into in vivo analgesic efficacy? Br J Pharmacol. 2022;179(14):3592–611.
18. Maverick EE, Tamkun MM. High spatial density is associated with non-conducting Kv channels from two families. Biophys J. 2022;121(5):755–68.
19. Higerd-Rusli GP, Alsaloum M, Tyagi S, SarveswaraN N, Estacion M, Akin EJ, et al. Depolarizing Na(V) and Hyperpolarizing K(V) Channels Are Co-Trafficked in Sensory Neurons. J Neurosci. 2022;42(24):4794–811.
20. Ong ST, Tyagi A, Chandy KG, Bhushan S. Mechanisms underlying C-type inactivation in Kv channels: Lessons from structures of human Kv1.3 and fly shaker-IR channels. Front Pharmacol. 2022;13:924289.
21. Ramirez-Franco J, Debreux K, Sangiardi M, Belghazi M, Kim Y, Lee SH, et al. The downregulation of Kv(1) channels in Lgi1(-/-)mice is accompanied by a profound modification of its interactome and a parallel decrease in Kv(2) channels. Neurobiol Dis. 2024;196:106513.
22. Sun H, Patil MJ, Ru F, Meeker S, Undem BJ. K(V) 1/D-type potassium channels inhibit the excitability of bronchopulmonary vagal afferent nerves. J Physiol. 2022;600(12):2953–71.
23. Seo MS, An JR, Kang M, Heo R, Park H, Han ET, et al. Mechanisms underlying the vasodilatory effects of canagliflozin in the rabbit thoracic aorta: Involvement of the SERCA pump and Kv channels. Life Sci. 2021;287:120101.
24. Hasan A, Hasan R. Empagliflozin relaxes resistance mesenteric arteries by stimulating multiple smooth muscle cell voltage-gated K(+) (K(V)) channels. Int J Mol Sci. 2021;22(19).
25. Tan XF, Bae C, Stix R, Fernandez-Marino AI, Huffer K, Chang TH, et al. Structure of the Shaker Kv channel and mechanism of slow C-type inactivation. Sci Adv. 2022;8(11):eabm7814.
26. Merk A, Fukumura T, Zhu X, Darling JE, Grisshammer R, Ognjenovic J, et al. 1.8 A resolution structure of beta-galactosidase with a 200 kV CRYO ARM electron microscope. IUCrJ. 2020;7(Pt 4):639–43.
27. Kalia J, Swartz KJ. Exploring structure-function relationships between TRP and Kv channels. Sci Rep. 2013;3:1523.
28. Lu J, Deutsch C. Secondary structure formation of a transmembrane segment in Kv channels. Biochemistry. 2005;44(23):8230–43.
29. Martinez AH, Mohiuddin SS. Biochemistry, chloride channels. StatPearls. Treasure Island (FL)2024.
30. Yamamura H. Physiological and pathological significance of chloride channels. Biol Pharm Bull. 2024;47(1):1–13.
31. Souza AJ, Freitas IS, Sharmin D, Cook JM, Guimaraes FS, Gomes FV. An alpha 5-GABA(A) receptor positive allosteric modulator attenuates social and cognitive deficits without changing dopamine system hyperactivity in rats exposed to valproic acid in utero. Autism Res. 2024;17(8):1534–44.
32. Sohns K, Kostenko A, Behrendt M, Schmelz M, Rukwied R, Carr R. Depolarization of mouse DRG neurons by GABA does not translate into acute pain or hyperalgesia in healthy human volunteers. PLoS One. 2024;19(8):e0307668.
33. Neumann E, Cramer T, Acuna MA, Scheurer L, Beccarini C, Luscher B, et al. gamma1 GABA(A) receptors in spinal nociceptive circuits. J Neurosci. 2024.
34. Pethe A, Hamze M, Giannaki M, Heimrich B, MedIna I, Hartmann AM, et al. K(+)/Cl(-) cotransporter 2 (KCC2) and Na(+)/HCO3- cotransporter 1 (NBCe1) interaction modulates profile of KCC2 phosphorylation. Front Cell Neurosci. 2023;17:1253424.
35. McMoneagle E, Zhou J, Zhang S, Huang W, Josiah SS, Ding K, et al. Neuronal K(+)-Cl(-) cotransporter KCC2 as a promising drug target for epilepsy treatment. Acta Pharmacol Sin. 2024;45(1):1–22.

36. Huang 黄玉莹 Y, Chen 陈红 H, Shao 邵建英 JY, Zhou 周京京 JJ, Chen 陈少瑞 SR, Pan 潘惠麟 HL. Constitutive KCC2 Cell- and synapse-specifically regulates NMDA receptor activity in the spinal cord. J Neurosci. 2024;44(4).
37. Hamze M, Brier C, BuhlEr E, Zhang J, MedIna I, Porcher C. Regulation of neuronal chloride homeostasis by pro- and mature brain-derived neurotrophic factor (BDNF) via KCC2 cation-chloride cotransporters in rat cortical neurons. Int J Mol Sci. 2024;25(11).
38. Cai J, Wu Z, Wang G, Zhao X, Wang X, Wang BH, et al. The suppressive effect of the specific KCC2 modulator CLP290 on seizure in mice. Epilepsy Res. 2024;203:107365.
39. Ando H, Shimizu-Okabe C, Okura N, Yafuso T, Kosaka Y, KobayaShi S, et al. Reduced gene expression of KCC2 accelerates axonal regeneration and reduces motor dysfunctions after tibial nerve severance and suturing. Neuroscience. 2024;551:55–68.
40. Ma Y, Chen J, Chen C, Wei B, Liu X. Suppression of HCN channels in the spinal dorsal horn restores KCC2 expression and attenuates diabetic neuropathic pain. Neurosci Lett. 2024;822:137626.
41. Zeng S, Zhu R, Wang Y, Yang Y, Li N, Fu N, et al. Role of GABA(A) receptor depolarization-mediated VGCC activation in sevoflurane-induced cognitive impairment in neonatal mice. Front Cell Neurosci. 2022;16:964227.
42. Altier C. GPCR and voltage-gated calcium channels (VGCC) signaling complexes. Subcell Biochem. 2012;63:241–62.
43. Lam A, Karekar P, Shah K, Hariharan G, Fleyshman M, Kaur H, et al. Drosophila voltage-gated calcium channel alpha1-subunits regulate cardiac function in the aging heart. Sci Rep. 2018;8(1):6910.
44. Hirano M, Takada Y, Wong CF, Yamaguchi K, Kotani H, Kurokawa T, et al. C-terminal splice variants of P/Q-type Ca (2+) channel Ca(V)2.1 alpha(1) subunits are differentially regulated by Rab3-interacting molecule proteins. J Biol Chem. 2017;292(22):9365–81.
45. Hirakawa T, Goto M, TaKahashi K, Iwasawa T, FujishimA A, MaKino K, et al. Na^+/K+ ATPase alpha1 and beta3 subunits are localized to the basolateral membrane of trophectoderm cells in human blastocysts. Hum Reprod. 2022;37(7):1423–30.
46. Herbertz M, Harder S, ScHluter H, Lohr C, Dobler S. Na,K-ATPase alpha1 and beta-subunits show distinct localizations in the nervous tissue of the large milkweed bug. Cell Tissue Res. 2022;388(3):503–19.
47. Song G, Li B, Yang Z, Lin H, Cheng J, Huang Y, et al. Regulation of cell membrane potential through supramolecular system for activating calcium ion channels. J Am Chem Soc. 2024.
48. Martin-Belmonte A, Aguado C, AlfaRo-Ruiz R, Kulik A, de La Ossa L, Moreno-Martinez AE, et al. Nanoarchitecture of Ca(V)2.1 channels and GABA(B) receptors in the mouse hippocampus: Impact of APP/PS1 pathology. Brain Pathol. 2024:e13279.
49. Salib AN, Crane MJ, Lee SH, Wainger BJ, Jamieson AM, Lipscombe D. Interleukin-1alpha links peripheral Ca(V)2.2 channel activation to rapid adaptive increases in heat sensitivity in skin. bioRxiv. 2024.
50. Nilsson M, Wang K, Minguez-Vinas T, Angelini M, Berglund S, Olcese R, et al. Electrical and G-protein regulation of CaV2.2 (N-type) Channels. bioRxiv. 2024.
51. Li X, Tae HS, Chen S, Yousuf A, Huang L, Zhang J, et al. Dual Antagonism of alpha9alpha10 nAChR and GABA(B) Receptor-Coupled Ca(V)2.2 Channels by an Analgesic alphaO-Conotoxin Analogue. J Med Chem. 2024;67(2):971–87.
52. Ferron L, Zamponi GW. A tale of two calcium channels: Structural pharmacology of Cav2.1 and Cav3.2. Cell Res. 2024;34(6):401–2.
53. Ferreira MA, Luckemeyer DD, Martins F, Schran RG, da Silva AM, Gambeta E, et al. Pronociceptive role of spinal Ca(v)2.3 (R-type) calcium channels in a mouse model of postoperative pain. Br J Pharmacol. 2024.
54. Sampedro-Castaneda M, Baltussen LL, Lopes AT, Qiu Y, Sirvio L, Mihaylov SR, et al. Epilepsy-linked kinase CDKL5 phosphorylates voltage-gated calcium channel Cav2.3, altering inactivation kinetics and neuronal excitability. Nat Commun. 2023;14(1):7830.

55. Gunnersen JM, Kuek A, Phipps JA, Hammond VE, PuThussery T, Fletcher EL, et al. Seizure-related gene 6 (Sez-6) in amacrine cells of the rodent retina and the consequence of gene deletion. PLoS One. 2009;4(8):e6546.
56. Zajaczkowska R, Mika J, Leppert W, Kocot-Kepska M, Malec-Milewska M, Wordliczek J. Mirogabalin-A novel selective ligand for the alpha2delta calcium channel subunit. Pharmaceuticals (Basel). 2021;14(2).
57. Khuong TM, Hamoudi Z, Manion J, Loo L, Muralidharan A, Neely GG. Peripheral straitjacket (alpha2delta Ca (2+) channel subunit) expression is required for neuropathic sensitization in Drosophila. Philos Trans R Soc Lond B Biol Sci. 2019;374(1785):20190287.
58. Chen X, An M, Ye S, Yang Z, Ding Z. The alpha (2) delta calcium channel subunit accessorily and independently affects the biological function of ditylenchus destructor. Int J Mol Sci. 2022;23(21).
59. Xiong X, Zhang L, Li Y, Guo S, Chen W, Huang L, et al. Calcium channel subunit alpha2delta-1 as a potential biomarker reflecting illness severity and neuroinflammation in patients with acute ischemic stroke. J Stroke Cerebrovasc Dis. 2021;30(8):105874.
60. Guo SJ, Shi YQ, Zheng YN, Liu H, Zheng YL. The voltage-gated calcium channel alpha2delta subunit in neuropathic pain. Mol Neurobiol. 2024.
61. Tian Y. The role of dopamine neurotransmitters in neurological diseases: New sight. Int J Mol Sci. 2024;25(14).
62. Strack R. Neurotransmitters at a glance. Nat Methods. 2024;21(7):1143.
63. Prescot A, Becerra L, Pendse G, Tully S, Jensen E, Hargreaves R, et al. Excitatory neurotransmitters in brain regions in interictal migraine patients. Mol Pain. 2009;5:34.
64. Parent AS, Matagne V, Bourguignon JP. Control of puberty by excitatory amino acid neurotransmitters and its clinical implications. Endocrine. 2005;28(3):281–6.
65. Lopez E, Hernandez J, ArCe C, CanadaS S, Oset-Gasque MJ, Gonzalez MP. Involvement of NMDA receptor in the modulation of excitatory and inhibitory amino acid neurotransmitters release in cortical neurons. Neurochem Res. 2010;35(9):1478–86.
66. Liang CL, Quang Nguyen T, Marks GA. Inhibitory and excitatory amino acid neurotransmitters are utilized by the projection from the dorsal deep mesencephalic nucleus to the sublaterodorsal nucleus REM sleep induction zone. Brain Res. 2014;1567:1–12.
67. Famiglietti EV, Sundquist SJ. Development of excitatory and inhibitory neurotransmitters in transitory cholinergic neurons, starburst amacrine cells, and GABAergic amacrine cells of rabbit retina, with implications for previsual and visual development of retinal ganglion cells. Vis Neurosci. 2010;27(1–2):19–42.
68. Boesmans W, Cirillo C, Van den Abbeel V, Van den Haute C, Depoortere I, Tack J, et al. Neurotransmitters involved in fast excitatory neurotransmission directly activate enteric glial cells. Neurogastroenterol Motil. 2013;25(2):e151–60.
69. Amantea D, Bagetta G. Excitatory and inhibitory amino acid neurotransmitters in stroke: from neurotoxicity to ischemic tolerance. Curr Opin Pharmacol. 2017;35:111–9.
70. Moore LA, Trussell LO. Corelease of inhibitory neurotransmitters in the mouse auditory midbrain. J Neurosci. 2017;37(39):9453–64.
71. Wei Y, Chen X, Li Y, Guo Y, Zhang S, Jin J, et al. Toxicological mechanism of cannabidiol (CBD) exposure on zebrafish embryonic development. Food Chem Toxicol. 2024:114929.
72. Pedrazzi JFC, Hassib L, Ferreira FR, Hallak JC, Del-Bel E, Crippa JA. Therapeutic potential of CBD in autism spectrum disorder. Int Rev Neurobiol. 2024;177:149–203.
73. Haghdoost M, Young S, Holloway AK, Roberts M, Zvorsky I, Bonn-Miller MO. CBD versus CBDP: Comparing in vitro receptor-binding activities. Int J Mol Sci. 2024;25(14).
74. Chang YC, Magnan RE, Cleveland MJ, Ladd BO. Event-level associations among THC, CBD, social context, and subjective effects during Cannabis use episodes. J Psychopharmacol. 2024:2698811241269800.
75. Wang J, Liu G, Xu K, Ai K, Huang W, Zhang J. The role of neurotransmitters in mediating the relationship between brain alterations and depressive symptoms in patients with inflammatory bowel disease. Hum Brain Mapp. 2023;44(16):5357–71.

76. Pauwels R, Joos G, Kips J, Van Der Straeten M. Interactions between neurotransmitters and inflammatory cells in the airways. Int Arch Allergy Appl Immunol. 1989;88(1–2):68–9.
77. Oshaghi M, Kourosh-Arami M, Roozbehkia M. Role of neurotransmitters in immune-mediated inflammatory disorders: A crosstalk between the nervous and immune systems. Neurol Sci. 2023;44(1):99–113.
78. Monday HR, Younts TJ, Castillo PE. Long-term plasticity of neurotransmitter release: Emerging mechanisms and contributions to brain function and disease. Annu Rev Neurosci. 2018;41:299–322.
79. Lazarevic V, Pothula S, Andres-Alonso M, Fejtova A. Molecular mechanisms driving homeostatic plasticity of neurotransmitter release. Front Cell Neurosci. 2013;7:244.
80. Kavalali ET. The mechanisms and functions of spontaneous neurotransmitter release. Nat Rev Neurosci. 2015;16(1):5–16.
81. Brunger AT, Choi UB, Lai Y, Leitz J, Zhou Q. Molecular mechanisms of fast neurotransmitter release. Annu Rev Biophys. 2018;47:469–97.
82. Williams DJ, Sidaway P, Cunnane TC, Brain KL. Mechanisms involved in nicotinic acetylcholine receptor-induced neurotransmitter release from sympathetic nerve terminals in the mouse vas deferens. PLoS One. 2011;6(12):e29209.
83. Fon EA, Edwards RH. Molecular mechanisms of neurotransmitter release. Muscle Nerve. 2001;24(5):581–601.
84. Zhang W, Zhang Y, Wang H, Sun X, Chen L, Zhou J. Animal models of chronic migraine: From the bench to therapy. Curr Pain Headache Rep. 2024.
85. Tang X, Chen H, Zhao M, Yang W, Shuang R, Xu S. alpha7nAChR-mediated astrocytic activation: A novel mechanism of Xiongzhi Dilong decoction in ameliorating chronic migraine. J Ethnopharmacol. 2024;334:118509.
86. Jantzen FT, Chaudhry BA, Younis S, Norgaard I, Cullum CK, Do TP, et al. Average steps per day as marker of treatment response with anti-CGRP mAbs in adults with chronic migraine: A pilot study. Sci Rep. 2024;14(1):18068.
87. Michaluk P, Heller JP, Rusakov DA. Rapid recycling of glutamate transporters on the astroglial surface. Elife. 2021;10.
88. Mejias R, Adamczyk A, Anggono V, Niranjan T, Thomas GM, Sharma K, et al. Gain-of-function glutamate receptor interacting protein 1 variants alter GluA2 recycling and surface distribution in patients with autism. Proc Natl Acad Sci U S A. 2011;108(12):4920–5.
89. Casse F, Bardou I, Danglot L, Briens A, Montagne A, Parcq J, et al. Glutamate controls tPA recycling by astrocytes, which in turn influences glutamatergic signals. J Neurosci. 2012;32(15):5186–99.
90. Cao P, Zhang J, Huang Y, Fang Y, Lyu J, Shen Y. The age-related changes and differences in energy metabolism and glutamate-glutamine recycling in the d-gal-induced and naturally occurring senescent astrocytes in vitro. Exp Gerontol. 2019;118:9–18.

6 Dorsal Horn Organization and Processing

Soun Sheen and Hemant Kalia

6.1 INTRODUCTION

Acute nociceptive pain, defined by Sherrington as a protective event secondary to "stimuli that become adequate as excitants of nociception when they are of such intensity as threatens damage," is essential for survival by triggering withdrawal and autonomic responses known as nociceptive reflex (Yaksh 2020). Acute high-threshold stimulus activates small primary afferents to project into the spinal dorsal horn, which is organized into layers with distinctive patterns of primary afferent input. The second-order dorsal horn neurons then process the incoming information and send supraspinal projections to relay both the sensory-discriminative and affective-motivational components of pain. This chapter will provide a brief overview of the basic anatomy of the primary afferent, spinal dorsal horn, and ascending projection pathways involved in acute nociceptive pain processing and review the properties of dorsal horn neurons that encode nociceptive information.

6.2 PRIMARY AFFERENTS: CLASSIFICATION

Acute nociceptive pain begins with the activation of primary afferent neurons. These neurons have cell bodies within the dorsal root ganglia (DRG) and send projections to the periphery and spinal cord (Cohen, S.A. 2020; Yaksh 2020). As shown in Table 6.1, primary afferent fibers are commonly classified by anatomical characteristics into three major classes—Aβ, Aδ, and C (Yaksh, Ramachandran, and Woller 2020). Aβ fibers are large and myelinated, with rapid conduction velocity greater than 40–50 m/s. Aβ fibers are low-threshold mechanoreceptors activated by low-threshold mechanical stimuli. Aδ fibers are small and unmyelinated, with conduction velocity between 10 and 40 m/s. Aδ fibers are activated by not only low-threshold mechanical or thermal stimuli but also by high-threshold mechanical and thermal stimuli. C fibers are small, unmyelinated fibers with low conduction velocities of less than 2 m/s. Unlike myelinated afferent axons with specialized nerve endings that define the characteristics of the stimulus, C fibers have no evidence of specialization and terminate as "free" nerve endings (Yaksh and Luo 2011). These fibers are known as polymodal nociceptors, as they respond to different modalities, including high-threshold thermal, mechanical, and chemical stimuli.

DOI: 10.1201/9781003094302-6

TABLE 6.1
Erlanger–Gasser Classification of Axons

Fiber Class	Diameter (µ dia)	Velocity (m/sec)	Effective Stimuli
Aβ (myelinated)	12–20	>40–50	Low-threshold mechanical Specialized nerve endings (Pacinian corpuscles)
Aδ (myelinated)	1–4	10–40	Low-threshold mechanical or thermal High-threshold mechanical or thermal Specialized nerve endings
C (unmyelinated)	0.5–1.5	<2	High-threshold thermal, mechanical, and chemical Free nerve endings

Source: Adapted from Bajwa, Wootton, and Warfield, *Principle and Practice of Pain Medicine, 3rd edition* (2017).

6.3 PRIMARY AFFERENTS: TRANSDUCTION

Sensory afferents can transduce modality-specific stimuli into action potentials based on their individual terminal transduction properties (Fisher et al. 2021). Initial depolarization is dependent upon specific transducer channels and the magnitude of the stimulus. Under normal conditions, sensory afferents have minimal, if any, spontaneous activities (Yaksh 2020). When the peripheral stimulus is applied, sensory afferents display a monotonic increase in discharge frequency in response to increasing stimulus intensities with different triggering thresholds, as shown in Figure 6.1 (Yaksh, Ramachandran, and Woller 2020). This means that increased stimulus intensity leads to a monotonic increase in discharge firing rate due to a greater depolarization of the terminal.

Different transducers expressed at distinct terminals define the response properties of specific axons (Fisher et al. 2021). For example, TRPV1 is one of many transducer channels on an afferent-free nerve ending terminal. It is a thermosensitive receptor that responds to thermal stimulus greater than 43°C but is also activated by chemical molecules such as capsaicin (Figure 6.2) (Yaksh 2020; Yaksh and Luo 2011). The sensation of heat with capsaicin occurs with the activation of the thermosensitive TRPV1 channel.

6.4 PRIMARY AFFERENTS: TERMINATION

The primary afferents extend through the DRG, where the excitatory neurotransmitters are synthesized, to the axon terminals of the spinal cord, where they terminate as the dorsal horn, where the first synapse in somatosensory processing occurs. The dorsal horn is constituted of a series of layers or laminae according to the Rexed lamination classification (Table 6.2; Figure 6.3) (Ringkamp, Dougherty, and Raja 2018). Specific primary afferents project to specific layers of the dorsal horn. High-threshold, small, unmyelinated C fibers terminate in the superficial layers of the

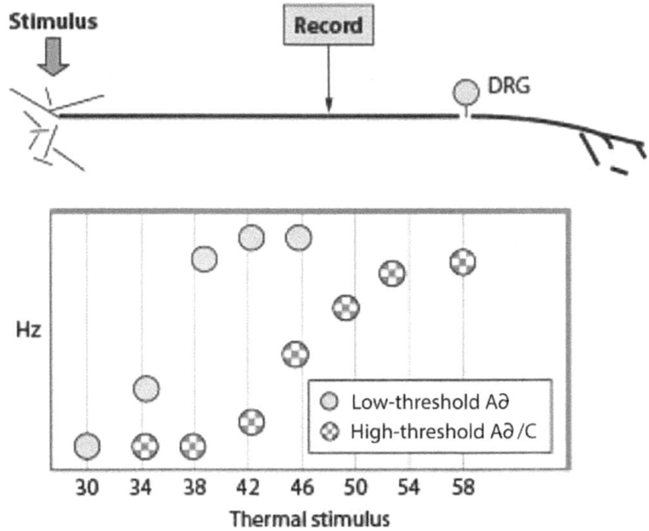

FIGURE 6.1 Stimulus–response curve. Both low-threshold and high-threshold fibers show little spontaneous activity. Both axons show a monotonic increase in discharge frequency in response to increasing stimulus intensities with different triggering thresholds. For high-threshold fibers, the temperature range greater than 42°C corresponds to temperatures that would psychophysically correspond to pain. In contrast, low-threshold fibers show responses that correspond to warmth sensation (34°C).

Source: Bajwa, Wootton, and Warfield, *Principle and Practice of Pain Medicine, 3rd edition* (2017).

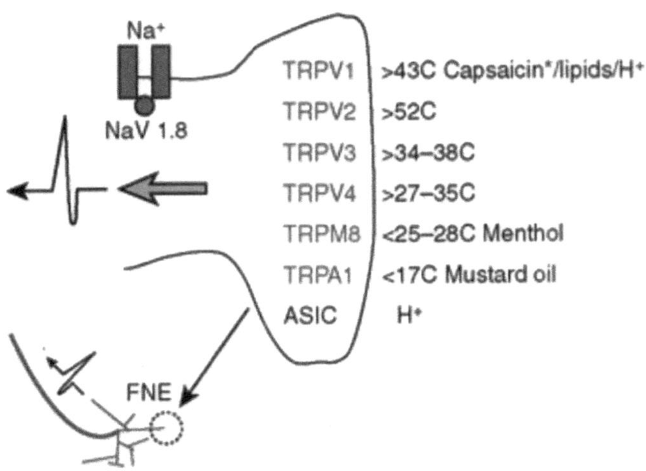

FIGURE 6.2 C fiber terminal transducer channels. Different terminals express different combinations of transducers, and this would define the thermal response properties of that sensory axon.

Source: Waldman, Pain Management (2011).

TABLE 6.2
Dorsal Horn Organization

Spinal Laminae		Afferent Terminals
Marginal	I	Aδ/C
Substantia gelatinosa	II	Aδ/C
Nucleus proprius	III, IV, V, VI	Aβ/Aδ
Motor horn	VII, VIII, IX	Aβ
Central canal	X	Aδ/C

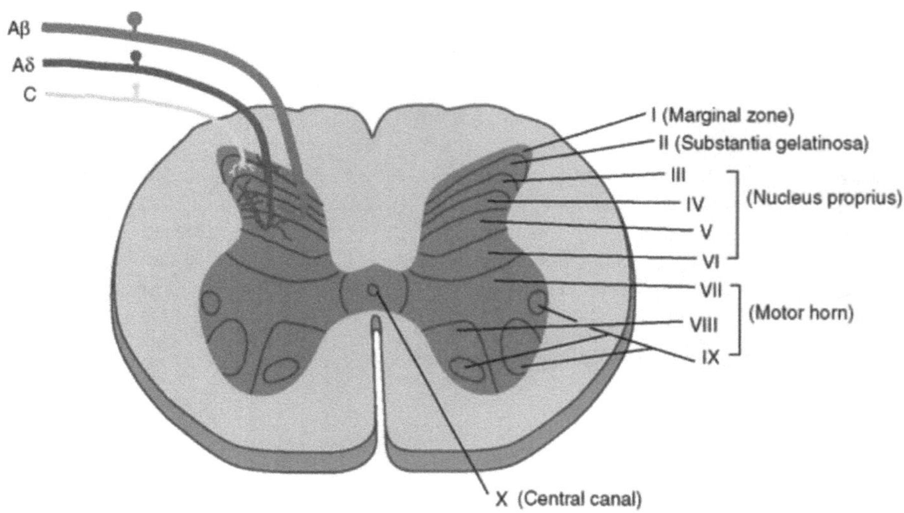

FIGURE 6.3 Organization of the dorsal horn. The dorsal horn is constituted of a series of layers referred to as spinal Rexed lamination. While Aδ and C fibers enter superficially in laminae I and II, large, myelinated Aβ fibers enter more deeply. See text for additional details.

Source: Waldman, *Pain Management* (2011).

dorsal horn, including the marginal zone (lamina I) and substantia gelatinosa (lamina II). Smaller, myelinated Aδ fibers also project to laminae I and II as well as the deeper nucleus proprius layers (laminae III–VI). Aδ and C fibers also project to the central canal (lamina X), which is the deepest layer of the dorsal horn. Low-threshold, large, myelinated Aβ afferents terminate in the nucleus propius (laminae III–VI) and motor horn layers (laminae VIII–IX).

As demonstrated in Figure 6.4, both A and C fibers send collateral axons rostrally and caudally in the dorsal columns and Lissauer tract, respectively (Yaksh and Luo 2011; Willis 2007). These collateralizations can be up to several segments above or below the entry point, but the density of terminal projections diminishes distally.

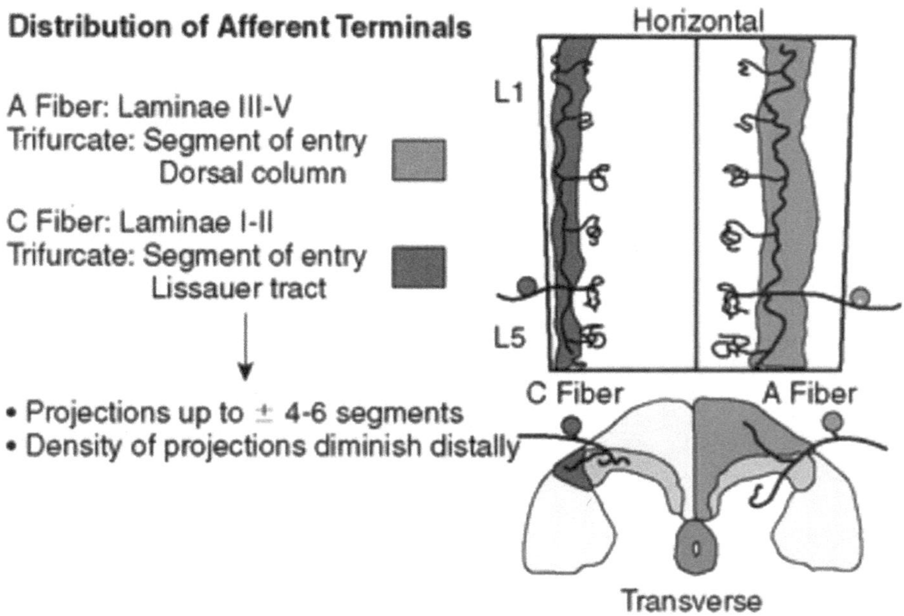

FIGURE 6.4 Distribution of afferent terminals. A and C fibers send collateral axons rostrally and caudally in the dorsal columns and Lissauer tract, respectively. The densest terminations occur within the segment of entry, and collateralizations at the more distal segments are less dense.

Source: Waldman, *Pain Management* (2011).

This concept of collateralization plays an important role in the expansion of receptive fields after tissue injury.

6.5 DORSAL HORN ANATOMY AND ORGANIZATION

The dorsal horn is primarily comprised of second-order neurons that send sensory information to supraspinal structures via the ascending spinal tracts. The second-order dorsal horn neurons can be classified by their functional characteristics and anatomic location within the dorsal horn (Fisher et al., 2021). The superficial marginal and substantia gelatinosa layers (laminae I–II) are where Aδ and C fibers terminate and have nociceptive-specific neurons that respond selectively to high-threshold stimulation (Fisher et al. 2021; Yaksh and Luo 2011; Sorkin and Wallace 1999). These nociceptive neurons send projections to the contralateral brain stem and thalamus through the ventrolateral tracts of the spinal cord, also known as the spinothalamic tracts. Lamina II also has local interneurons that project from the superficial dorsal horn to the deeper nucleus proprius layers (laminae III–VI), which serve to regulate the excitability of dorsal horn neurons (Fisher et al. 2021).

The deeper nucleus proprius layers (laminae III–VI) are rich in Aβ axons but also have distal dendrites that receive input from Aδ and C afferents in the upper laminae,

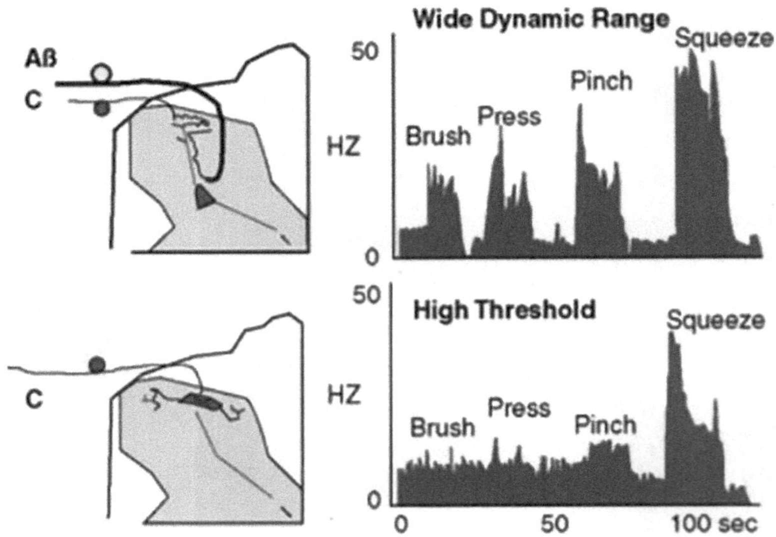

FIGURE 6.5 Firing patterns of dorsal horn neurons. Graphs present the neuronal responses to graded intensities of mechanical stimulation. While wide dynamic range (WDR) neurons respond to a wide range of stimuli, nociceptive-specific neurons respond selectively to high-threshold stimulation.

Source: Waldman, *Pain Management* (2011).

thus receiving significant fiber convergence (Yaksh 2020; Woller et al. 2017). The second-order neurons of the deeper layers are also known as wide dynamic range (WDR) neurons and respond to a wide range of stimuli (Figure 6.5). The WDR neurons encode the stimulus intensity as a function of discharge frequency, which enables them to increase discharge rates with increasing stimulus intensities and differentiate a noxious stimulus from a non-adverse stimulus (Yaksh 2020).

6.6 ASCENDING SPINAL TRACTS

Activity evoked in the spinal cord by high-threshold stimuli reaches supraspinal sites by several long tract systems within the ventrolateral quadrant of the spinal cord, including the spinoreticulothalamic, spinomesencephalic, spinoparabrachial, and spinothalamic pathways (Figure 6.6) (Yaksh and Luo 2010; Dostrovsky and Craig 2006). It has been established that pain is a crossed pathway, as unilateral ventrolateral lesions result in contralateral pain and temperature deficits, indicating that pain is a crossed pathway.

The spinoreticulothalamic tract originates from the deeper dorsal horn layers (laminae V–VIII) and projects into the brain stem reticular formation along the ipsilateral and contralateral ventrolateral quadrant. The spinomesencephalic tract originates primarily in lamina I and then travels into the contralateral lateral periaqueductal gray matter. The spinoparabrachial tract also primarily originates from

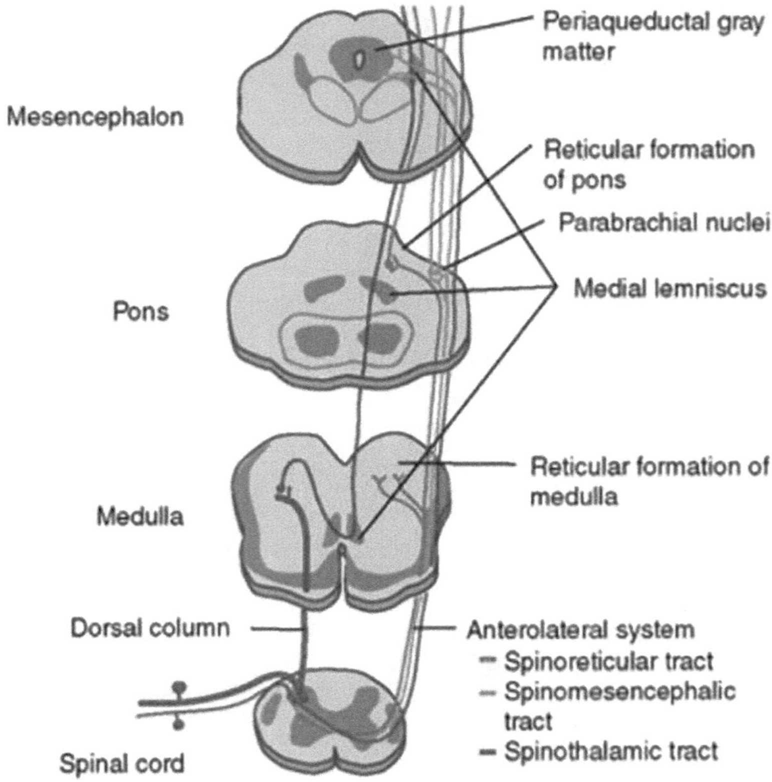

FIGURE 6.6 Summary of ascending spinal tracts. See text for details.

Source: Waldman, *Pain Management* (2011).

lamina I neurons and then sends projections to the parabrachial nucleus pons through the contralateral ventrolateral quadrant.

The spinothalamic tract neurons are located throughout the dorsal horn, with the greatest concentration in laminae I and V. The spinothalamic tract crosses through the ventral spinal commissures within a few segments rostral to the origin and ascend to the contralateral thalamus along the ventrolateral tract. The spinothalamic axons divide into medial and lateral components as they travel rostrally. The majority of the lamina V neurons project to the classical somatosensory thalamus, known as the ventroposterolateral (VPL) thalamus (Fisher et al. 2021). Neurons in this region then project to the somatosensory cortex, and this pathway is characterized by the retention of a precise mapping of the body surface (Dostrovsky 2000; Dostrovsky and Craig 2006). The nociceptive-specific lamina I neurons largely make medial projections to the posterior ventral medial (VMpo) and ventral caudal portion of the medial dorsal (MDvc) nuclei of the thalamus (Yaksh and Luo 2011; Fisher et al. 2021). These neurons then project to the inferior insula and anterior cingulate, respectively. This pathway is characterized by a poor somatotopic map and is involved in the affect and emotionality of pain (Dostrovsky and Craig 2006; Cohen, R.I. 2020). These different projections reflect the encoding information that is related to the "sensory-discriminative" and "affective-motivational" aspects of the pain experience.

6.7 CONCLUSION

The pain pathway begins with the activation of transducer channels located in the peripheral terminal, leading to the conduction of peripheral stimulus through the primary afferents to the second-order neurons. The nociceptive-specific neurons of the superficial dorsal horn and polymodal WDR neurons of the deeper layers send ascending projections to the thalamus through the contralateral ventrolateral tracts along two principal tracts. It is important to note that different supraspinal projection targets reflect the encoding information related to the sensory-discriminative and affective-motivational aspects of the pain experience.

REFERENCES

Cohen, R.I. 2020. Anatomy and Physiology of Pain. In *Principles and Practice of Pain Medicine,* Ed. Z.H. Bajwa, R.J. Wootton, and C.A. Warfield. 3rd edition. Chapter 2. McGraw Hill.

Cohen, S.A. 2020. Pathophysiology of Pain. In *Principles and Practice of Pain Medicine,* Ed. Z.H. Bajwa, R.J. Wootton, and C.A. Warfield. 3rd edition. Chapter 3. McGraw Hill.

Dostrovsky, J.O. 2000. Role of Thalamus in Pain. *Progress in Brain Research* 129: 245–257.

Dostrovsky, J.O. and A.D. Craig. 2006. Ascending Projection Systems. In *Wall & Melzack's Text of Pain,* Ed. S.B. McMahon, M. Koltzengurb, I. Tracey, and D.C. Turk. 6th edition. 182–197. Elsevier.

Fisher, C.J., T.L. Yaksh, K. Bruno, and K.A. Eddinger. 2021. Basic Science of Pain. In *Pain Care Essentials and Innovations*, Ed. S. Pangarkar, Q.G. Pham, and B.C. Eapen. 1–14. Elsevier. https://doi.org/10.1016/b978-0-323-72216-2.00001-6.

Ringkamp, M., P.M. Dougherty, and S.N. Raja. 2018. Anatomy and Physiology of the Pain Signaling Process. In *Essentials of Pain Medicine*, Ed. H.T. Benzon, S.N. Raja, S.S. Liu, S.M. Fishman, S.P. Cohen. 4th edition. 1–10. Elsevier.

Sorkin, L.S., and M.S. Wallace. 1999. Acute Pain Mechanism. *Surgical Clinics of North America* 79 (2): 213–229.

Willis, W.D. 2007. The Somatosensory System, with Emphasis on Structures Important for Pain. *Brain Research Reviews* 55: 297–313.

Woller, S.A., K.A. Eddinger, M. Corr, and T.L. Yaksh. 2017. An Overview of Pathways Encoding Nociception. *Clinical and Experimental Rheumatology* 35: 40–46.

Yaksh, T.L., and Z.D. Luo. 2010. Pain Pathways. In *Wall and Melzack's Textbook of Pain*, Ed. S.B. McMahon, M. Koltzenburg, I. Tracey, and D.C. Turk. 5th edition. 65–91. Elsevier.

Yaksh, T.L. and Z.D. Luo. 2011. Anatomy of the Pain Processing System. In *Pain Management,* Ed. S.D. Waldman. 2nd edition. Elsevier.

Yaksh, T.L. 2020. Biology of Pain Processing. Presentation at the University of California, San Diego.

Yaksh, T.L., R. Ramachandran, and S.A. Woller. 2020. Molecular Biology of Pain. In *Principles and Practice of Pain Medicine,* Ed. Z.H. Bajwa, R.J. Wootton, and C.A. Warfield. 3rd edition. Chapter 1. McGraw Hill.

7 The Psychophysiology of Pain

Fadel Zeidan

7.1 INTRODUCTION

Psychophysiology is a field of study that seeks to relate subjective awareness and behavior to physiologic events.[1–3] As a field of scientific inquiry, it concerns itself with central mechanisms of perception, cognition, and behavior, including learning, emotions, and the relationship of brain activity to consciousness. As a clinical area, psychophysiology has classically addressed somatoform disorders, stress (most recently posttraumatic stress disorders), and affective disorders in general. As a domain, psychophysiology is an important resource for the pain field for two primary reasons. On one hand, it offers a framework for understanding how stress contributes to pain, including the persistence of chronic pain; on the other hand, it uncovers links between cognitive processes (attention, expectancy, meaning, belief) and pain, as well as pain relief through psychological intervention.

Most physicians and pain researchers consider pain an unpleasant sensation originating from traumatized or inflamed tissues; however, pain encompasses more than just sensory information about the body's condition. *Affect* is an intrinsic dimension of pain. Any reasonable and unbiased observer studying mammals, particularly humans, would have to conclude that pain's affective features, rather than its sensory properties, govern behavioral responses to injury. People who experience pain do not quietly report the fact; they express negative emotions.

Is the affective dimension of pain as important as its sensory aspect? The linguist Elaine Scarry,[4] described pain's qualities as comprising extreme aversiveness, an ability to annihilate complex thoughts and other feelings, an ability to destroy language, and a strong resistance to objectification. Her perspective resonates with the lessons of everyday life: Although pain has sensory features and lends itself to sensory description, it is, above all else, a powerful negative feeling state. One cannot evaluate and address the suffering of a person in pain without an appreciation of its emotional nature.

The International Association for the Study of Pain (IASP) acknowledged the central role of emotion in its keystone definition: "Pain [is] an unpleasant sensory and *emotional* [emphasis added] experience associated with actual or potential tissue damage or described in terms of such damage."[5] This definition clearly emphasizes the role of affect as an intrinsic component of pain. Emotion is not a consequence of pain sensation that occurs after a noxious sensory message arrives at sensory cortices; rather, it is an integral part of the pain experience.

DOI: 10.1201/9781003094302-7

Psychophysiology has revealed that emotion and cognition are interdependent. Strong emotions can alter thought processes, perceptions, beliefs, attitudes, and expectancies. Conversely, thoughts can generate negative or positive emotional states, and the physiologic changes associated with such states can interact with tissue injury or inflammation and alter both the sensory and affective aspects of pain. Because pain states rarely exist in isolation, it is important to consider the psychophysiological context of a pain problem. The cognitive, emotional, and physiologic state of the patient presenting with pain is potentially very important for both assessment and intervention. I propose here that the best framework for characterizing this state is stress theory.

The purpose of this chapter is to describe the psychophysiological mechanisms underlying the subjective experience of pain and to explore their importance in the assessment and management of pain patients. The psychophysiology of pain requires an incursion into mind–body issues, consideration of the nature of emotion and its interdependence with cognition, and the overarching influence of stress. In this chapter, we show that (1) pain (awareness of tissue trauma) has intrinsic affective properties, including negative emotional arousal; (2) the brain creates bodily states of arousal (negative emotions) in response to threats to biological and psychological integrity; and (3) the affective dimension of pain is intrinsically linked to the related processes of defense and stress, and the physiologic mechanisms of these processes shape the affective dimension of pain.

7.2 HISTORICAL PERSPECTIVE: MIND–BODY ISSUES

Through most of the 20th century, our understanding of the relationship between mental processes and the body stemmed directly from Cartesian notions of mind–body dualism. For Descartes, a 17th-century philosopher and mathematician, human beings are dualistic: The mind and body are separate entities. Descartes described the life processes of the body as though they were clockwork mechanisms. The actions of the mind were, in his thinking, the workings of the soul.

Descartes believed that the awareness of pain, like awareness of other bodily sensations, must take place in a specific location where the mind observes the body. Dennett[6] termed this hypothetical seat of the mind the *Cartesian theater*. In this theater, the mind observes and interprets the array of multimodality signals that the body produces. The body is a passive environment; the mind is the nonphysical activity of the soul.

Today, most people will agree that such a theater of the mind cannot exist. Scientifically, the activity of the brain and that of the mind are inseparable, yet Cartesian dualism is endemic in Western thought and culture. Classical approaches to psychophysiology stemmed from Cartesian thinking, as did psychophysics. Early work on psychosomatic disorders focused on the mind–body relationships. Today, much of the popular movement favoring integrative medicine emphasizes the "mind–body connection," keeping oneself healthy through health-promoting cognitive approaches to better regulate immune responses. It is hard to avoid Cartesian thinking when the very fabric of our language carries it along as we reason and speak.

Cartesian assumptions are a subtle but powerful barrier for someone seeking to understand the affective dimension of pain. Relegating emotions to the realm of the mind and their physiologic consequences for the body is classical Descartes. It prevents us from appreciating the intricate interdependence of subjective feelings and physiology, and it detracts from our ability to comprehend how the efferent properties of autonomic nervous function can contribute causally to the realization of an emotional state. This chapter emphasizes the interdependence of mental processes and physiology. What we call the mind is consciousness, and consciousness is an emergent property of the activity of the brain. In a feedback-dependent manner, the brain regulates the physiologic arousal of the body, and emotion is a part of this process.

7.2.1 What Are Emotions?

The first step in understanding the nociceptive experience as an affective response is to appreciate the origins and purposes of emotion. Many physicians regard *emotions* as epiphenomenal feeling states associated with mental activity, subjective in character, and largely irrelevant to the state of a patient's physical health. Emotions are primarily physiologic and only secondarily subjective. Because they can strongly affect cardiovascular function, visceral motility, genitourinary function, and immune competence, patient emotions can have an important role in health overall and especially in pain management. Simple negative emotional arousal can exacerbate certain pain states, such as sympathetically maintained pain, angina, headache, neuropathic pain, and fibromyalgia. It contributes significantly to musculoskeletal pain, pelvic pain, and other pain problems in some patients.

Emotions are complex states of physiologic arousal and awareness that impute positive or negative hedonic qualities to a stimulus (event) in the internal or external environment. The objective aspect of emotion is autonomically and hormonally mediated physiologic arousal. The subjective aspects of emotion and *feelings* are phenomena of consciousness. Emotion represents in consciousness the biological importance or meaning of an event to the perceiver.

Emotion has two defining features: valence and arousal. *Valence* refers to the hedonic quality associated with an emotion—the positive or negative feeling attached to perception. *Arousal* refers to the degree of heightened activity in the central nervous system and autonomic nervous system (ANS) associated with perception.

Although emotions as a whole can be either positive or negative in valence, pain research addresses only negative emotions. Viewed as an emotion, pain signals a threat to the biological, psychological, or social integrity of an individual. In this respect, the emotional aspect of pain is a protective response that normally contributes to adaptation and survival. If uncontrolled or poorly managed in patients with severe or prolonged pain, it produces suffering.

7.2.2 Emotion in a Sociobiologic Perspective

Psychologists have many frameworks for studying emotion. Nature has equipped us with the capability of negative emotion for a purpose; bad feelings are not simply accidents of human consciousness. They are protective mechanisms that normally serve us well, but like uncontrolled pain, sustained and uncontrolled negative emotions can become pathologic states that can produce both maladaptive behavior and physiologic pathology.

By exploring the emotional dimension of pain from the sociobiologic perspective, the reader may gain some insight into how to prevent or control the negative affective aspect of pain, which fosters suffering. Unfortunately, implementing this perspective requires that we change conventional language habits that involve describing pain as a transient sensory event. *Pain is a compelling and emotionally negative state of the individual that has as its primary defining feature awareness of and adaptive adjustment to tissue trauma or disease.*

7.2.3 Adaptive Functions of Emotion

Emotions, including the emotional dimension of pain, characterize mammals exclusively, and they foster mammalian adaptation by making possible complex behaviors and adaptations. Importantly, they play a strong role in consciousness, producing and summarizing information that is important for the selection of alternative behaviors. According to MacLean,[7] emotions "impart subjective information that is instrumental in guiding behavior required for self-preservation and preservation of the species. The subjective awareness that is an affect consists of a sense of bodily pervasiveness or by *feelings localized to certain parts of the body* [emphasis added]." Because negative emotions, such as fear, evolved to facilitate adaptation and survival, emotion plays an important defensive role. The ability to experience threat when encountering injurious events protects against life-threatening injury.

The strength of emotional arousal associated with an injury indicates and expresses the magnitude of the perceived threat to the biological integrity of the person. Within the contents of consciousness, threat is a strong negative feeling state and not a pure informational appraisal. In humans, threatening events, such as injuries that are not immediately present, can exist as emotionally colored somatosensory images.

Phenomenal awareness consists largely of the production of images. Visual images are familiar to everyone: We can readily imagine seeing things. We can also produce auditory images by imagining a familiar tune, a birdsong, or the sound of a friend's voice. Similarly, we can generate somatosensory images. We can, for example, imagine the feeling of a full bladder, the sensation of a particular shoe on a foot, or a familiar muscle tension or ache. Cognition operates largely on images and plays a strong role in the experience of symptoms.

Patients can react emotionally to the mental image of a painful event before it happens (e.g., venipuncture), or for that matter, they can respond emotionally to the sight of another person's injury. The emotional intensity of such a feeling marks the adaptive significance of the event that produced the experience for the perceiver. In general, the threat of a minor injury normally provokes less feeling than one that incurs a risk of death. *The emotional magnitude of pain is the internal representation of the threat associated with the event that produced the pain.*

7.2.4 Emotions and Behavior

Negative emotions compel action, such as fight or flight, along with expression through vocalization, posture, variations in facial musculature patterns, and alterations of activity. This represents communication and often elicits social support, thus contributing to survival. Darwin,[8] observing animals, noted that emotions enable communication through vocalization, startle, posture, facial expression, and specific behaviors. He held that emotions must be inborn rather than learned tendencies. Darwin[8] pursued this issue by comparing the facial and other emotional expressions of children born blind with those of other children, reasoning that blind children would express emotion differently if the emotion is primarily a learned behavior. As others have since confirmed,[9] Darwin[8] learned that the basic blueprints for human emotional expression are innate.

Contemporary investigators who study emotions and human or animal social behavior emphasize that communication is a fundamental adaptive function of emotional expression.[10, 11] Social mammals, including humans, depend on one another or their social group as resources for adaptation and survival. The emotional expression of pain in the presence of supportive persons is socially powerful; it draws on a fundamental sociobiologic imperative: communicating threats and summoning assistance.

7.2.5 The Central Neuroanatomy of Emotion

7.2.5.1 Limbic Structures

The limbic brain represents an anatomical common denominator across mammalian species,[7] and emotion is a common feature of mammals. Consequently, investigators can learn much about human emotion by studying mammalian laboratory animals. Humans and animals differ in that the limbic brain is more developed in humans, the frontal lobes are unique to our species, and the interdependence of cognition and emotion is greatest in humans.

Early investigators focused on the role of olfaction in limbic function, and this led them to link the limbic brain to emotion. Emotion may have evolutionary roots in olfactory perception. MacLean[12] introduced the somewhat-controversial term "limbic system" and characterized its functions. He identified three main subdivisions of the limbic brain: amygdala, septum, and thalamocingulate,[7] which represent sources of afferents to parts of the limbic cortex. He also postulated that the limbic brain responds to two basic types of input: interoceptive and exteroceptive. These refer to sensory information from internal and external environments, respectively. Figure 7.1 summarizes and extends this concept. Noxious signaling can arise from an injurious event in the external environment or from a pathologic condition in the internal environment.

Over the last decade, numerous studies have employed functional brain imaging to investigate how the human brain responds to painful laboratory stimulation as well as how it behaves in chronic pain conditions. These studies reveal unequivocally that limbic structures involved in emotion and cognition are active during pain. In addition, related studies show that cognitive processes such as threat appraisal and perceived control are related to pain modulation. Early brain imaging studies have shown that the following brain structures are consistently active during states of

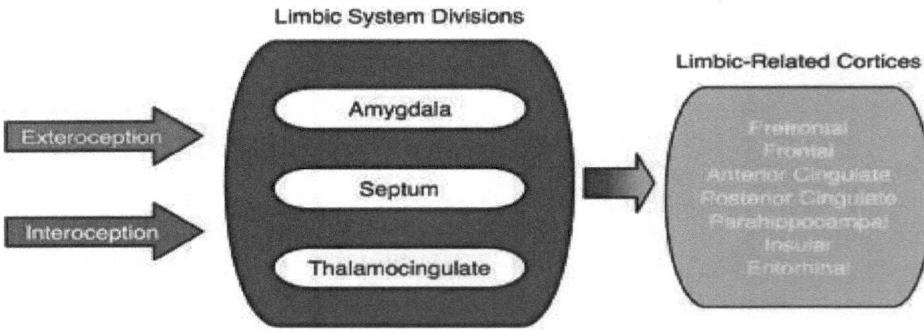

FIGURE 7.1

pain: the thalamus, primary and secondary somatosensory cortices, insular cortex, anterior cingulate, and the prefrontal cortices (PFC), as well as deactivation of the posterior cingulate cortex and medial prefrontal cortex,[13–15] which compose of the default mode network involved in self-referential processing.[16] The thalamus and the somatosensory cortices played a prominent role in early neurophysiologic models of pain and processing of ascending nociceptive information. The insular cortex may play a role in the somatosensory representation of the body, and it appears to integrate multimodal sensory information.[17] PFC controls the executive functions of the brain and the sense of self. They are involved in threat appraisal, meaning, and the integration of information from the internal and external environment.

7.2.6 Peripheral Neuroanatomy of Emotion

7.2.6.1 The Autonomic Nervous System

The ANS plays a major role in regulating the constancy of the internal environment, and it does so in a feedback-regulated fashion under the direction of the hypothalamus, the solitary nucleus (nucleus tractus solitarius), and ventral lateral medulla, the amygdala, and other brain structures.[18, 19] In general, it regulates activities that are not normally under voluntary control. The hypothalamus is the principal integrator of autonomic activity. Stimulation of the hypothalamus elicits highly integrated patterns of response that involve the limbic system and other structures.[20]

Many researchers hold that the ANS has three divisions: the sympathetic, the parasympathetic, and the enteric.[21, 22] Others subsume the enteric under the other two divisions. Broadly, the sympathetic nervous system makes possible the arousal needed for fight-and-flight reactions, whereas the parasympathetic system governs basal heart rate, metabolism, and respiration. The enteric nervous system innervates the viscera via a complex network of interconnected plexuses.

The sympathetic and parasympathetic systems are largely mutual physiologic antagonists—if one system inhibits a function, the other typically augments it. There are, however, important exceptions to this rule that demonstrate complementary or integratory relationships. The mechanism most heavily involved in the affective response to tissue trauma is the sympathetic nervous system.

During an emergency or injury to the body, the hypothalamus uses the sympathetic nervous system to increase cardiac output, respiration rate, and blood glucose. It also regulates the body temperature, causes piloerection, alters muscle tone, provides compensatory responses to hemorrhage, and dilates pupils. These responses are part of a coordinated, well-orchestrated response pattern called the defense response.[23–25] It resembles the better-known orienting response in some respects, but it can only occur following a strong stimulus that is noxious or, frankly, painful. It sets the stage for escape or confrontation, thus serving to protect the organism from danger. In an awake cat, both electrical stimulation of the hypothalamus and infusion of norepinephrine into the hypothalamus elicit a rage reaction with hissing, snarling, and attack posture with claw exposure, and a pattern of sympathetic nervous system arousal accompanies this.[26–28] Circulating epinephrine and norepinephrine produced by the adrenal medulla during activation of the sympathoadrenomedullary (SAM) axis accentuate the defense response, fear responses, and aversive emotional arousal in general.

7.2.6.2 Autonomic Arousal and Subjective Experience

Because the defense response and related changes are involuntary, we generally perceive them as something that the environment does to us. We typically describe such physiologic changes not as the bodily responses that they are but rather as feelings. We might describe a threatening and physiologically arousing event by saying, "It scared me" or "It made me really mad."

Phenomenologically, feelings seem to happen to us; we do not "do" them in the sense that we think thoughts or choose actions. Emotions are who we are in a given circumstance rather than the choices we make, and we commonly interpret events and circumstances in terms of the emotions that they elicit. ANS arousal, therefore, plays a major role in the complex psychological experience of injury and is a part of that experience.

Early views of the ANS followed the lead of Cannon[23] and held that emergency responses and all forms of intense aversive arousal are undifferentiated, diffuse patterns of sympathetic activation. Although this is broadly true, research has shown that definable patterns characterize emotional arousal and that these are related to the emotion involved, the motor activity required, and perhaps the context.[18, 19] An investigator attempting to understand how humans experience emotions must remember that the brain not only recognizes patterns of arousal but also creates them.

7.2.7 The Role of Feedback

One of the primary mechanisms involved in the generation and regulation of emotion is feedback. Feedback refers to the process by which information about a system's output is transmitted back to its input, shaping future responses. The subjective experience of emotion arises from patterns of physiological signals rather than existing as a separate entity within the mind, independent of the body. Similarly, in a medical context, a patient expressing emotional distress during a painful procedure or experiencing uncontrolled post-operative pain is not only reacting to the sensory features of pain but also to the overwhelming background of sympathetic arousal and neuroendocrine stress responses. These physiological changes amplify the perception of pain, reinforcing the emotional and physical experiences.

7.2.7.1 Relationship of Central and Peripheral Mechanisms

Figure 7.2 illustrates that noxious signaling undergoes parallel processing at the cognitive, affective, and sensory levels. An event representing a threat to biological

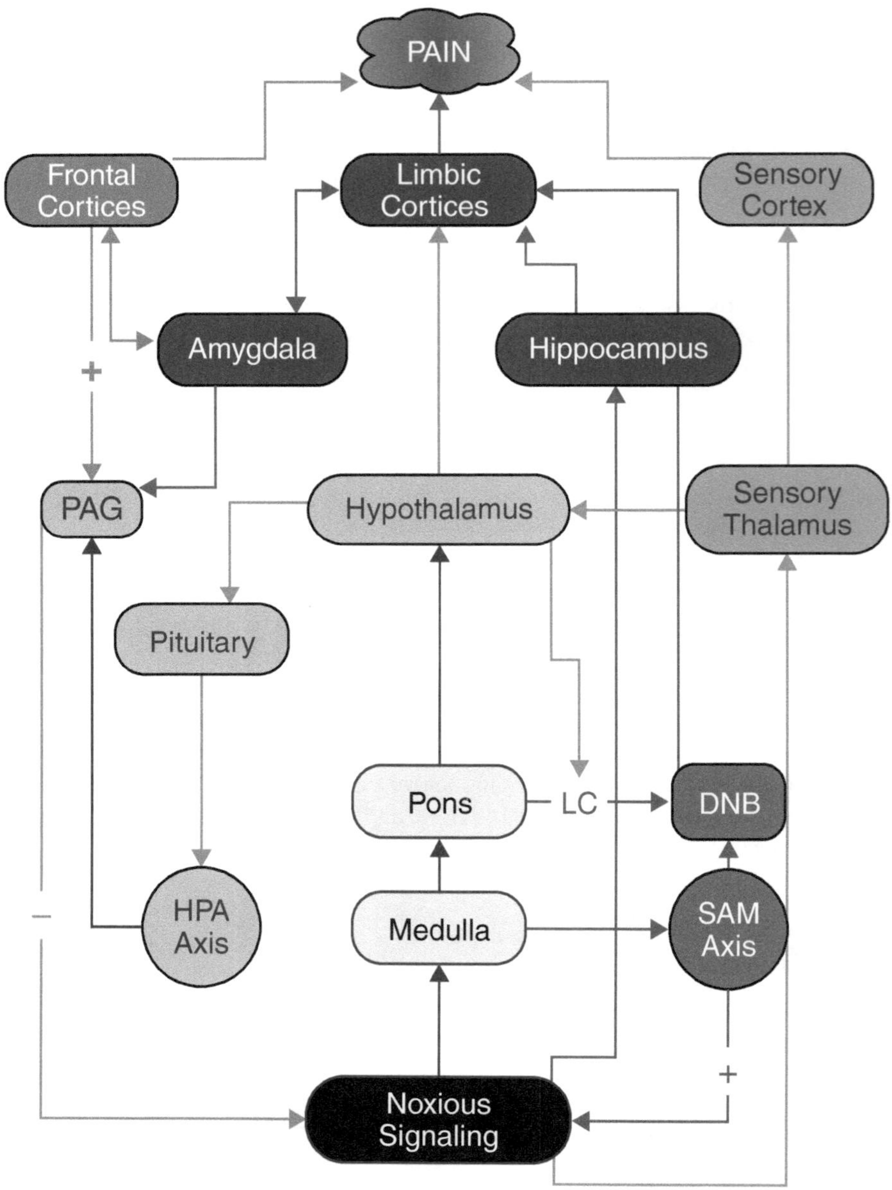

FIGURE 7.2 Noxious signaling undergoes parallel processing at the cognitive, affective, and sensory levels.

integrity elicits strong patterns of sympathetic and neuroendocrine response. These, in turn, contribute to the awareness of the perceiver. Sensory processing provides information about the environment, but this information exists in awareness against a background of emotional arousal, either positive or negative, and that arousal may vary from mild to extreme.

The transition from acute to chronic pain may involve complex changes in these pathways. The hypothalamic–pituitary–adrenocortical (HPA) and SAM axes are vulnerable to dysregulation with prolonged exposure to a stressor or series of stressors. This can include prolonged noxious signaling, as might occur with a degenerative disease or unrelenting noxious neuropathic signaling. Dysregulation in these systems may cause sensitization or impair normal inhibitory modulation.

Neural networks associated with threat, dysphoria, and other cognitive and emotional states play a crucial role in responding to acute threats with defensive arousal. Each mode of operation has adaptive value as a short-term response to specific types of injury or danger. These neural systems dynamically regulate the level of output, allowing for flexible responses to environmental demands.

System self-regulation and self-organization rely on feedback mechanisms, which also govern self-direction. Feedback loops can be either negative or positive. Negative feedback maintains stability by counteracting deviations from a set point, ensuring homeostasis and allostasis. In contrast, positive feedback amplifies changes, leading to escalation and rapid acceleration, which can be critical for mounting emergency responses. Homeostatic and allostatic regulatory processes primarily rely on negative feedback to preserve equilibrium. In contrast, positive feedback occurs when a variable changes and the system amplifies that change in the same direction, leading to instability rather than stability. From an adaptive perspective, positive feedback loops enable the body to rapidly adjust to acute challenges, but excessive activation can contribute to dysregulated physiological and psychological states.

In general, defensive reactions involve a pattern of rapid arousal created through positive feedback that prepares the body and the brain for emergency response, followed by a negative feedback–controlled transition to recovery and return to normalcy. Because smaller physiologic systems are nested within larger physiologic systems, higher-order systems typically limit positive feedback processes in smaller systems. In some cases, top-down regulation of positive feedback fails, for example, in a panic attack. In other cases, the event that triggered the emotion terminates, and the positive feedback process then stops. Sustained periods of positive feedback have the potential for destructive consequences.

Feedback is the basis of neuroendocrine regulation, as we describe it in the following discussion. Neuroendocrine feedback depends on blood-borne messengers that are typically hormones or peptides. The ANS uses feedback for afferent and efferent functions. The afferent mechanisms signal changes in the viscera and other organs, whereas efferent activity conveys commands to those organs. Consequently, the ANS can maintain feedback loops related to viscera, muscle, blood flow, and other responses. The visceral feedback system exemplifies this process.

The feedback concept is central to the field of psychophysiology: Awareness of physiologic changes elicited by a stimulus is a primary mechanism of emotion. The patient presents with panic attacks, phobia, or anxiety in a mental health setting.

Sensory transmission follows spinothalamic pathways, and transmission destined for affective processing takes place in spinoreticular pathways.

Noxious centripetal transmission engages multiple pathways: spinoreticular, spinomesencephalic, spinolimbic, spinocervical, and spinothalamic tracts,[30, 31] as Figure 7.3 indicates. The spinoreticular tract contains somatosensory and viscerosensory afferent pathways that arrive at different levels of the brain stem. Spinoreticular axons possess receptive fields that resemble those of spinothalamic tract neurons projecting to medial thalamus, and like their spinothalamic counterparts, they transmit tissue injury information.[32, 33] Most spinoreticular neurons carry noxious signals, and many of them respond preferentially to noxious activity.[34, 35] The spinomesencephalic tract comprises several projections that terminate in multiple midbrain nuclei, including the periaqueductal gray (PAG), the red nucleus, nucleus cuneiformis, and the Edinger–Westphal nucleus.[31] Spinolimbic tracts include the spinohypothalamic tract, which reaches both lateral and medial hypothalamus,[36, 37] and the spinoamygdalar tract that extends to the central nucleus of the amygdala.[38] The spinocervical tract, like the spinothalamic tract, conveys signals to the thalamus. All these tracts transmit tissue trauma signals rostrally.

Negative emotions, such as those regulated by the frontal–amygdalar system, may strengthen and become self-sustaining, persisting even in the absence of ongoing

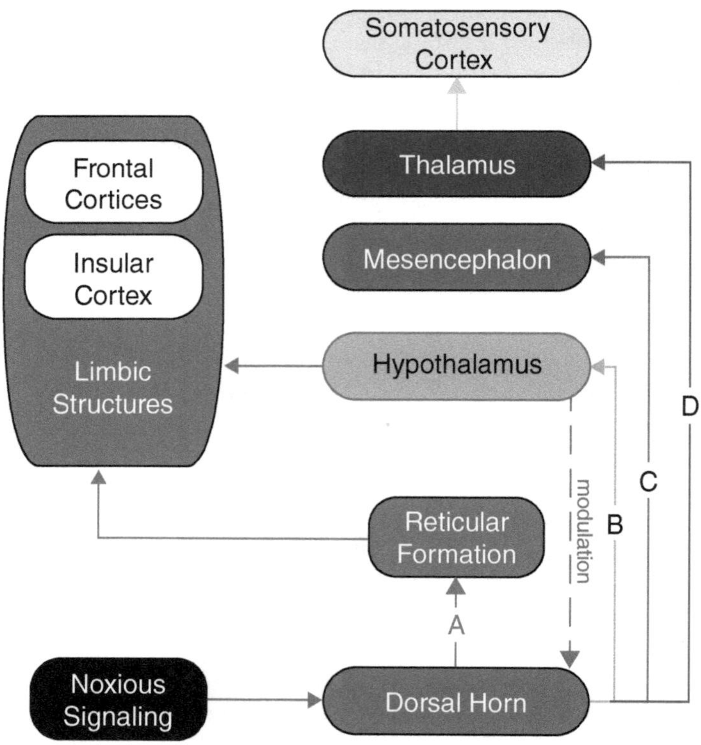

FIGURE 7.3 Noxious centripetal transmission engages multiple pathways: spinoreticular, spinomesencephalic, spinolimbic, spinocervical, and spinothalamic tracts.

noxious signaling. This persistent activation can lead to maladaptive emotional states, reinforcing anxiety, hypervigilance, and depressive symptoms. Duric and McCarson[39] demonstrated that prolonged noxious signaling can induce stress-like neurotoxic effects on the hippocampus, a region crucial for mood regulation and cognitive processing, contributing to the pathogenesis of depression. These findings suggest that chronic pain and stress-related disorders share overlapping neurobiological mechanisms, with persistent nociceptive input exacerbating emotional dysregulation through hippocampal dysfunction.

7.2.8 Noxious Signaling and the Central

7.2.8.1 Limbic Processing

Central sensory and affective pain processes share common sensory mechanisms in the periphery. As other chapters in this book describe, Aδ and C fibers serve as tissue trauma transducers (nociceptors) for both; the chemical products of inflammation sensitize these nociceptors, and peripheral neuropathic mechanisms, such as ectopic firing, excite both processes. In some cases, neuropathic mechanisms may substitute for transduction as we classically define it, producing afferent signal volleys that appear to the central nervous system like signals originating in nociceptors. Differentiation of sensory and affective processing begins at the level of the spinal cord and brainstem, where nociceptive signals are relayed to distinct neural pathways that separately encode the sensory-discriminative and affective-motivational aspects of pain. From the spinal cord, sensory information is transmitted via the spinothalamic and spinoreticular tracts to the thalamus, which further projects to the somatosensory cortex for localization and intensity coding. In parallel, affective processing is mediated through pathways that engage the limbic system, including the amygdala, anterior cingulate cortex, and insular cortex, integrating pain perception with emotional and autonomic responses. This early segregation of sensory and affective components allows the nervous system to generate appropriate behavioral and physiological reactions to pain, reinforcing both protective withdrawal reflexes and adaptive coping strategies.

7.2.8.1.1 Central Neurotransmitter Systems

Central processing of noxious signals to produce affect undoubtedly involves multiple neurotransmitter systems. Four extrathalamic afferent pathways project to neocortex: the dorsal noradrenergic bundle (DNB) originating in the locus coeruleus (LC), the serotonergic fibers that arise in the dorsal and median raphe nuclei, the dopaminergic pathways of the ventral tegmental tract that arise from substantia nigra, and the acetylcholinergic (ACh) neurons that arise principally from the nucleus basalis of the substantia innominata.[40] Of these, the noradrenergic and serotonergic pathways link most closely to negative emotional states.[41–43] The set of structures receiving projections from this complex and extensive network corresponds to the classic definition of the limbic brain.[7, 43–45]

Although other processes governed predominantly by other neurotransmitters almost certainly play important roles in the complex experience of emotion during pain, we emphasize the role of central noradrenergic processing here. This limited

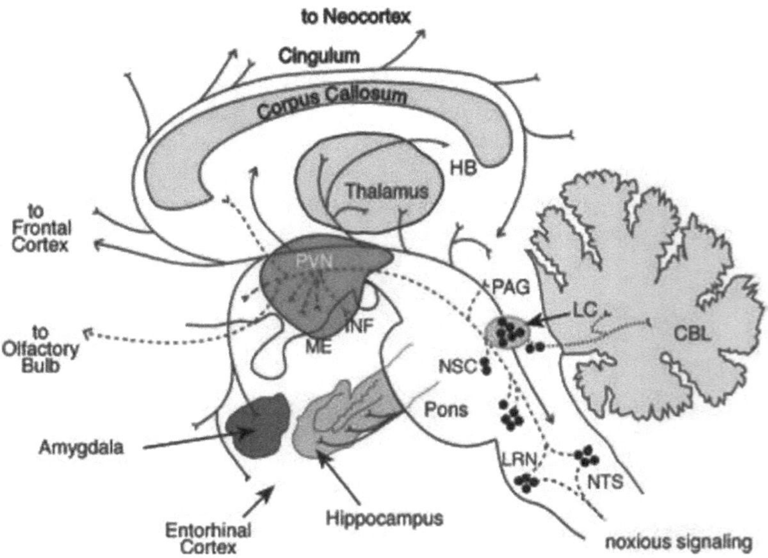

FIGURE 7.4 The role of central noradrenergic processing. This processing involves two central noradrenergic pathways: the dorsal and ventral noradrenergic bundles (VNBs) as illustrated in the figure.

perspective offers the advantage of simplicity, and the literature on the role of central noradrenergic pathways in anxiety, panic, stress, and posttraumatic stress disorder provides a strong basis.[41, 46] This processing involves two central noradrenergic pathways: the dorsal and ventral noradrenergic bundles (VNBs) (Figure 7.4).

7.2.9 Locus Coeruleus and the Dorsal

7.2.9.1 Noradrenergic Bundle

Substantial evidence supports the hypothesis that noradrenergic brain pathways are major mechanisms of anxiety and stress.[41] The majority of noradrenergic neurons originate in the LC. This pontine nucleus resides bilaterally near the wall of the fourth ventricle. The locus has three major projections: ascending, descending, and cerebellar. The ascending projection, the DNB, is the most extensive and important pathway for our purposes.[47] Projecting from the LC throughout the limbic brain and to all the neocortex, the DNB accounts for about 70% of all brain norepinephrine.[48] The LC gives rise to most central noradrenergic fibers in the spinal cord, hypothalamus, thalamus, and hippocampus,[49] and in addition, it projects to the limbic cortex and neocortex. Consequently, the LC exerts a powerful influence on higher-level brain activity.

The *noradrenergic stress response hypothesis* holds that any stimulus that threatens the biological, psychological, or psychosocial integrity of the individual increases the firing rate of the LC, and this, in turn, results in increased release and turnover of norepinephrine in the brain areas involved in noradrenergic innervation. Studies show that the LC reacts to signaling from sensory stimuli that potentially threaten the biological integrity of the individual or signal damage to that integrity.[48] Spinal cord lamina I cells terminate in the LC.[33] The major sources of LC afferent input are the paragigantocellularis and prepositus hypoglossal nuclei in the medulla, but the destruction of these nuclei does not block LC response to somatosensory stimuli.[50, 51] Other sources of afferent input to the locus include the lateral hypothalamus, the amygdala, and the solitary nucleus. Whether noxious signaling stimulates the LC directly or indirectly is still uncertain.

It is quite clear that noxious signaling inevitably and reliably increases activity in neurons of the LC, and LC excitation appears to be a consistent response to noxious signaling.[48, 52–54] Notably, this does not require cognitively mediated attentional control, because it occurs in anesthetized animals. Foote et al.[55] reported that slow, tonic spontaneous activity at the locus in rats changed under anesthesia in response to noxious stimulation. Experimentally induced phasic LC activation produces alarm and apparent fear in primates,[56, 57] and lesions of the LC eliminate normal heart rate increases to threatening stimuli.[58] In a resting animal, LC neurons discharge in a slow, phasic manner.[59]

The LC reacts consistently, but not exclusively, to noxious signaling. LC firing rates increase following non-noxious but threatening events, such as strong cardiovascular stimulation,[53, 60,] and certain visceral events, such as distention of the bladder, stomach, colon, or rectum.[48, 61] Highly novel and sudden stimuli that could represent potential threats, such as loud clicks or light flashes, can also excite the LC in experimental animals.[59] Thus, the LC responds to biologically threatening or potentially threatening events, of which tissue injury is a significant subset. Amaral and Sinnamon[62] described the LC as a central analog of the sympathetic ganglia. Viewed in this way, it is an extension of the autonomic protective mechanism described earlier.

Invasive studies confirm the linkage between LC activity and threat. Direct activation of the DNB and associated limbic structures in laboratory animals produces a sympathetic nervous system response and elicits emotional behaviors, such as defensive threat, fright, enhanced startle, freezing, and vocalization.[63] This indicates that enhanced activity in these pathways corresponds to negative emotional arousal and behaviors appropriate to the perceived threat. LC firing rates increase two- to threefold during the defense response elicited in a cat that has perceived a dog.[26] Moreover, infusion of norepinephrine into the hypothalamus of an awake cat elicits a defensive rage reaction that includes activation of the LC noradrenergic system. In general, the mammalian defense response involves increased regional turnover and release of norepinephrine in the brain regions that the LC innervates. The LC response to threat, therefore, may be a component of the partly "prewired" patterns associated with the defense response.

Increased alertness is a key element in the early stages of the defense response. Normally, activity in the LC increases alertness. Tonically enhanced LC and DNB discharge corresponds to hypervigilance and emotionality.[41, 55, 64] The DNB is the mechanism for vigilance and defensive orientation to affectively relevant and novel stimuli. It also regulates attentional processes and facilitates motor responses.[40, 43, 48, 65] In this sense, the LC influences the stream of consciousness on an ongoing basis and readies the individual to respond quickly and effectively to threats when they occur.

LC and DNB support biological survival by making possible global vigilance for threatening and harmful stimuli. Siegel and Rogawski[66] hypothesized a link between the LC noradrenergic system and vigilance, focusing on rapid eye movement (REM) sleep. They noted that LC noradrenergic neurons maintain continuous activity in both normal waking state and non-REM sleep, but during REM sleep, these neurons virtually cease discharge activity. Moreover, an increase in REM sleep ensues after either a lesion of the DNB or following administration of clonidine, an alpha-2 adrenoceptor agonist. Because LC inactivation during REM sleep permits the rebuilding of noradrenergic stores, REM sleep may be a necessary preparation for sustained periods of high alertness during subsequent waking. Siegel and Rogawski[66(p226)] contended that "a principal function of NE in the CNS is to facilitate the excitability of target neurons to specific high priority signals." Conversely, reduced LC activity periods (REM sleep) allow time for suppression of sympathetic tone.

Both adaptation and sensitization can alter the LC response to threat. Abercrombie and Jacobs[67, 68] demonstrated a noradrenergically mediated increase in heart rate in cats exposed to white noise. Elevated heart rate decreased with repeated exposure, as did LC activation and circulating levels of norepinephrine. Libet and Gleason[69] found that stimulation via permanently implanted LC electrodes did not elicit indefinite anxiety. This indicates that the brain either adapts to locus excitation or engages in a compensatory response to excessive LC activation under some circumstances. In addition, central noradrenergic responsiveness changes as a function of learning. In the cat, pairing a stimulus with a noxious air puff results in increased LC firing with subsequent presentations of the stimulus, but the previous pairing of that stimulus with a food reward produces no alteration in LC firing rates with repeated presentation.[59] These studies show that, despite its apparently "prewired" behavioral subroutines, the noradrenergic brain shows substantial neuroplasticity. The emotional response of animals and people to a painful stimulus can adapt, and it can change as a function of experience.

From a different perspective, Bremner et al.[41] postulated that chronic stress can affect regional norepinephrine turnover and thus contribute to the *response sensitization* evident in panic disorder and posttraumatic stress disorder. Chronic exposure to a stressor (including perseverating noxious signaling) could create a situation in which noradrenergic synthesis cannot keep up with demand, thus depleting brain norepinephrine levels. Animals exposed to inescapable shock demonstrate greater LC responsiveness to an excitatory stimulus than animals who have experienced escapable shock.[70] In addition, such animals display "learned helplessness" behaviors—they cease trying to adapt to or cope with the source of shock.[71] From an evolutionary perspective, this is a failure of the defense response as adaptation; it represents surrender to suffering. Extrapolating this and related observations to patients, Bremner and colleagues[41] suggested that persons who have once encountered overwhelming stress and suffered exhaustion of central noradrenergic resources may respond excessively to similar stressors that they encounter at a later time.

7.2.10 The Ventral Noradrenergic Bundle and the Hypothalamic–Pituitary–Adrenocortical Axis

The VNB originates in the LC and enters the medial forebrain bundle. Neurons in the medullary reticular formation project to the hypothalamus via the VNB.[72]

Sawchenko and Swanson[73] identified two VNB-linked noradrenergic and adrenergic pathways to the paraventricular hypothalamus in the rat: the A1 region of the ventral medulla (lateral reticular nucleus [LRN]) and the A2 region of the dorsal vagal complex (the nucleus tractus solitarius, or solitary nucleus), which receives visceral afferents. These medullary neuronal complexes supply 90% of catecholaminergic innervation to the paraventricular hypothalamus via the VNB.[74] Regions A5 and A7 contribute in a comparatively minor way to the VNB.

The noradrenergic axons in the VNB respond to noxious stimulation,[48] as does the hypothalamus itself.[75] Moreover, noxious-signaling neurons at all segmental levels of the spinal cord project to medial and lateral hypothalamus and several telencephalic regions.[32,37,38] These projections link tissue injury and the hypothalamic response, as do hormonal messengers in some circumstances.

The hypothalamic paraventricular nucleus (PVN) coordinates the HPA axis. Neurons of the PVN receive afferent information from several reticular areas, including the ventrolateral medulla, dorsal raphe nucleus, nucleus raphe magnus, LC, dorsomedial nucleus, and the nucleus tractus solitarius.[73,76,77] Still, other afferents project to the PVN from the hippocampus, septum amygdala.[78] Nearly all hypothalamic and preoptic nuclei send projections to the PVN. This suggests that limbic connections mediate endocrine responses during stress. Feldman et al.[78] note that limbic stimulation always increases adrenocortical activity in rats.

In responding to potentially or frankly injurious stimuli, the PVN initiates a complex series of events regulated by negative feedback mechanisms, as Figure 7.5 indicates. These processes ready the organism for extraordinary behaviors that will maximize its chances to cope with the threat at hand,[79] but they must limit overshooting and return to recover when the stressor has passed. Although laboratory

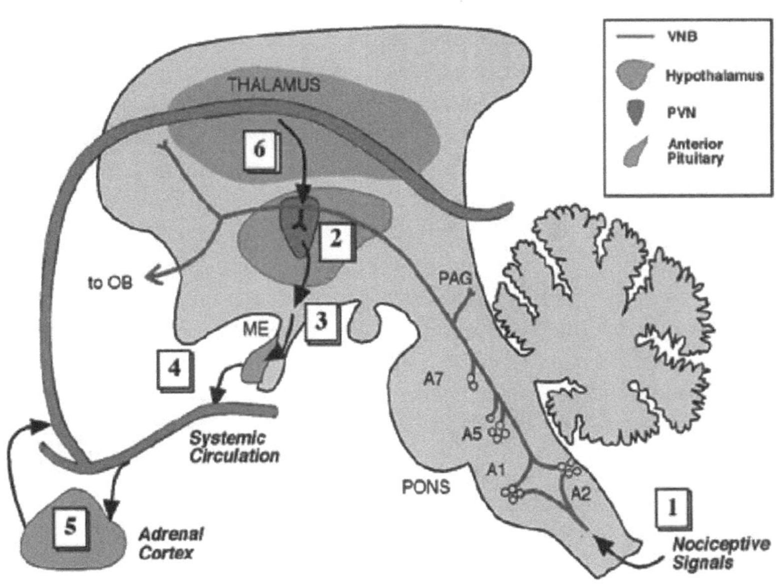

FIGURE 7.5 Summary of complex pathway signaling and negative feedback mechanisms in regards to hypothalamic paraventricular nucleus (PVN) response to potential or frank injurious stimuli.

studies often involve highly controlled and specific noxious stimulation, real-life tissue trauma usually involves a spectrum of afferent activity, and the pattern of activity may be a greater determinant of the stress response than the specific receptor system involved.[80] Traumatic injury, for example, might involve complex signaling from the site of injury, including inflammatory mediators, baroreceptor signals from blood volume changes, and hypercapnia. Tissue trauma normally initiates much more than noxious signaling.

Diminished, noxious signal transmission during stress or injury helps people and animals cope with threats without the distraction of pain. The medullary mechanisms involved in this are complex and include the response of the solitary nucleus to baroreceptor stimulation.[81] Laboratory studies with rodents indicate that animals placed in restraint or subjected to cold water develop analgesia.[82–84] Lesioning the PVN attenuates such stress-induced analgesia.[85]

Some investigators[86, 87] emphasize that neuroendocrine arousal mechanisms are not limited to emergencies, even though most research emphasizes that such situations elicit them. In complex social contexts, submission, dominance, and other transactions can elicit neuroendocrine and autonomic responses, modified perhaps by learning and memory. This suggests that neuroendocrine processes accompany all sorts of emotion-eliciting situations.

The hypothalamic PVN supports stress-related autonomic arousal through neural as well as hormonal pathways. It sends direct projections to the sympathetic intermediolateral cell column in the thoracolumbar spinal cord and the parasympathetic vagal complex, both sources of preganglionic autonomic outflow.[88] In addition, it signals the release of epinephrine and norepinephrine from the adrenal medulla. Adrenocorticotrophic hormone (ACTH) release, although not instantaneous, is quite rapid: It occurs within about 15 seconds.[89] These considerations implicate the HPA axis in the neuroendocrinologic and autonomic manifestations of emotion associated with tissue trauma.

In addition to controlling neuroendocrine and ANS reactivity, the HPA axis coordinates emotional arousal with behavior.[90] As noted earlier, stimulation of the hypothalamus in animals can elicit well-organized action patterns, including defensive threat behaviors and autonomic arousal.[91] The existence of demonstrable behavioral subroutines in animals suggests that the hypothalamus plays a key role in matching behavioral reactions and bodily adjustments to challenging circumstances or biologically relevant stimuli.

Moreover, stress hormones at high levels may affect central emotional arousal, lowering startle thresholds and influencing cognition.[89] Saphier[92] observed that cortisol altered the firing rate of neurons in the limbic forebrain. Stress regulation is a complex, feedback-dependent, and coordinated process. The hypothalamus appears to coordinate behavioral readiness with physiologic capability, awareness, and cognitive function.

7.2.11 Primary and Secondary Features of the Affective Dimension of Pain

The physiology of emotion suggests that the affective dimension of pain involves a two-stage mechanism. The primary mechanism generates an immediate experience akin to hypervigilance or fear. In nature, this rapid response to injury serves to disrupt ongoing attentional and behavioral patterns. At the same time, efferent messages from the hypothalamus, amygdala, and other limbic structures excite the ANS, and this, in turn, alters bodily states. Cardiac function, muscle tension, altered visceral function, respiration rate, and trembling all occur, and awareness of these reactions creates a strong negative subjective experience. This body state awareness is the second mechanism of the affective dimension of pain.

Damasio[93] contended that visceral and other event-related, autonomically mediated body state changes constitute "somatic markers." That is, they serve as messengers, delivering affective evaluations of perceptual experiences that either confirm or deny the potential threat inherent in an event. A somatic marker is essentially a somatic image. Perceptually, the brain operates on images that are symbolic representations of external and internal objects or events. Just as it is more efficient for a listener to work with words in language as opposed to phonemes, cognition is more efficient when it uses images rather than simple sensations. The somatic marker images associated with tissue trauma are often complex patterns of physiologic arousal. They serve as symbolic representations of threats to the biological (and sometimes the psychological or social) integrity of the person. Like other images, they can enter into complex patterns of association. Because the secondary stage of the affective response involves images and symbols, it represents cognition as well as emotion.

7.2.12 Summary of the Construction and Modulation of Pain

Pain is a complex and subjective conscious experience constructed and modulated by a constellation of sensory, cognitive, and affective factors, including mood, psychological disposition, meaning-related cognitions (e.g., suffering), learning, desires, and pre-pain cognitive states (e.g., expectations, anxiety) to provide a continually changing experience. Feedback connections between low-level afferent and higher-order neural processes foster the cultivation of a distributed, multidimensional network associated with the subjective experience of pain. Nociceptive sensory events are first *registered* by peripheral primary afferents (first pain, Aδ; second pain, C fibers) at the site of injury/tissue damage that then relay said nociceptive information to the dorsal horn of the spinal cord. From the spinal cord, nociceptive information ascends contralateral to the site of pain to the brain largely through the spinothalamic pathway. Nociceptive input is subsequently processed through feedback connections between lower-level sensory regions, including the parabrachial nucleus, PAG matter, thalamus, and primary and secondary somatosensory cortices.[13–15, 94–97] Ascending nociceptive information is then transmitted to the posterior and anterior insular cortices, where it is "fine-tuned" to foster the subsequent evaluation of pain.[98, 99] The contextual meaning of pain is then facilitated through the activation of higher-order brain regions, including the dorsal anterior cingulate cortex (dACC), the anterior cingulate cortex (ACC), and the PFC.[99–101] Yet the subjective experience of pain is highly influenced by the context in which it occurs. That is, previous experiences, expectations, mood, conditioning, desires, sensitization/habituation, and other cognitive factors can dramatically amplify and/or attenuate pain.[97, 102–106]

Nonpharmacologic-based pain manipulations attenuate the subjective experience of pain through a common final pathway, including overlapping endogenously driven and neural systems. Although the cognitive modulation of pain is mediated through a host of endogenous modulatory systems, including cannabinoid, serotonergic, dopaminergic, cholecystokinin, adrenergic, and other neurochemical systems (i.e., vasopressin), the endogenous opioidergic system is the most understood (and studied) pain modulatory system.[107] Endogenous opioidergic mechanisms have been repeatedly demonstrated to mediate analgesia produced by placebo,[108–112] conditioned pain modulation,[113] acupuncture,[114] hypnosis,[115] and attentional control.[116] Pain relief produced by said cognitive techniques is associated with significant reductions in pain-related brain activation (i.e., primary and secondary somatosensory cortices, posterior insula, and parietal operculum) and activation in higher-order brain regions, such as the ACC, PFC, and insula.[105, 108, 117–129] Importantly, the PFC, insula, and ACC contain high concentrations of opioid receptors and are associated with producing analgesia through descending inhibitory systems.[124, 130–134] The ACC and PFC project to the PAG matter,[135] a structure that can be directly activated by opioids. The PAG projects to the rostral ventral medulla,[136–138] which, in turn, projects to the spinal dorsal horn and can inhibit nociceptive processing through multiple neurotransmitter systems.[139]

Negative emotions and somatic markers are much more than reactions to undesirable events; in nature, they help an organism determine which things benefit and which things threaten survival, and they compel behavior consistent with such evaluations. Moreover, emotional expression communicates this judgment to others and thus sets up group approach or avoidance behaviors. MacLean[7] described *emotion* as a process that imparts subjective information. In these respects, our feelings approximate crude intelligence. How we feel about something is often as important as, or more important than, what we know about it. If emotion is a proto-intelligence, then evolutionarily newer structures, namely, the later stages of cortical development, should have demonstrable links with limbic structures and functions.

Such interconnections exist. Parts of the frontal lobe (the dorsal trend) appear to have developed from rudimentary hippocampal formation, whereas other parts (the paleocortical trend) originated in the olfactory cortex. Although these two areas interconnect anatomically, the former analyzes sensory information, whereas the latter contributes emotional tone to that sensory information.[68, 69, 140] Pribram,[141] noting that limbic function involves the frontal and temporal cortex, offered a bottom-up concept for how cognition relates to feelings, that is, emotion determines cognition. However, the multimodal neocortical association areas project corticofugal to limbic structures,[142] which suggests that cognitions may drive emotions.

The debate on whether emotion or cognition is primary may never be resolved. For immediate purposes, it seems best to conclude that *knowing* and *feeling* are closely interrelated. Still, these processes are not identical. We can know something about our feelings, and we can have emotional responses to what we know. The brain is a complex, dynamic organ, constantly constructing its internal model of reality from sensory input and memory storage. Feeling and thinking are major processes in this construction.

7.2.13 Cognitive Perspective

Pain informs the brain of injury to bodily integrity, and its emotional aspect reflects the importance of that injury to the individual. An injury does not just cause objective harm; it harms "me." That is, it harms what I consider myself. Similarly, a social affront harms what I consider myself, and I might metaphorically describe the incident as something that "hurt" me. What constitutes the self? What would happen if an injured person had an altered or poorly developed sense of self? Clinical observations of schizophrenic patients and other psychiatric patients indicate that they sometimes mutilate themselves horribly and apparently with little or no pain.[143] This suggests that the sense of self may be an intrinsic part of the complex experience of pain because it is the focal point around which perceptions form and from which cognitions arise.

7.2.14 Multiple Perspectives on the Self

The *self* is a hierarchical construct that has different meanings at different levels of the neuraxis. Multiple levels of the self exist, and each level becomes a precondition for the existence of higher levels. At least two biological definitions merit inclusion in the construct. At the level of the human genome, the self is the unique genetic code that makes each of us an individual. It sets the basic rules of life by defining sex, size and features, and basic abilities.

At a higher biological level, the self is what the immune system recognizes as "me" versus "not me." The immunologic self is an enigma because "me" and my genetic code are not identical. Our bodies host elaborate microbial ecosystems, and disturbing or damaging these systems (e.g., via antibiotic use) compromises health. Various microorganisms in our digestive tracts, in our oropharyngeal passages, and on our skin qualify as self to our immune systems; we live comfortably with them in a symbiotic relationship. Our microbial floras are us, even though they do not carry our genetic code. For the immune system, neither is there a single chemical marker that defines individuality nor is self limited to certain biological structures. Thus, even at this basic level, the boundaries of the self are fuzzy.

At a neurologic level, the self exists as a central representation of the body. Melzack termed this the *body neuromatrix*.[144–146] The brain maintains a detailed map of the body at several levels of the neuraxis. A study of phantom limb patients and patients born without limbs reveals that the brain has an elaborate internal representation of the body. If a person loses a leg, the brain maintains its representation of the leg, and the person experiences a phantom limb. Even patients born without limbs have an internal sense or representation of the absent body parts. Thus, humans and, almost certainly, higher-order animals carry within them a phenomenal representation of a body self.

These biological selves exist below the level of consciousness. They are very much a part of every person, but they normally play little or no part in what we think of as "me." Humans and animals do not differ about themselves at this level.

Multiple psychological dimensions of the self also exist. At the most fundamental level, there is the self-as-agent, which engages in biological adaptation and survival. From an evolutionary perspective, it is the agent that struggles to survive.

The self-as-agent sets goals, chooses among alternatives, and engages in behaviors. Animals and humans share self-as-agent, and this self is, in part, social. That is, it exists not alone but in relation to others of its kind. Animals, including humans, engage in social dominance and submission. In this respect, each organism defines its relationship to others, often via struggle or conflict. The defined relationship often determines the extent of one's opportunity to reproduce or one's access to the resources necessary for survival. The self-as-agent is primitive and does not require cognition. It is something that the individual does, not something that the individual experiences as a phenomenal reality. In other words, this is a self of behavior. It does not entail subjective awareness.

At a higher, and perhaps uniquely human, level, the psychological self is also a point of view (self-as-perspective). It is the center of experiential gravity about which the brain organizes present circumstances, history, future goals, and expectations. This is an inevitable outcome of the higher-order, self-organizing processes of the brain. This aspect of the self stems from the recognition of one's physical being as an entity in the environment, and it becomes a frame of reference for all that happens to the person.

On still another level, the self represents the individual's complex sense of identity, to which we have referred earlier as "me" *vide supra*. This self-as-identity resembles the self-as-agent in some respects, but it is an age-dependent, autobiographically based narrative and interpretation, modified by the immediate circumstances and surroundings. Unlike the self-as-agent, the self-as-identity is the product of a developmental process, and it changes over time.

Finally, every human has a sociologic self. That is, we have an identity defined by our relationships with social groups and society and culture as a whole. Gender roles, social class, education level, age roles, and our culture constrain who we are. To some degree, we are the roles that we play in our families, vocational settings, recreational pursuits, and elsewhere.

7.2.15 Basic Definitions: Stress, Homeostasis, and Allostasis

Human life entails repeated adverse physical and psychosocial events, and these challenges require an adaptive response. The brain mounts a coordinated, adaptive reaction characterized by physiologic arousal. This response is often associated psychologically with the experience of threat or other negative affect. The term for this arousal reaction is the *stress response*, and any event that triggers such a response is a *stressor*. Some stressors are singular events, such as traffic accidents or surgery. Other stressors are constellations of vexing problems that never end. Examples include dysfunctional family relationships and vocational problems. Stress and negative emotions feed one another, and the processes involved affect pain.

We have discussed the defense response earlier. It resembles the stress response and shares common mechanisms. The defense response and stress have historically different origins in science but seem to be different perspectives on a common adaptive mechanism. To integrate relevant information in these two fields, we consider the stress response to be a subset of the more general defense response. This position has the shortcoming of potentially obscuring an important distinction. Classically, the defense response pertained to threats appearing in the external environment and not the internal environment. However, the concept applies equally well to threatening internal events. The pain of a kidney stone, angina, or a migraine headache is threatening and can function as a stressor and elicit the physiologic changes common to the defense response and the stress response.

In everyday life, *stress* is the resource-intensive process of mounting adaptive coping responses to challenges that occur in the external or internal environment. A *stressor* may be a physical or social event, an invading microorganism, or in the case of chronic pain, patient pain itself. Selye[79] first described this response as a syndrome produced by "diverse nocuous agents." He eventually characterized the stress response as having three stages: alarm reaction, resistance, and if the stressor does not relent, exhaustion. The normal stress responses of daily living consist of the alarm reaction, resistance, and recovery. Stressors have as their primary features intensity, duration, and frequency. The impact of a stressor is the magnitude of the response it elicits. This impact involves cognitive mediation (thought processes) because it is a function of both the predictability and the controllability of the stressor.

A stressor can threaten homeostasis,[147] which strictly means a limited set of systems concerned with maintaining the essentials of the internal milieu. Homeostasis represents the control of internal processes truly necessary for life, such as thermoregulation, blood gases, acid–base balance, fluid levels, metabolite levels, and blood pressure. Generic threats to homeostasis include environmental extremes, extreme exercise, depletion of essential resources, abnormal feedback processes, aging, and disease. Of course, various defensive processes must exist to protect homeostasis.

The term for the general adaptive process that protects against threats to homeostasis is *allostasis*. Allostatic processes dynamically adapt multiple internal systems to changes in the environment and coordinate their responses.[147, 148] Allostasis exists when changes in the external or internal environment trigger physiologic coping mechanisms, such as autonomic arousal. These mechanisms ensure that the processes sustaining homeostasis stay within normal range. Allostasis is the essence of the stress response because it mobilizes internal resources to meet the challenge that a stressor represents. When a stressor, such as neuropathic signaling, persists for a long period, or when repeated stressors occur in rapid succession, allostasis may burn resources faster than the body can replenish them. The cost to the body of allostatic adjustment, whether in response to extreme acute challenges or lesser challenges over an extended period, is called *allostatic load.*

7.2.16 Physiologic Mechanisms of Stress

The major mechanisms of the stress response are the HPA axis, based in the hypothalamic PVN[149] and the SAM axis,[150] which includes the LC noradrenergic system (see Figure 7.1). The peripheral effectors of these mechanisms are the ANS, the SAM circulating hormones, principally the catecholamines epinephrine and norepinephrine, together with the sympathetic cotransmitter neuropeptide Y (NPY),[151] all of which originate in the chromaffin cells of the adrenal medulla. Circulating catecholamines increase blood pressure and heart rate, dilate pupils, and increase skin conductance, thereby initiating arousal for the fight-or-flight response. The stress response involves the hypothalamically induced release of peptides derived from pro-opiomelanocortin (POMC) at the anterior pituitary. The POMC-related family of anterior pituitary hormones includes ACTH, β-lipotropin, α-melanocyte–stimulating hormone, and β-endorphin.

The hypothalamic PVN initiates the HPA stress response and controls it through negative feedback mechanisms. Corticotropin-releasing hormone (CRH) produced at the PVN initiates the stress response. CRH initializes and coordinates the stress response at many levels,[152] including the LC.[153] It is the key excitatory central neurotransmitter and regulator in the endocrine response to injury.

The PVN triggers another aspect of the stress response in the SAM axis by recruiting catecholaminergic cells in the rostral ventrolateral medulla. This structure is a cardiovascular regulatory area involved, along with the solitary nucleus, in the control of blood pressure. The rostral ventrolateral medulla activates the solitary nucleus and, together with it, provides tonic excitatory drive to sympathetic vasoconstrictor nerves that maintain resting blood pressure levels. A normal stress response involves a complex pattern of autonomic arousal that includes increased blood pressure, followed by a period of recovery. when blood pressure and other aspects of arousal return to normal.

7.2.16.1 Neural Substrates

Viewing stress as a mechanism of defense brings additional neural substrates into focus. Chief among them are the medial hypothalamus, amygdala, and dorsal PAG. These structures respond reliably, but not exclusively, to noxious signaling, interact with one another, and actively integrate cognitive, sensory, and emotional processes. Some pain researchers have begun to address the issue of integration. Tracey et al.,[117] for example, employed functional brain imaging to study subjects attending to or distracting themselves from painful stimuli cued with colored lights. Distraction and pain reduction occurred in conjunction with activation of the PAG, linking cortical control and the PAG and the role of endogenous opioids to attenuate pain.

Frontal–amygdalar circuits are a well-studied aspect of the defense response.[154–156] Cognitive variables such as interpretation, attention, and anticipation can influence amygdalar response through the frontal–amygdalar circuit. The amygdala, in turn, can influence the HPA axis.[157–159] Frontal influences also affect patterns of activity at the LC, which is a part of the SAM axis.

An important implication of viewing stress within the defense response framework is that endogenous cognitive activity (thoughts) generated during anticipation or memory reconstruction can activate complex neural circuits that mobilize the stress response in the absence of tissue trauma. In other words, mental activity may have direct and deleterious physiologic consequences. Patients with chronic pain can stress themselves through negative thought processes, termed *catastrophizing*, and, in so doing, exacerbate and perpetuate their pain.[160]

The central nucleus of the amygdala projects to the PAG, which coordinates defensive behaviors.[161] In general, the amygdala is proving to be a key mechanism of conditioned fear.[162,163] It communicates with the hypothalamus via neural circuitry,[164,165] as well as the frontal cortices.

A second and underestimated aspect of the defense response depends predominantly on the immune system. The brain controls the immune system via the actions of the sympathetic nervous system and the hypothalamic secretion of releasing factors into the bloodstream. These messenger substances activate the anterior pituitary via the HPA axis.[166] The pituitary body releases peptides related to POMC, such as ACTH and #-endorphin, and these, in turn, trigger the release of glucocorticoids. Because the cells and organs of the immune system express receptors for these hormones, they can respond to humoral messenger molecules of central origin. In this way, the brain enlists the immune system in the defense response.

7.2.16.2 Immune Mechanisms

Just as the nervous system is the primary agent for detecting and defending against threats arising in the external environment, the immune system is the primary agent of defense for the internal environment. Kohl[167] described the *immune system* as "a network of complex danger sensors and transmitters." This interactive network of lymphoid organs, cells, humoral factors, and cytokines works interdependently with the nervous and endocrine systems to protect homeostasis.

Physical trauma produces specific tissue breakdown, triggering the release of nitric oxide (NO), bradykinin, histamine, and peptides, some of which are immunostimulatory. The neuropeptides substance P (SP) and neurokinin A (NKA) activate T cells and cause them to increase production of the pro-inflammatory cytokine interferon (IFN)-$.[168] In addition, another pro-inflammatory cytokine, interleukin (IL)1-#, stimulates the release of SP from primary afferent neurons.[169] Thus, the neurogenic inflammatory response contributes to the immune defense response and, at the same time, is, in part, a product of that response.[170]

The immune system detects an injury event in at least three ways: (1) through blood-borne immune messengers originating at the site of injury, (2) through nociceptor-induced sympathetic activation and subsequent stimulation of immune tissues, and (3) through SAM endocrine signaling. Immune messaging begins with the acute phase reaction in the injured tissues.[171] Local macrophages, neutrophils, and granulocytes produce and release into intracellular space and circulation the pro-inflammatory cytokines IL-1, IL-6, IL-8, and tumor necrosis factor (TNF-α) This alerts and activates other immune tissues and cells that have a complex systemic impact.

The acute phase reaction to tissue trauma is the immune counterpart to noxious signaling in the nervous system in that it encompasses transduction, transmission, and effector responses. This is a feedback-dependent process. Sympathetic outflow following tissue injury can directly modulate many aspects of immune activity and provide feedback. This can occur because all lymphoid organs have sympathetic nervous system innervation[172] and because many immune cells express adrenoceptors.[173–175]

In addition to the familiar acute phase reaction, the immune system manifests several complex response patterns to tissue injury. In a primitive world, microbial invasion normally accompanies any breach of the skin, and when the microorganisms reach the bloodstream, sepsis occurs. Resultant inflammation, therefore, assists the immune system in defense. Redness, pain, heat, and swelling are its cardinal signs. The inflammatory process creates a barrier against the invading microorganisms and activates a variety of cells, including macrophages and lymphocytes, that find and destroy invaders. It also sensitizes the injured tissue and thereby minimizes the risk of further injury. Inflammation reduces function and increases pain by sensitizing nociceptors. Tracey[176] described the "inflammatory reflex" as an ACh-mediated process by which the nervous system recognizes the presence of and exerts influence on peripheral inflammation. Through vagal and glossopharyngeal bidirectional processes, the nervous system modulates circulating cytokine levels.[177] Put another way, the nervous system can sense the activities of the immune system.

7.2.16.3 The Sickness Response

The immune system can mount a system-wide defense response characterized by fatigue, fever, and sickness with associated pain.[178–183] This is the "sickness response," and although it is cytokine-mediated, it depends on the central nervous system. Macrophages and other cells release pro-inflammatory cytokines, including IL-1β, IL-6, IL-8, IL-12, IFN-γ, and TNF-α in response to tissue trauma. These substances act on the vagus nerve, the glossopharyngeal nerve, the hypothalamus, and elsewhere to trigger a cascade of unpleasant, activity-limiting symptoms.[180, 184]

Subjectively, the sickness response is a vivid and dysphoric experience characterized by fever, malaise, fatigue, difficulty concentrating, excessive sleep, decreased appetite and libido, stimulation of the HPA axis, and hyperalgesia. The sickness-related hyperalgesia may reflect the contributions of spinal cord microglia and astrocytes.[182] Functionally, this state is adaptive; it minimizes risk by limiting normal behavior and social interactions and forces recuperation. Curiously, this response does not always resolve with physical healing.

7.2.16.4 The Sickness Response and Depression

Mounting evidence supports the hypothesis that the sickness response and depression are related to immune response patterns. This hypothesis derives from evidence that pro-inflammatory cytokines are agents of depression. The specific mechanisms are still at issue,[185] but pro-inflammatory cytokines instigate the behavioral, neuroendocrine, and neurochemical features of depressive disorders.[186–189] The therapeutic use of pro-inflammatory cytokines IFN-γ and IL-2 for cancer treatment produces depression,[190, 191] and their administration generates hyperactivity and dysregulation in the HPA axis. These are common features of severe depression. The sickness response and depression overlap in that many of the behavioral manifestations of sickness are also manifestations of a depressive disorder. Whether sickness and depression constitute separate states of the system is still uncertain. It is becoming clear, however, that the immune defense responses associated with tissue damage contribute to bodily awareness and the complex, multidimensional experience of pain.

7.2.17 Summary of the Physiologic

This review of mechanisms reveals that the emotional aspects of pain are the product of the defensive and stress responses that tissue trauma, a related stressor, or a constellation of stressors evokes. These responses comprise two forms of allostasis. At the neuroendocrine level, the defense response is an adaptive reaction characterized by sympathetic arousal, hypervigilance, and a sense of threat. However, a coordinated immune system adaptive defense response also occurs at the immune level. Mediated by pro-inflammatory cytokines, it produces a sense of sickness and curtails normal activity. The sickness response produces fatigue, general malaise, fever, and hyperalgesia, typically experienced as musculoskeletal pain. Depression is related to the sickness response in that both are the product of pro-inflammatory cytokines. Thus, the defensive responses generate negative emotions in the general domains of anxiety/threat, depression, fatigue, and sickness.

7.2.18 Stress and Chronic Pain

Stress and related defensive responses can promote chronic pain and related disability in at least three ways.

First, noxious somatic or neuropathic signaling or a central mechanism generating the perception of pain can function as stressors, thereby triggering a defense response and stress. As the mechanism discussion indicates, this can lead to negative emotional states, depressed mood, general sickness, and fatigue. If this is prolonged, patients typically undergo physical deconditioning that makes the pain worse.

Second, psychosocial stressors, such as dysfunctional family relationships or poor vocational adjustment, can trigger the stress response and lead to all the consequences noted earlier.

Third, comorbid disorders and associated interventions are stressors and can contribute to pain by producing negative affective states, the sickness response, and ultimately, physical deconditioning. Immunologic diseases, cancer, diabetes, neurologic disorders, and other disease states can increase patient vulnerability to chronic pain through these mechanisms.

The three mechanisms are not mutually exclusive; they can exist in any combination. The normal course of a stress response or defense response is immediate arousal with subsequent slow recovery to normalcy. When stressors confront a patient as a chain of events, the recovery process to the first mechanism may not finish before the second sets off another arousal pattern. A chain of stressors can dysregulate one or another feedback-dependent aspect of the stress response system, such as the HPA axis. Hypercortisolemia, for example, characterizes almost half of severely depressed patients. Stress-induced chronobiologic dysregulation is perhaps more common. Patients with chronic pain often complain of disturbed sleep patterns.

Psychophysiology is a rapidly expanding domain of inquiry. We have been able to cover only a small fraction of the field in this review. Other relevant areas include sleep and sleep disorders, chronobiology, physiologic mechanisms of learning and memory, somatic representation, and psychoneuroimmunology. Painful conditions influence these various domains and, in turn, change in response to changes within these domains. Furthermore, functional brain imaging has opened new opportunities for pursuing the relationship of brain activity to physical and psychological manipulations and subjective experience. Building an interdisciplinary scientific evidence base in the domain of psychophysiology should be a priority in pain research because this field bridges psychological states and physiologic health.

Multisymptom syndromes such as fibromyalgia syndrome, irritable bowel syndrome, and temporomandibular disorder pose major challenges in pain medicine and other medical areas. It is clear that these problems are related to stress, but the causal mechanisms of such disorders and their resistance to treatment remain ill-defined. These disorders are mind–body problems that refuse to yield to either purely physiologic or purely psychological intervention. Psychophysiology is the only approach formally organized to pursue such mechanisms from an integrated body–mind perspective. Future research on the nature of multisymptom disorders and the development of management strategies or curative interventions can benefit from a psychophysiological approach.

Finally, psychophysiology as a field offers unique tools and methods for research that can address the mechanisms and benefits of interdisciplinary pain management. It is no surprise to experienced pain clinicians that psychological interventions and events have physiologic consequences and, conversely, physiologic events and interventions have psychological consequences. Psychophysiology as a field is well positioned to characterize such phenomena and also to optimize interdisciplinary intervention through the coordinated examination of subjective and objective outcomes.

REFERENCES

1. Andreassi JL. *Psychophysiology: Human Behavior and Physiological Response*. 2nd ed. Hillsdale, NJ: Lawrence Erlbaum Associates; 1989.
2. Cacioppo JT, Tassinary LG. Psychophysiology and psychophysiological inference. In: Cacioppo JT, Tassinary LG, eds. *Principles of Psychophysiology: Physical, Social, and Inferential Elements*. New York: Cambridge University Press; 1990:3–33.
3. Hugdahl K. *Psychophysiology: The Mind-Body Perspective*. Cambridge, MA: Harvard University Press; 1995.
4. Scarry E. *The Body in Pain: The Making and Unmaking of the World*. New York: Oxford University Press; 1985.
5. Merskey H. Pain terms: a list with definitions and a note on usage. Recommended by the IASP Subcommittee on Taxonomy. *Pain* 1979;6:249–252.
6. Dennett D. *Consciousness Explained*. Boston, MA: Little Brown; 1991.
7. MacLean PD. Phenomenology of psychomotor epilepsy: basic and specific affects. In: *The Triune Brain in Evolution: Role in Paleocerebral Functions*. New York: Plenum Press; 1990:425.
8. Darwin C. *The Expression of the Emotions in Man and Animals*. London: John Murray; 1872.
9. Thompson J. Development of facial expression of emotion in blind and seeing children. *Arch Psychol* 1941;37:264.
10. Ploog D. Biological foundations of the vocal expressions of emotions. In: Plutchik R, Kellerman H, eds. *Emotion: Theory, Research, and Experience*. New York: Academic Press; 1986:173–198.
11. Ploog D. Human neuroethology of emotion. *Prog Neuropsychopharmacol Biol Psychiatry* 1989;13(suppl):S15–S22.
12. MacLean PD. Some psychiatric implications of physiological studies on frontotemporal portion of limbic system (visceral brain). *Electroencephalogr Clin Neurophysiol* 1952;4:407–418.
13. Coghill RC, Sang CN, Maisog JM, et al. Pain intensity processing within the human brain: a bilateral, distributed mechanism. *J Neurophysiol* 1999;82(4): 1934–1943.

14. Coghill RC, McHaffie JG, Yen YF. Neural correlates of interindividual differences in the subjective experience of pain. *Proc Natl Acad Sci U S A* 2003;100(14):8538–8542.
15. Derbyshire SW, Jones AK, Gyulai F, et al. Pain processing during three levels of noxious stimulation produces differential patterns of central activity. *Pain* 1997;73(3):431–445.
16. Raichle ME, MacLeod AM, Snyder AZ, et al. A default mode of brain function. *Proc Natl Acad Sci U S A* 2001;98(2):676–682.
17. Nagai M, Kishi K, Kato S. Insular cortex and neuropsychiatric disorders: a review of recent literature. *Eur Psychiatry* 2007;22(6):387–394.
18. Ledoux JE. The neurobiology of emotion. In: Ledoux JE, Hirst W, eds. *Mind and Brain: Dialogs in Cognitive Neuroscience.* Cambridge, MA: Cambridge University Press; 1986:301–354.
19. Ledoux JE. *The Emotional Brain: The Mysterious Underpinnings of Emotional Life.* New York: Simon and Shuster; 1996.
20. Morgane PJ. Historical and modern concepts of hypothalamic organization and function. In: Morgan PJ, Panksepp J, eds. *Handbook of the Hypothalamus.* New York: Marcel Dekker Inc; 1981:1–64.
21. Burnstock G, Hoyle CHV, eds. *Autonomic Neuroeffector Mechanisms.* Philadelphia: Harwood Academic Publishers; 1992.
22. Dodd J, Role LW. The anatomic nervous system. In: Kandel ER, Schwartz JH, Jessell TM, eds. *Principles of Neural Science.* 3rd ed. New York: Elsevier; 1991:761–775.
23. Cannon WB. *Bodily Changes in Pain, Hunger, Fear, and Rage.* New York: Appleton; 1929.
24. Sokolov EN. *Perception and The Conditioned Reflex.* Oxford, United Kingdom: Pergamon Press; 1963.
25. Sokolov EN. The orienting response, and future directions of its development. *Pavlov J Biol Sci* 1990;25(3):142–150.
26. Barrett JA, Shaikh MB, Edinger H, et al. The effects of intrahypothalamic injections of norepinephrine upon affective defense behavior in the cat. *Brain Res* 1987;426(2):381–384.
27. Hess WR. Hypothalamus und die zantren des autonomen nervensystems: physiologie. *Archiv Psychiatr Nervenkr* 1936;104(548–557).
28. Hilton SM. Hypothalamic regulation of the cardiovascular system. *Br Med Bull* 1966;22:243–248.
29. Ferrell JE Jr. Self-perpetuating states in signal transduction: positive feedback, double-negative feedback and bistability. *Curr Opin Cell Biol* 2002;14(2):140–148.
30. Villanueva L, Bing Z, Bouhassira D, et al. Encoding of electrical, thermal, and mechanical noxious stimuli by subnucleus reticularis dorsalis neurons in the rat medulla. *J Neurophysiol* 1989;61:391–402.
31. Willis WD, Westlund KN. Neuroanatomy of the pain system and of the pathways that modulate pain. *J Clin Neurophysiol* 1997;14(1):2–31.
32. Craig AD. Spinal and trigeminal lamina I input to the locus coeruleus anterogradely labeled with *Phaseolus vulgaris* leucoagglutinin (PHA-L) in the cat and the monkey. *Brain Res* 1992;584(1–2):325–328.
33. Villanueva L, Cliffer KD, Sorkin LS, et al. Convergence of heterotopic nociceptive information onto neurons of caudal medullary reticular formation in monkey (*Macaca fascicularis*). *J Neurophysiol* 1990;63:1118–1127.
34. Bing Z, Villanueva L, Le Bars D. Ascending pathways in the spinal cord involved in the activation of subnucleus reticularis dorsalis neurons in the medulla of the rat. *J Neurophysiol* 1990;63:424–438.
35. Bowsher D. Role of the reticular formation in responses to noxious stimulation. *Pain* 1976;2:361–378.
36. Burstein R, Cliffer KD, Giesler GJ. The spinohypothalamic and spinotelecephalic U+xU tracts: direct nociceptive projections from the spinal cord to the hypothalamus and telencephalon. In: Dubne R, Gebhart GF, Bond MR, eds. *Proceedings of the 5th World Congress on Pain.* New York: Elsevier; 1988:548–554.

37. Burstein R, Dado RJ, Cliffer KD, et al. Physiological characterization of spinohypothalamic tract neurons in the lumbar enlargement of rats. *J Neurophysiol* 1991;66(1):261–284.
38. Bernard JF, Besson JM. The spino(trigemino)pontoamygdaloid pathway: electrophysiological evidence for an involvement in pain processes. *J Neurophysiol* 1990;63(3):473–490.
39. Duric V, McCarson KE. Persistent pain produces stress-like alterations in hippocampal neurogenesis and gene expression. *J Pain* 2006;7(8):544–555.
40. Foote SL, Morrison JH. Extrathalamic modulation of corticofunction. *Annu Rev Neurosci* 1987;10:67–95.
41. Bremner JD, Krystal JH, Southwick SM, et al. Noradrenergic mechanisms in stress and anxiety: I. Preclinical studies. *Synapse* 1996;23(1):28–38.
42. Gray JA. *The Neuropsychology of Anxiety: An Enquiry into the Functions of the Septo-Hippocampal System*. New York: Oxford University Press; 1982.
43. Gray JA. *The Psychology of Fear and Stress*. 2nd ed. Cambridge, United Kingdom: Cambridge University Press; 1987.
44. Isaacson RL. *The Limbic System*. 2nd ed. New York: Plenum Press; 1982.
45. Papez JW. A proposed mechanism of emotion. *Arch Neurol Psych* 1937;38:725–743.
46. Charney DS, Deutch A. A functional neuroanatomy of anxiety and fear: implications for the pathophysiology and treatment of anxiety disorders. *Crit Rev Neurobiol* 1996;10(3–4):419–446.
47. Fillenz M. *Noradrenergic Neurons*. Cambridge, United Kingdom: Cambridge University Press; 1990.
48. Svensson TH. Peripheral, autonomic regulation of locus coeruleus noradrenergic neurons in brain: putative implications for psychiatry and psychopharmacology. *Psychopharmacology (Berl)* 1987;92:1–7.
49. Aston–Jones G, Foote SL, Segal M. Impulse conduction properties of noradrenergic locus coeruleus axons projecting to monkey cerebrocortex. *Neuroscience* 1985;15:765–777.
50. Rasmussen K, Aghajanian GK. Withdrawal-induced activation of locus coeruleus neurons in opiate-dependent rats: attenuation by lesions of the nucleus paragigantocellularis. *Brain Res* 1989;505(2):346–350.
51. Rasmussen K, Aghajanian GK. Failure to block responses of locus coeruleus neurons to somatosensory stimuli by destruction of two major afferent nuclei. *Synapse* 1989;4(2):162–164.
52. Korf J, Bunney BS, Aghajanian GK. Noradrenergic neurons: morphine inhibition of spontaneous activity. *Eur J Pharmacol* 1974;25:165–169.
53. Morilak DA, Fornal CA, Jacobs BL. Effects of physiological manipulations on locus coeruleus neuronal activity in freely moving cats. II. Cardiovascular challenge. *Brain Res* 1987;422:24–31.
54. Stone EA. Stress and catecholamines. In: Friedhoff AJ, ed. *Catecholamines and Behavior*. New York: Plenum Press; 1975:31–72.
55. Foote SL, Bloom FE, Aston-Jones G. Nucleus locus ceruleus: new evidence of anatomical and physiological specificity. *Physiol Rev* 1983;63:844–914.
56. Redmond DE Jr, Huang YH. Current concepts. II. New evidence for a locus coeruleus–norepinephrine connection with anxiety. *Life Sci* 1979;25:2149–2162.
57. Grant SJ, Aston-Jones G, Redmond DE Jr. Responses of primate locus coeruleus neurons to simple and complex sensory stimuli. *Brain Res Bull* 1988;21(3):401–410.
58. Redmond DE Jr. Alteration in the functions of the nucleus locus coeruleus: a possible model for studies of anxiety. In: HannIn I, Usdin E, eds. *Animal Models in Psychiatry and Neurology*. New York: Pergamon Press; 1977:293–306.
59. Rasmussen K, Morilak DA, Jacobs BL. Single unit activity of locus coeruleus neurons in the freely moving cat. I. During naturalistic behaviors and in response to simple and complex stimuli. *Brain Res* 1986;371(2):324–334.

60. Elam M, Svensson TH, Thoren P. Differentiated cardiovascular afferent regulation of locus coeruleus neurons and sympathetic nerves. *Brain Res* 1985;358:77–84.
61. Elam M, Thorén P, Svensson TH. Locus coeruleus neurons and sympathetic nerves: activation by visceral afferents. *Brain Res* 1986;375:117–125.
62. Amaral DB, Sinnamon HM. The locus coeruleus: neurobiology of a central noradrenergic nucleus. *Prog Neurobiol* 1977;9:147–196.
63. McNaughton N, Mason ST. The neuropsychology and neuropharmacology of the dorsal ascending noradrenergic bundle—a review. *Prog Neurobiol* 1980;14:157–219.
64. Butler PD, Weiss JM, Stout JC, et al. Corticotropin-releasing factor produces fear-enhancing and behavioral activating effects following infusion into the locus coeruleus. *J Neurosci* 1990;10:176–183.
65. Elam M, Svensson TH, Thorén P. Locus coeruleus neurons and sympathetic nerves: activation by cutaneous sensory afferents. *Brain Res* 1986;366:254–261.
66. Siegel JM, Rogawski MA. A function for REM sleep: regulation of noradrenergic receptor sensitivity. *Brain Res Rev* 1988;472:213–233.
67. Abercrombie ED, Jacobs BL. Single-unit response of noradrenergic neurons in the locus coeruleus of freely moving cats. I. Acutely presented stressful and nonstressful stimuli. *J Neurosci* 1987;7(9):2837–2843.
68. Abercrombie ED, Jacobs BL. Single-unit response of noradrenergic neurons in the locus coeruleus of freely moving cats. II. Adaptation to chronically presented stressful stimuli. *J Neurosci* 1987;7(9):2844–2848.
69. Libet B, Gleason CA. The human locus coeruleus and anxiogenesis. *Brain Res* 1994;634(1):178–180.
70. Weiss JM, Simson PG. Depression in an animal model: focus on the locus ceruleus. *Ciba Found Symp* 1986;123:191–215.
71. Seligman ME, Weiss J, Weinraub M, et al. Coping behavior: learned helplessness, physiological change and learned inactivity. *Behav Res Ther* 1980;18(5):459–512.
72. Sumal KK, Blessing WW, Joh TH, et al. Synaptic interaction of vagal afference and catecholaminergic neurons in the rat nucleus tractus solitarius. *J Brain Res* 1983;277:31–40.
73. Sawchenko PE, Swanson LW. The organization of noradrenergic pathways from the brain stem to the paraventricular and supraoptic nuclei in the rat. *Brain Res* 1982;257(3):275–325.
74. Assenmacher I, Szafarczyk A, Alonso G, et al. Physiology of neuropathways affecting CRH secretion. In: Ganong WF, Dallman MF, Roberts JL, eds. *The Hypothalamic–Pituitary–Adrenal Axis Revisited* 1987:149–161.
75. Kanosue K, Nakayama T, Ishikawa Y, et al. Responses of hypothalamic and thalamic neurons to noxious and scrotal thermal stimulation in rats. *J Thermobiol* 1984;9:11–13.
76. Peschanski M, Weil–Fugacza J. Aminergic and cholinergic afferents to the thalamus: experimental data with reference to pain pathways. In: Besson JM, Guilbaud G, Paschanski M, eds. *Thalamus and Pain*. Amsterdam, The Netherlands: Excerpta Medica; 1987:127–154.
77. Lopez JF, Young EA, Herman JP, et al. Regulatory biology of the HPA axis: an integrative approach. In: RiSCh SC, ed. *Central Nervous System Peptide Mechanisms in Stress and Depression*. Washington, DC: American Psychiatric Press; 1991:1–52.
78. Feldman S, Conforti N, Weidenfeld J. Limbic pathways and hypothalamic neurotransmitters mediating adrenocortical responses to neural stimuli. *Neurosci Biobehav Rev* 1995;19(2):235–240.
79. Selye H. *The Stress of Life*. New York: McGraw–Hill; 1978.
80. Lilly MP, Gann DS. The hypothalamic–pituitary–adrenal-immune axis. A critical assessment. *Arch Surg* 1992;127(12):1463–1474.
81. Ghione S. Hypertension-associated hypalgesia. Evidence in experimental animals and humans, pathophysiological mechanisms, and potential clinical consequences. *Hypertension* 1996;28(3):494–504.

82. Amir S, Amit Z. The pituitary gland mediates acute and chronic pain responsiveness in stressed and non-stressed rats. *Life Sci* 1979;24:439–448.
83. Kelly DD, Silverman AJ, Glusman M, et al. Characterization of pituitary mediation of stress-induced antinociception in rats. *Physiol Behav* 1993;53:769–775.
84. Bodnar RJ, Glusman M, Brutus M, et al. Analgesia induced by cold-water stress: attenuation following hypophysectomy. *Physiol Behav* 1979;23:53–62.
85. Truesdell LS, Bodner RJ. Reduction in cold-water swim analgesia following hypothalamic paraventricular nucleus lesions. *Physiol Behav* 1987;39:727–731.
86. Henry JP. Neuroendocrine patterns of emotional response. In: Plutchik R, Kellerman H, eds. *Emotion: Theory, Research and Practice*. Orlando, FL: Academic Press; 1986:37–60.
87. LeDoux JE, Iwata J, Cicchetti P, et al. Different projections of the central amygdaloid nucleus mediate autonomic and behavioral correlates of conditioned fear. *J Neurosci* 1988;8:2517–2529.
88. Krukoff TL. Neuropeptide regulation of autonomic outflow at the sympathetic preganglionic neuron. Anatomical and neurochemical specificity. *Ann N Y Acad Sci* 1990;579:160–167.
89. Sapolsky RM. *Stress, the Aging Brain, and the Mechanisms of Neuron Death*. Cambridge, MA: The MIT Press; 1992.
90. Panksepp J. The anatomy of emotions. In: Plutchik R, Kellerman H, eds. *Emotion: Theory, Research and Experience*. Orlando, FL: Academic Press; 1986:91–124.
91. Jänig W. Systemic and specific autonomic reactions in pain: efferent, afferent and endocrine components. *Eur J Anaesthesiol* 1985;2:319–346.
92. Saphier D. Cortisol alters firing rate and synaptic responses of limbic forebrain units. *Brain Res Bull* 1987;19:519–524.
93. Damasio AR. *Descartes' Error: Emotion and Reason in the Human Brain*. New York: Grosset/Putnam; 1994.
94. Basbaum AI, Fields HL. Endogenous pain control systems: brainstem spinal pathways and endorphin circuitry. *Annu Rev Neurosci* 1984;7:309–338.
95. Coghill RC, Talbot JD, Evans AC, et al. Distributed processing of pain and vibration by the human brain. *J Neurosci* 1994;14(7):4095–4108.
96. Tracey I, Mantyh PW. The cerebral signature for pain perception and its modulation. *Neuron* 2007;55(3):377–391.
97. Wiech K, Ploner M, Tracey I. Neurocognitive aspects of pain perception. *Trends Cogn Sci* 2008;12(8):306–313.
98. Oshiro Y, Quevedo AS, McHaffie JG, et al. Brain mechanisms supporting spatial discrimination of pain. *J Neurosci* 2007;27(13):3388–3394.
99. Oshiro Y, Quevedo AS, McHaffie JG, et al. Brain mechanisms supporting discrimination of sensory features of pain: a new model. *J Neurosci* 2009;29(47):14924–14931.
100. Lobanov OV, Quevado AS, Hadsel MS, et al. Frontoparietal mechanisms supporting attention to location and intensity of Painful stimuli. *Pain* 2013;154(9):1758–1768.
101. Lobanov OV, Zeidan F, McHaffie JG, et al. From cue to meaning: brain mechanisms supporting the construction of expectations of pain. *Pain* 2014;155(1):129–136.
102. Bushnell MC, Ceko M, Low LA. Cognitive and emotional control of pain and its disruption in chronic pain. *Nat Rev Neurosci* 2013;14(7):502–511.
103. Kong J, White NS, Kwong KK, et al. Using fMRI to dissociate sensory encoding from cognitive evaluation of heat pain intensity. *Hum Brain Mapp* 2006;27(9):715–721.
104. Petrovic P, Ingvar M. Imaging cognitive modulation of pain processing. *Pain* 2002;95(1–2):1–5.
105. Seminowicz DA, Mikulis DJ, Davis KD. Cognitive modulation of pain- related brain responses depend on behavioral strategy. *Pain* 2004;112(1–2):
106. Villemure C, Bushnell MC. Cognitive modulation of pain: how do attention and emotion influence Pain processing? *Pain* 2002;95(3):195–199.

107. Millan MJ. Descending control of pain. *Prog Neurobiol* 2002;66(6):355–474.
108. Eippert F, Bingel U, Schoell ED, et al. Activation of the opioidergic descending pain control system underlies placebo analgesia. *Neuron* 2009;63(4):533–543.
109. Grevert P, Albert LH, Goldstein A. Partial antagonism of placebo analgesia by naloxone. *Pain* 1983;16(2):129–143.
110. Levine JD, Gordon NC, Fields HL. The mechanism of placebo analgesia. *Lancet* 1978:2 (8091):654–657.
111. Zubieta JK, Bueller JA, Jackson LR, et al. Placebo effects mediated by endogenous opioid activity on mu-opioid receptors. *J Neurosci* 2005;25(34):7754–7762.
112. Amanzio M, Benedetti F. Neuropharmacological dissection of placebo analgesia: expectation-activated opioid systems versus conditioning-activated specific subsystems. *J Neurosci* 1999;19(1):484–494.
113. King CD, Goodin B, Kinder LL, et al. Reduction of conditioned pain modulation in humans by naltrexone: an exploratory study of the effects of pain catastrophizing. *J Behav Med* 2013;36(3):315–327.
114. Harris RE, Zubieta JK, Scott DJ, et al. Traditional Chinese acupuncture and placebo (sham) acupuncture are differentiated by their effects on mu-opioid receptors (MORs). *Neuroimage* 2009;47(3):1077–1085.
115. Stephenson JB. Reversal of hypnosis-induced analgesia by naloxone. *Lancet* 1978;2(8097):991–992.
116. Sprenger C, Eippert F, Finsterbusch J, et al. Attention modulates spinal cord responses to pain. *Curr Biol* 2012;22(11):1019–1022.
117. Tracey I, Ploghaus A, Gati JS, et al. Imaging attentional modulation of pain in the periaqueductal gray in humans. *J Neurosci* 2002;22(7):2748–2752.
118. Valet M, Sprenger T, Boecker H, et al. Distraction modulates connectivity of the cingulo-frontal cortex and the midbrain during pain—an fMRI analysis. *Pain* 2004;109(3):399–408.
119. Koyama T, McHaffie JG, Laurienti PJ, et al. The subjective experience of pain: where expectations become reality. *Proc Natl Acad Sci U S A* 2005;102(36):12950–12955.
120. Zeidan F, Lobanov OV, Kraft RA, et al. Brain mechanisms supporting violated expectations of pain. *Pain* 2015;156(9):1772–1785.
121. Salomons TV, Johnstone T, Backonja MM, et al. Individual differences in the effects of perceived controllability on pain perception: critical role of the prefrontal cortex. *J Cogn Neurosci* 2007;19(6):993–1003.
122. Wager TD, Atlas LY, Leotti LA, et al. Predicting individual differences in placebo analgesia: contributions of brain activity during anticipation and pain experience. *J Neurosci* 2011;31(2):439–452.
123. Wager TD, Rilling JK, Smith EE, et al. Placebo-induced changes in FMRI in the anticipation and experience of pain. *Science* 2004;303(5661):1162–1167.
124. Wager TD, Scott DJ, Zubieta JK. Placebo effects on human mu-opioid activity during pain. *Proc Natl Acad Sci U S A* 2007;104(26):11056–11061.
125. Rainville P. Brain mechanisms of pain affect and pain modulation. *Curr Opin Neurobiol* 2002;12(2):195–204.
126. Rainville P, Carrier B, Hofbauer RK, et al. Dissociation of sensory and affective dimensions of Pain using hypnotic modulation. *Pain* 1999;82(2):159–171.
127. Rainville P, Duncan GH, Price DD, et al. Pain affect encoded in human anterior cingulate but not somatosensory cortex. *Science* 1997;277(5328):968–971.
128. Roy M, Lebuis A, Peretz I, et al. The modulation of pain by attention and emotion: a dissociation of perceptual and spinal nociceptive processes. *Eur J Pain* 2011;15(6):641.e10.
129. Roy M, Piché M, Chen JI, et al. Cerebral and spinAl modulAtion of pAin by emotions. *Proc NAtl Acad Sci U S A* 2009;106(49):20900–20905.

130. Casey KL, Svensson P, Morrow TJ, et al. Selective opiate modulation of nociceptive processing in the human brain. *J Neurophysiol* 2000;84(1):525–533.
131. Willoch F, Schindler F, Wester HJ, et al. Central poststroke pain and reduced opioid receptor binding within pain processing circuitries: a [11C] diprenorphine PET study. *Pain* 2004;108(3):213–220.
132. Adler LJ, Gyulai FE, Diehl DJ, et al. Regional brain activity changes associated with fentanyl analgesia elucidated by positron emission tomography. *Anesth Analg* 1997;84(1):120–126.
133. Willoch F, Tölle TR, Wester HJ, et al. Central pain after pontine infarction is associated with changes in opioid receptor binding: a PET study with 11C-diprenorphine. *AJNR Am J Neuroradiol* 1999;20(4):686–690.
134. Jones AK, Qi LY, Fujiwara T, et al. In vivo distribution of opioid receptors in man in relation to the cortical projections of the medial and lateral pain systems measured with positron emission tomography. *Neurosci Lett* 1991;126(1):25–28.
135. Floyd NS, Price JL, Ferry AT, et al. Orbitomedial prefrontal cortical projections to distinct longitudinal columns of the periaqueductal gray in the rat. *J Comp Neurol* 2000;422(4):556–578.
136. Beitz AJ. The organization of afferent projections to the midbrain periaqueductal gray of the rat. *Neuroscience* 1982;7(1):133–159.
137. Mantyh PW. Connections of midbrain periaqueductal gray in the monkey. II. Descending efferent projections. *J Neurophysiol* 1983;49(3):582–594.
138. Mantyh PW. Connections of midbrain periaqueductal gray in the monkey. I. Ascending efferent projections. *J Neurophysiol* 1983;49(3):567–581.
139. Liebeskind JC, Guilbaud G, Besson JM, et al. Analgesia from electrical stimulation of the periaqueductal gray matter in the cat: behavioral observations and inhibitory effects on spinal cord interneurons. *Brain Res* 1973;50(2):441–446.
140. Pandya DN, Barnes CL, Panksepp J. Architecture and connections of the frontal lobe. In: Perecman E, ed. *The Frontal Lobes Revisited.* Hillsdale, NJ: Lawrence Erlbaum Associates; 1987:41–72.
141. Pribram KH. The biology of emotions and other feelings. In: Plutchik R, Kellerman H, eds. *Emotion: Theory, Research, and Experience.* New York: Academic Press; 1980:245–269.
142. Turner BH, Mishkin M, Knapp M. Organization of the amygdalopedal projections from modality-specific cortical association areas in the monkey. *J Comp Neurol* 1980;19:515–543.
143. Dworkin RH. Pain insensitivity in schizophrenia: a neglected phenomenon and some implications. *Schizophr Bull* 1994;20(2):235–248.
144. Melzack R. Phantom limbs and the concept of a neuromatrix. *Trends Neurosci* 1990;13:88–92.
145. Melzack R. Phantom limbs. *Sci Am* 1992;266(4):120–126.
146. Melzack R, Israel R, Lacroix R, et al. Phantom limbs in people with congenital limb deficiency or amputation in early childhood. *Brain* 1997;120(pt 9):1603–1620.
147. McEwen BS. The neurobiology of stress: from serendipity to clinical relevance. *Brain Res* 2000;886(1–2):172–189.
148. Korte SM, Koolhaas JM, Wingfield JC, et al. The Darwinian concept of stress: benefits of allostasis and costs of allostatic load and the trade-offs in health and disease. *Neurosci Biobehav Rev* 2005;29(1):3–38.
149. Tsigos C, Chrousos GP. Hypothalamic–pituitary–adrenal axis, neuroendocrine factors and stress. *J Psychosom Res* 2002;53(4):865–871.
150. Padgett DA, Glaser R. How stress influences the immune response. *Trends Immunol* 2003;24(8):444–448.

151. Zukowska Z, Pons J, Lee EW, et al. Neuropeptide Y: a new mediator linking sympathetic nerves, blood vessels and immune system? *Can J Physiol Pharmacol* 2003;81(2):89–94.
152. Elenkov IJ. Glucocorticoids and the Th1/Th2 balance. *Ann N Y Acad Sci* 2004;1024:138–146.
153. Rassnick S, Sved AF, Rabin BS. Locus coeruleus stimulation by corticotropin- releasing hormone suppresses in vitro cellular immune responses. *J Neurosci* 1994;14(10):6033–6040.
154. Davidson RJ, Irwin W. The functional neuroanatomy of emotion and affective style. *Trends Cogn Sci* 1999;3(1):11–21.
155. Hariri AR, Mattay VS, Tessitore A, et al. Neocortical modulation of the amygdala response to fearful stimuli. *Biol Psychiatry* 2003;53(6):494–501.
156. Likhtik E, Pelletier JG, Paz R, et al. Prefrontal control of the amygdala. *J Neurosci* 2005;25(32):7429–7437.
157. Merali Z, Michaud D, McIntosh J, et al. Differential involvement of amygdaloid CRH system(s) in the salience and valence of the stimuli. *Prog Neuropsychopharmacol Biol Psychiatry* 2003;27(8):1201–1212.
158. Herman JP, Figueiredo H, Mueller NK, et al. Central mechanisms of stress integration: hierarchical circuitry controlling hypothalamic-pituitary– adrenocortical responsiveness. *Front Neuroendocrinol* 2003;24(3):151–180.
159. Pessoa L, Padmala S, Morland T. Fate of unattended fearful faces in the amygdala is determined by both attentional resources and cognitive modulation. *Neuroimage* 2005;28(1):249–255.
160. Keefe FJ, Rumble ME, Scipio CD, et al. Psychological aspects of persistent pain: current state of the science. *J Pain* 2004;5(4):195–211.
161. Misslin R. The defense system of fear: behavior and neurocircuitry. *Neurophysiol Clin* 2003;33(2):55–66.
162. Rosen JB. The neurobiology of conditioned and unconditioned fear: a neurobehavioral system analysis of the amygdala. *Behav Cogn Neurosci Rev* 2004;3(1):23–41.
163. Pare D, Quirk GJ, Ledoux JE. New vistas on amygdala networks in conditioned fear. *J Neurophysiol* 2004;92(1):1–9.
164. Forray MI, Gysling K. Role of noradrenergic projections to the bed nucleus of the stria terminalis in the regulation of the hypothalamic-pituitary-adrenal axis. *Brain Res Rev* 2004;47(1–3):145–160.
165. Xu Y, Day TA, Buller KM. The central amygdala modulates hypothalamic–pituitary–adrenal axis responses to systemic interleukin-1beta administration. *Neuroscience* 1999;94(1):175–183.
166. Sternberg EM. Neuroendocrine factors in susceptibility to inflammatory disease: focus on the hypothalamic–pituitary–adrenal axis. *Horm Res* 1995; 43(4):159–161.
167. Kohl J. The role of complement in danger sensing and transmission. *Immunol Res* 2006;34(2):157–176.
168. Lambrecht BN. Immunologists getting nervous: neuropeptides, dendritic cells and T cell activation. *Respir Res* 2001;2(3):133–138.
169. Inoue A, Ikoma K, Morioka N, et al. Interleukin-1beta induces substance P release from primary afferent neurons through the cyclooxygenase-2 system. *J Neurochem* 1999;73(5):2206–2213.
170. Eskandari F, Webster JI, Sternberg EM. Neural immune pathways and their connection to inflammatory diseases. *Arthritis Res Ther* 2003;5(6):251–265.
171. Gruys E, Toussaint M, Niewold T, et al. Acute phase reaction and acute phase proteins. *J Zhejiang Univ SCI* 2005;6(11):1045–1056.
172. Elenkov IJ, Wilder RL, Chrousos GP, et al. The sympathetic nerve—an integrative interface between two supersystems: the brain and the immune system. *Pharmacol Rev* 2000;52(4):595–638.

173. Vizi ES, Elenkov IJ. Nonsynaptic noradrenaline release in neuro-immune responses. *Acta Biol Hung* 2002;53(1–2):229–244.
174. Kin NW, Sanders VM. It takes nerve to tell T and B cells what to do. *J Leukoc Biol* 2006;79(6):1093–1104.
175. Oberbeck R. Catecholamines: physiological immunomodulators during health and illness. *Curr Med Chem* 2006;13(17):1979–1989.
176. Tracey KJ. The inflammatory reflex. *Nature* 2002;420(6917):853–859.
177. Maier SF, Goehler LE, Fleshner M, et al. The role of the vagus nerve in cytokine-to-brain communication. *Ann N Y Acad Sci* 1998;840:289–300.
178. Dantzer R. Cytokine-induced sickness behavior: mechanisms and implications. *Ann N Y Acad Sci* 2001;933:222–234.
179. Elenkov IJ, Iezzoni DG, DAly A, et al. Cytokine dysregulation, inflammation and well-being. *Neuroimmunomodulation* 2005;12(5):255–269.
180. Watkins LR, Maier SF. Immune regulation of central nervous system functions: from sickness responses to pathological pain. *J Intern Med* 2005;257(2):139–155.
181. Watkins LR, Maier SF. Implications of immune-to-brain communication for sickness and pAin. *Proc NAtl Acad Sci U S A* 1996;96(14):7710–7713.
182. Wieseler–Frank J, Maier SF, Watkins LR. Immune-to-brain communication dynamically modulates pain: physiological and pathological consequences. *Brain Behav Immun* 2005;19(2):104–111.
183. Steinman L. Elaborate interactions between the immune and nervous systems. *Nat Immunol* 2004;5(6):575–581.
184. Romeo HE, Tio DL, Rahman SU, et al. The glossopharyngeal nerve as a novel pathway in immune-to-brain communication: relevance to neuroimmune surveillance of the oral cavity. *J Neuroimmunol* 2001;115(1–2):91–100.
185. Reiche EM, Morimoto HK, Nunes SM. Stress and depression-induced immune dysfunction: implications for the development and progression of cancer. *Int Rev Psychiatry* 2005;17(6):515–527.
186. Wichers M, Maes M. The psychoneuroimmuno-pathophysiology of cytokine-induced depression in humans. *Int J Neuropsychopharmacol* 2002;5(4):375–388.
187. Anisman H, Merali Z. Cytokines, stress and depressive illness: brain- immune interactions. *Ann Med* 2003;35(1):2–11.
188. Pucak ML, Kaplin AI. Unkind cytokines: current evidence for the potential role of cytokines in immune-mediated depression. *Int Rev Psychiatry* 2005;17(6):477–483.
189. Schiepers OJ, Wichers MC, Maes M. Cytokines and major depression. *Prog Neuropsychopharmacol Biol Psychiatry* 2005;29(2):201–217.
190. Wood LJ, Nail LM, Gilster A, et al. Cancer chemotherapy-related symptoms: evidence to suggest a role for proinflammatory cytokines. *Oncol Nurs Forum* 2006;33(3):535–542.
191. Raison CL, Capuron L, Miller AH. Cytokines sing the blues: inflammation and the pathogenesis of depression. *Trends Immunol* 2006;27(1):24–31.

8 Post–Tissue Injury Pain State

Primary Afferent

Soun Sheen and Hemant Kalia

8.1 INTRODUCTION

The afferent C fibers are referred to as silent nociceptors because they have minimal spontaneous activity in the absence of injury (Woller et al. 2017; Yaksh and Luo 2011a). In the presence of tissue injury, these silent afferents develop persistent spontaneous activity beyond the removal of the originating stimulus and enhanced sensitivity of the peripheral terminal through sensitization in the periphery and at the dorsal horn (Yaksh 2014; Yaksh et al. 1999; Baumann et al. 1991). This chapter reviews the inflammatory response secondary to tissue injuries and its role in the sensitization of the primary afferents.

8.2 TISSUE INJURY

An acute high-threshold stimulus evokes a pain sensation that resolves when the stimulus is removed. Ongoing exposure to high-threshold stimuli results in tissue injury, which leads to a pain state due to persistent afferent discharges beyond the removal of the originating stimulus (Yaksh 2020, 2014; Xu and Yaksh 2011). In rat models, the injection of an irritant, such as carrageenan, causes local inflammation and edema, as demonstrated by the increased paw thickness shown in Figure 8.1 (Yaksh 2010). Local inflammation also resulted in reduced thermal escape latency and tactile threshold, as well as increased discrepancy in limb weight-bearing (Yaksh 2010, 2020). The decreased stimulus threshold leads to an enhanced sensitivity to otherwise moderately noxious stimuli at the site of tissue injury, referred to as primary hyperalgesia, and a nociceptive response to a normally innocuous stimulus (allodynia) (Nouri et al. 2018; Ringkamp, Dougherty, and Raja 2018; Yaksh 2010). In addition, sensitization of the non-injured tissue adjacent to the injury site may produce pain, referred to as secondary hyperalgesia or allodynia (Yaksh 2010, 2020).

8.3 PERIPHERAL SENSITIZATION

As demonstrated in Figure 8.2, non-injurious pinch results in a brief stimulus-linked discharge noted in the sural C fiber. In contrast, crush stimulus resulting in tissue injury leads to a prolonged ongoing discharge which continues long after the crushing

DOI: 10.1201/9781003094302-8

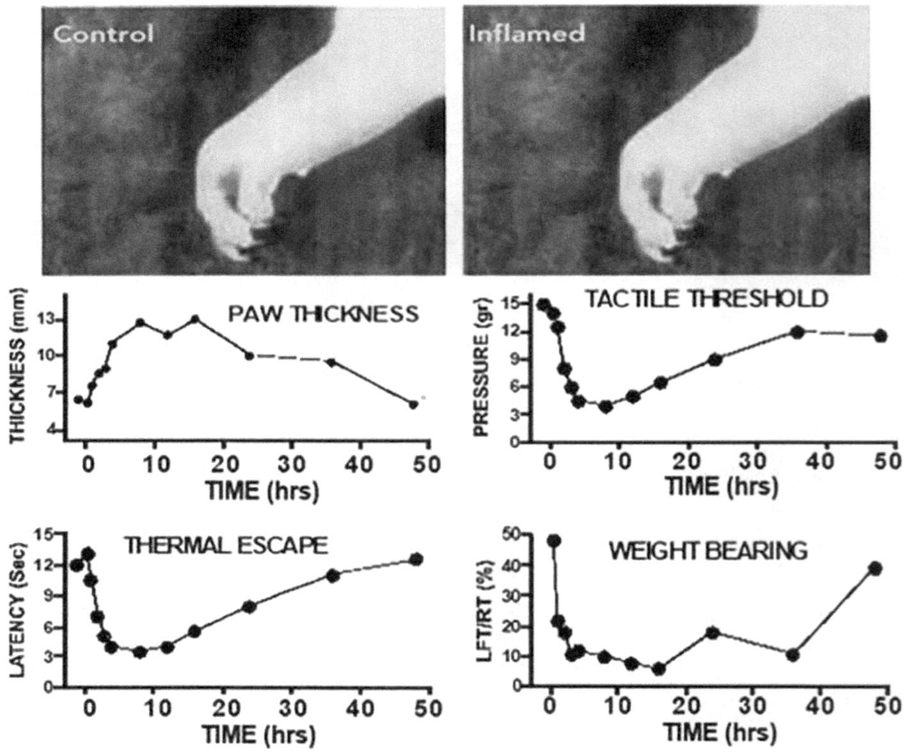

FIGURE 8.1 Preclinical model of inflammation leading to hyperalgesia and tactile allodynia. Injection of an irritant such as carrageenan will lead to local inflammation and edema, which persist for 24–48 hours before resolution. In addition to increased paw thickness, there is a decrease in the thermal escape latency and a reduction in the tactile stimulus required to evoke an escape response (allodynia). There is also a shift to contralateral weight-bearing.

Source: Modified from Yaksh, *Biology of Pain Processing* (2020).

FIGURE 8.2 Discharge of a single afferent in response to tissue pinch vs. crush. A brief pinch results in a transient, stimulus-linked discharge. In contrast, local injury due to a crush results in a prolonged ongoing discharge beyond the removal of the crushing stimulus.

Source: Modified from Yaksh, *Biology of Pain Processing* (2020).

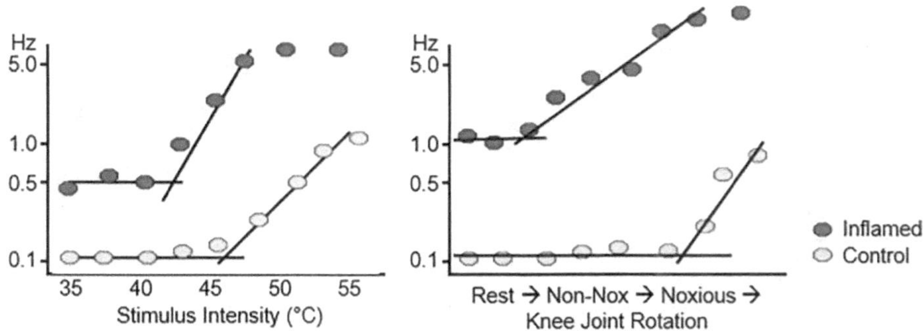

FIGURE 8.3 Response phenotype of an inflamed afferent. *Left,* frequency firing of small afferents in the skin occurs with increasing stimulation temperature. Following carrageenan injection, the afferent shows increasing spontaneous activity (left shift) and an increase in the slope of the stimulus–response curve, indicating a facilitated response to the thermal stimulus. *Right,* firing of knee joint afferent under normal state and in the presence of non-noxious, then noxious, rotation of the knee. There is an increased spontaneous activity and enhanced sensitivity to mild knee rotation.

Source: Serhan, Ward, and Gilroy, Fundamentals of Inflammation (2010).

stimulus has been removed as a result of the inflammatory cascade leading to the release of inflammatory markers and migration of inflammatory cells (Yaksh 2020; Yaksh et al. 1999). The ongoing traffic in tissue injury yields a persistent pain sensation. Such pain typically resolves with the resolution of the injury and inflammatory state.

The stimulus–response curve (Figure 8.3) demonstrates a significant augmentation in discharge frequency with tissue injury noted in both cutaneous and articular primary afferents (Yaksh 2010, 2020). In the absence of injury, there is minimal spontaneous activity in uninjured C fibers to a certain threshold, with a monotonic increase in the discharge frequency with increasing stimulus intensities (Yaksh 2020; Yaksh and Luo 2011b). The stimulus threshold also typically reflects the presumed role of each specific population of afferents. Local inflammation following tissue injury leads to increased levels of spontaneous afferent activity, a left shift, and an increased slope of the stimulus–response curve, indicating a facilitated response of the primary afferents and a reduction in the nociceptor threshold (Yaksh 2020; Campbell and Meyer 1986).

8.4 INFLAMMATORY MILIEU

Tissue injury activates an immune response, yielding both orthodromic and antidromic activities on the primary afferent terminal, innervating the injury site (Figure 8.4). Activation of the primary afferent terminals leads to not only orthodromic potentials to the spinal cord but also antidromic action potentials, resulting in the release of neurogenic peptides, such as substance P (sP) and calcitonin gene–related peptide (CGRP) (Sorkin et al. 2018; Yaksh 2010, 2014, 2020; Fisher et al. 2021; Cohen, S.A. 2020). These peptides result in a significant dilation of local blood

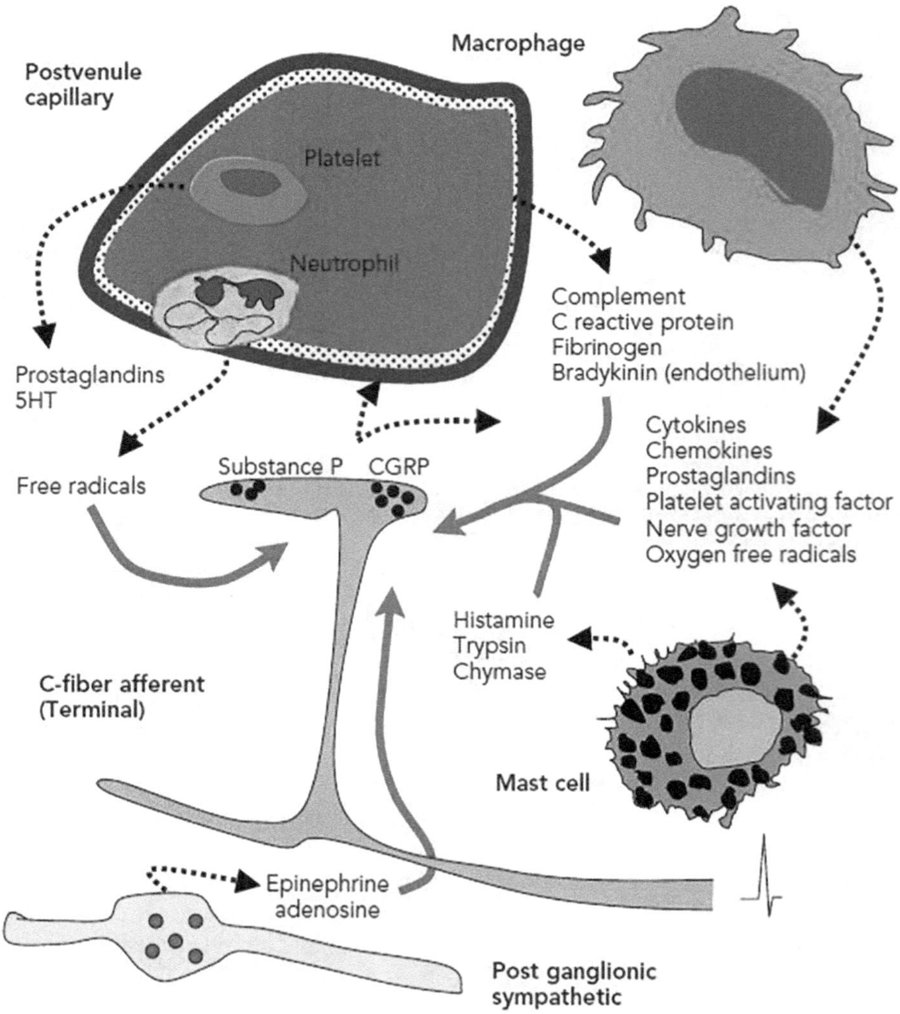

FIGURE 8.4 Summary of the inflammatory milieu of the primary afferent. See text for additional details.

Source: Serhan, Ward, and Gilroy, *Fundamentals of Inflammation* (2010).

vessels and plasma extravasation, which leads to further activation of mast cells and macrophages. These inflammatory cells then secrete a large number of inflammatory factors, such as histamine, cytokines, bradykinin, prostaglandins, nerve growth factors, potassium and hydrogen ions, that further promote the local inflammatory cascade and facilitate the excitability of free nerve endings (Yaksh 2010, 2020; Yaksh and Luo 2011b; Cohen, S.A. 2020). All these extracellular products interact with specific (eponymous) receptors or channels found on C fibers (Yaksh 2010, 2020). The activation of these receptors induces an influx of calcium and sodium, which leads

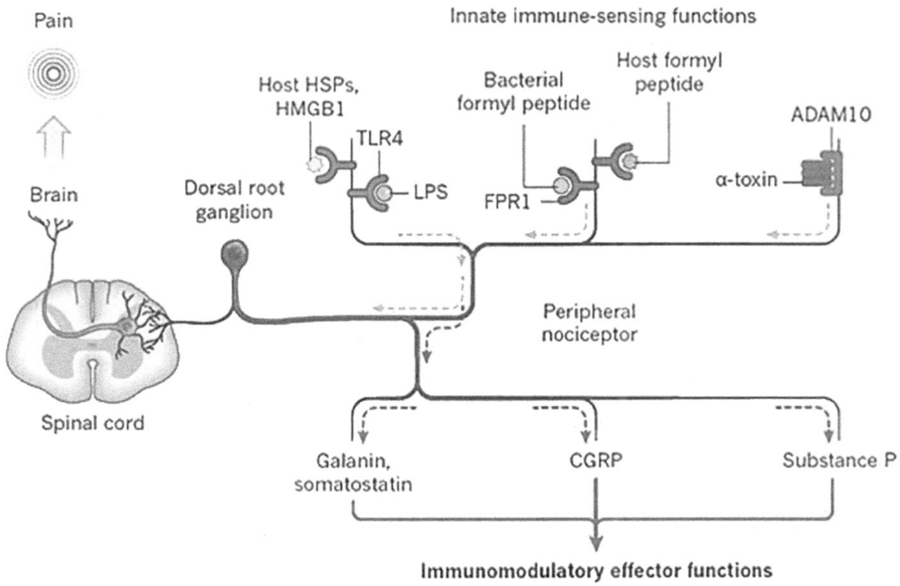

FIGURE 8.5 Immune-related functions of peripheral nociceptors. Peripheral afferent terminals express receptors that detect bacterial toxins (ADAM10), formal peptides (FPR1), and lipopolysaccharides (TLR4). In addition to pain signal transduction to the central nervous system through the dorsal root ganglion (yellow arrows), this activation also leads to the local release of bioactive peptides, such as substance P, CGRP, galanin, and somatostatin. This antidromic signal modulates the local inflammatory response.

Source: Nizet and Yaksh (2013).

to a depolarization of the terminals and the activation of a variety of intracellular enzymes, including protein kinases. The terminal kinases then phosphorylate channels and receptors, including voltage-gated sodium channels (NaV), which will then open at a lower voltage and stay open longer (Yaksh 2010, 2014, 2020). This results in stimulation and sensitization of free nerve endings, thus producing persistent afferent activity and enhanced response to any given stimulus.

In recent years, the concept of infectious microbes directly activating pain receptors, rather than indirectly through an immune cell intermediary, has emerged (Figure 8.5) (Nizet and Yaksh 2013). Sensory afferent nociceptors express receptors that detect bacteria and their toxins, formyl peptides, and lipopolysaccharides (LPS), leading to signal transduction and the local release of vasoactive and immunomodulatory peptides (Yaksh 2020; Nizet and Yaksh 2013). This is concurrent with the axonal propagation of action potentials and the subjective pain experience.

It is important to realize that while studies focus on local afferent terminals and antidromic invasion, the antidromic input to the peripheral terminals can also arise from the neuraxis based on extensive work with the phenomena of dorsal root reflexes (DRR) (Yaksh 2020; Willis 1999). It can be reasonably speculated that neuraxial events leading to such DRRs may influence the local immune response, and events regulating dorsal horn primary afferent terminal excitability may alter the peripheral innate immune response.

8.5 DORSAL ROOT GANGLIA

Following tissue inflammation, a variety of changes may occur in the dorsal root ganglia (DRG) (Fisher et al. 2021; Cohen, R.I. 2020). It has been shown that DRG displays an increased number of macrophages that secrete pro-inflammatory products, leading to ectopic DRG activities and axon collaterals that release neurotransmitters in the DRG (Yaksh 2010, 2014, 2020). The DRG also expresses the receptors and channels expressed on the peripheral terminals and responds to the same mediators that act on these terminals. Pro-inflammatory products may also increase DRG transcription and transport of a variety of proteins to further promote the excitability of primary afferents (Yaksh 2010, 2020).

8.6 CONCLUSION

A tissue injury activates an innate immune response and subsequent events, leading to stimulation and sensitization of free nerve endings, thus resulting in ongoing pain and primary hyperalgesia. It is important to identify the peripheral consequences of tissue injuries to understand what initiates the post–tissue injury pain state.

REFERENCES

Baumann, T.K., D.A. Simone, C.N. Shain, and R.H. Lamotte. 1991. Neurogenic Hyperalgesia: The Search for the Primary Cutaneous Afferent Fibers That Contribute to Capsaicin-Induced Pain and Hyperalgesia. *Journal of Neurophysiology*. 66: 212–227.

Campbell, J.N. and R.A. Meyer. 1986. Primary Afferents and Hyperalgesia. In *Spinal Afferent Processing,* Ed. T.L. Yaksh. 59–79. Springer Science+Business Media, LLC.

Cohen, R.I. 2020. Anatomy and Physiology of Pain. In *Principles and Practice of Pain Medicine,* Ed. Z.H. Bajwa, R.J. Wootton, and C.A. Warfield. 3rd edition. Chapter 2. McGraw Hill.

Cohen, S.A. 2020. Pathophysiology of Pain. In *Principles and Practice of Pain Medicine,* Ed. Z.H. Bajwa, R.J. Wootton, and C.A. Warfield. 3rd edition. Chapter 3. McGraw Hill.

Fisher, C.J., T.L. Yaksh, K. Bruno, and K.A. Eddinger. 2021. Basic Science of Pain. In *Pain Care Essentials and Innovations*, Ed S. Pangarkar, Q.G. Pham, and B.C. Eapen, 1–14. Elsevier. https://doi.org/10.1016/b978-0-323-72216-2.00001-6.

Nizet, V. and T.L. Yaksh. 2013. Bacteria get on your nerves. *Nature*. 501: 43–44.

Nouri, K.H., U. Osuagwu, J. Boyette-Davis, M. Ringkamp, S.N. Raja, and P.M. Dougherty. 2018. Neurochemistry of Somatosensory and Pain Processing. In *Essentials of Pain Medicine*, Ed H.T. Benzon, S.N. Raja, S.S. Liu, S.M. Fishman, S.P. Cohen. 4th edition. 11–20. Elsevier.

Ringkamp, M., P.M. Dougherty, and S.N. Raja. 2018. Anatomy and Physiology of the Pain Signaling Process. In *Essentials of Pain Medicine*, Ed H.T. Benzon, S.N. Raja, S.S. Liu, S.M. Fishman, S.P. Cohen. 4th edition. 1–10. Elsevier.

Sorkin, L.S., K.A. Eddinger, S.A. Woller, and T.L. Yaksh. 2018. Origins of Antidromic Activity in Sensory Afferent Fibers and Neurogenic Inflammation. *Seminars in Immunopathology*. 40(3): 237–247. https://doi.org/10.1007/s00281-017-0669-2.

Willis, W.D. 1999. Dorsal Root Potentials and Dorsal Root Reflexes: A Double-Edged Sword. *Experimental Brain Research*. 124: 395–421.

Woller, S.A., K.A. Eddinger, M. Corr, and T.L. Yaksh. 2017. An Overview of Pathways Encoding Nociception. *Clinical Experimental Rheumatology*. 35: 40–46.

Xu, Q., and T.L. Yaksh. 2011. A Brief Comparison of the Pathophysiology of Inflammatory versus Neuropathic Pain. *Current Opinion in Anaesthesiology* 24 (4): 400–407. https://doi.org/10.1097/ACO.0b013e32834871df.

Yaksh, T.L., X.Y. Hua, I. Kalcheva, N. Nozaki-Taguchi, and M. Marsala. 1999. The spinal biology in humans and animals of pain states generated by persistent small afferent input. *Proceedings of the National Academy of Sciences of the United States of America*. 95: 7680–7686.

Yaksh, T.L. 2010. Mediators and Mechanisms of Inflammatory Pain. In *Fundamentals of Inflammation,* Ed. C.N. Serhan, P.A. Ward, and D.W. Gilroy, 217–233.

Yaksh, T.L. 2014. A Review of Pain-Processing Pharmacology. In *Practical Management of Pain,* Ed. H.T Benzon, J.P. Rathmell, C.L. Wu, D.C. Turk, C.E. Argoff, and R.W. Hurley. 5th Edition. Elsevier.

Yaksh, T.L. 2020. *Biology of Pain Processing*. Presentation at University of California, San Diego.

Yaksh, T.L. and Z.D. Luo. 2011a. Anatomy of the pain processing system. In *Pain Management,* Ed. S.D. Waldman. 2nd Edition. Elsevier.

Yaksh, T.L. and Z.D. Luo. 2011b. Dynamics of the pain processing system. In *Pain Management,* Ed. S.D. Waldman. 2nd Edition. Elsevier.

9 Post–Tissue Injury Pain State
Spinal Cord

Soun Sheen and Hemant Kalia

9.1 INTRODUCTION

In the presence of tissue injury, primary afferents become sensitized and exhibit hyperexcitability to noxious and non-noxious stimuli, which is termed peripheral sensitization.

These activated primary afferents project into the spinal dorsal horn and induce a post-synaptic excitation at the level of the second-order neurons (Yaksh 2010, 2014, 2020; LaMotte 1986). Ongoing afferent traffic due to peripheral sensitization results in the development of central sensitization through different facilitatory cascades. This chapter will review the mechanism of pain transmission through the dorsal horn and brain stem in the setting of tissue injury.

9.2 DORSAL HORN SENSITIZATION

In the absence of tissue injury, the afferent input activates specific populations of the spinal dorsal horn neurons with an adequate stimulus. These second-order neurons can be broadly classified into the marginal neurons lying superficially in lamina I and the wide dynamic range (WDR) neurons lying more deeply in lamina V (Sorkin and Wallace 1999). The response of the dorsal horn neurons is related to the frequency of the afferent input, which typically correlates with the stimulus intensity in a graded manner (Yaksh and Luo 2011; Yaksh 2020). However, in the setting of persistent afferent traffic in the setting of tissue injury, the dorsal horn neurons display enhanced excitability and susceptibility to afferent input. As previously reviewed, WDR neurons receive fiber convergence of full spectrum input from Aβ, Aδ, and C afferent fibers (Yaksh 2020; Woller et al. 2017; Willis 2007). Thus, WDR neurons can encode both innocuous and noxious stimuli over a wide range of stimulus intensities. Persistent discharges from small-diameter afferents facilitate dorsal horn activity.

9.3 WINDUP PHENOMENON

Persistent small afferent discharges result in a facilitation of dorsal horn activity. In animal models, WDR neurons in the dorsal horn display a stimulus-dependent response to discrete activation of afferent C fibers (Li, Simone, and Larson 1999; Yaksh 2020; Yaksh, Ramachandran, and Woller 2020). Repetitive stimulation of C,

DOI: 10.1201/9781003094302-9

but not A, fibers at a moderately faster rate results in a progressively facilitated discharge (Figure 9.1) (Yaksh and Luo 2011; Yaksh 2020). This exaggerated C fiber–evoked discharge in response to repetitive activation of C fibers was named *windup* by Lorne Mendell and Pat Wall in 1966 (Li, Simone, and Larson 1999; Yaksh and Luo 2011). Intracellular recording in the WDR neuron indicated that a progressive and long-sustained partial depolarization of the cell leads the membrane to be increasingly susceptible to afferent input, thus indicating the facilitated state (Yaksh and Luo 2011; Yaksh 2020; Fisher et al. 2021).

The WDR neurons, under normal conditions, are activated by a natural stimulus applied to a small discrete region. After C fiber conditioning, stimuli sufficient to produce windup will also result in an expansion of the receptive field (Yaksh and Luo 2011). Therefore, a natural stimulus applied over a larger area of the leg now displays the ability to activate the same WDR neurons, as seen in Figure 9.1. The increased receptivity with local tissue injury reflects two mechanisms. It is believed that the dorsal horn receptive field depends upon its segmental input.

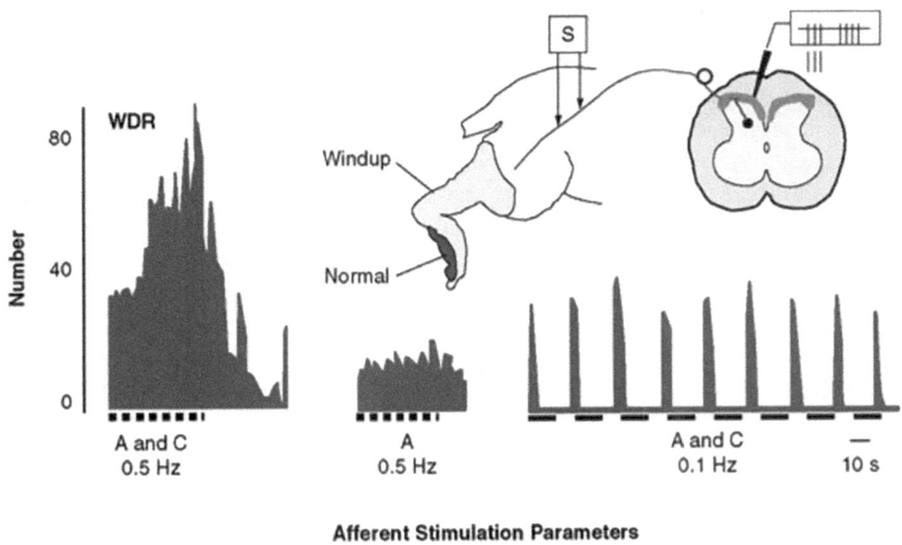

FIGURE 9.1 *The right lower* Schematic shows a single unit recording from a wide dynamic range (WDR) neuron of an anesthetized rat in response to an electrical stimulus, activating A and C fibers, delivered at 0.1 Hz. A reliable, stimulus-linked response is evoked at this frequency. *Left,* in contrast, when the stimulation rate is increased to 0.5 Hz, there is a progressive increase in the magnitude of the response generated by stimulation. *Middle,* facilitation resulting from the C fiber input, but not A, is called windup. *Right upper,* the WDR under normal conditions may be activated by a natural stimulus applied to a small discrete region on the bottom of the paw, shown in red. After C fiber conditioning, a natural stimulus is applied over a large area of the leg (yellow), which now displays the ability to activate the same WDR neuron.

Source: Waldman, *Pain Management* (2011).

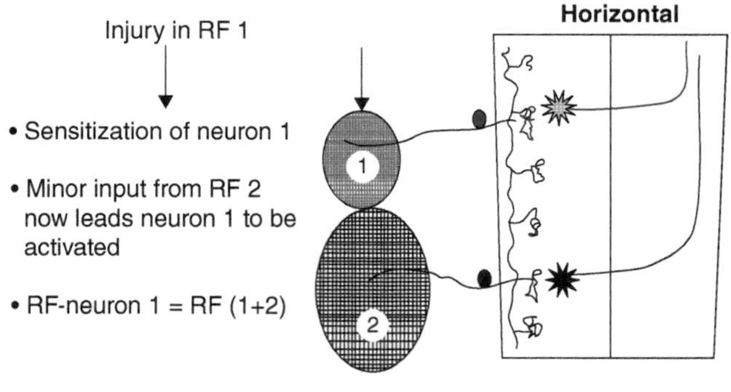

FIGURE 9.2 The receptive field (RF) of the dorsal horn neuron depends upon its segmental input and the input from other segments that can activate it. After an injury in RF 1, neuron 1 becomes sensitized. Collateral input from RF 2 normally is unable to initiate sufficient excitatory activity to activate neuron 1. However, after sensitization, RF 2 input is sufficient, and the RF of neuron 1 is now effectively RF 1 + RF 2. Thus, local injury by spinal mechanisms acutely leads to increased RFs such that stimuli applied to a non-injured RF can contribute to the post–tissue injury sensation.

Source: Waldman, *Pain Management* (2011).

In the presence of a tissue injury, the distant dorsal horn neuron becomes sensitized and activated by input from the proximal dermatome that was previously insufficient to activate the distant neuron (Yaksh and Luo 2011). Thus, local injury can lead to increased receptive fields that stimuli applied to a non-injured receptive field can contribute to post–tissue injury pain (Figure 9.2) (Yaksh and Luo 2011; Yaksh 2020). It is also important to remember that the afferents collateralize upon entering the spinal cord, sending fibers rostrally and caudally up to several segments in Lissauer's tract (C fibers) or in the dorsal column (A fibers) (Yaksh and Luo 2011; Willis 2007). This ramification of afferent fibers indicates that distal neurons will also receive excitatory input. The concept of enhanced receptive fields after injury also applies to visceral somatic convergence. Laird et al. demonstrated that activation of visceral afferents by intracolonic injection of capsaicin led to increased somatic sensitization (Laird et al. 2002; Latremoliere and Woolf 2009).

LaMotte et al. demonstrated that the intradermal injection of capsaicin leads to local C fiber activation, resulting in immediate pain (LaMotte, Lundberg, and Torebjork 1991). Although the initial pain resolves within 20 to 30 minutes, persistent secondary tactile allodynia occurs. Interestingly, secondary allodynia was prevented by a transient effect of local anesthetic given before the capsaicin. This suggested that increased sensitization depended upon the persistent effect of C fiber input to the spinal cord generated by capsaicin. Moreover, animal studies have demonstrated that windup occurs in anesthetized animals (Yaksh 2020). This observation implies the basis for the consideration of preemptive analgesics to prevent small afferent input (LaMotte, Lundberg, and Torebjork 1991).

9.4 LOCAL SPINAL NEURONAL CIRCUITS

Primary afferent C fibers release neuropeptides, such as substance P (sP) and calcitonin gene–related peptide (CGRP), and excitatory amino acids, such as glutamate, that activate second-order neurons within seconds to minutes (Yaksh 2010). Glutamate binds to receptors located on the post-synaptic dorsal horn neurons, including amino-3-hydroxy-5-methyl-4-isoxazole propionate (AMPA) and *N*-methyl-D-aspartate (NMDA) receptors (Figure 9.3). Acute activation leads to primary depolarization largely mediated by AMPA receptor sodium ionophore, which produces a powerful

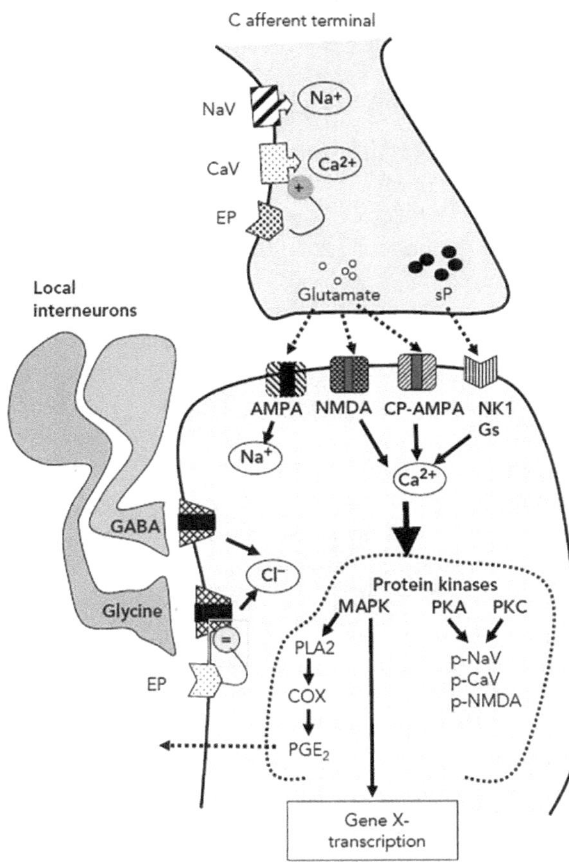

FIGURE 9.3 First-order synapse for a small afferent axon in the spinal dorsal horn. As indicated, there is the release of small afferent transmitters which depolarize the second-order neurons through glutamate and sP receptors. These serve to depolarize the membrane, which, in turn, activates downstream cascades to sensitize the membrane to additional depolarization through a variety of mechanisms.

Source: Serhan, Ward, and Gilroy, *Fundamentals of Inflammation* (2010).

but transient membrane depolarization (Yaksh 2010, 2020). This initial activation leads to a complex cascade.

In the face of repetitive stimulation, the AMPA receptors become calcium-permeable, and there is an increased expression of calcium-permeable AMPA (CP-AMPA) receptors (Yaksh 2020). It is important to note that the NMDA receptors do not appear to mediate acute excitation. Under normal resting membrane potentials, despite the presence of glutamate, the NMDA receptors are inactive due to a magnesium block (Yaksh 2010, 2020; Yaksh and Luo 2011). With repetitive stimulation, the NMDA receptors then become depolarized, resulting in the removal of the magnesium block and increased calcium influx. Moreover, the activation of neurokinin 1 (NK1) receptors, also referred to as the metabotropic sP receptors, leads to increased intracellular calcium (Westlund 2006).

9.5 PHOSPHORYLATION AND LIPID CASCADES

The marked increase in intracellular calcium activates a variety of phosphorylating enzymes, including protein kinases A and C (PKA and PKC) and P38 mitogen-activated protein kinase (P38 MAPK) (Yaksh 2010, 2020). When PKA and PKC are activated by increased intracellular calcium, they phosphorylate a variety of proteins, including the NMDA receptors. This NMDA receptor phosphorylation reduces its threshold for activation and enhances its functionality, resulting in a further increase in calcium passage. Inhibition of PKA and PKC has been shown to reduce behaviorally defined hyperalgesia observed after tissue injury (Yaksh 2020; Jones and Sorkin 2005).

Activation of P38 MAPK leads to phosphorylation of phospholipase A2 (PLA2), which initiates the downstream release of arachidonic acid and provides the substrate for cyclooxygenase (COX) to synthesize prostaglandins (Yaksh 2010, 2020). P38 MAPK activation also leads to increased gene transcription of specific proteins, including COX-2 and nitric oxide synthase (NOS) (Yaksh 2010, 2020). Therefore, in the presence of persistent afferent stimulation, increased intracellular calcium in dorsal horn neurons leads to the activation of a cascade that results in prostaglandin production. Prostaglandins act on both pre-synaptic and post-synaptic receptors. Prostaglandins act pre-synaptically to enhance primary afferent transmitter release by increasing the opening of voltage-sensitive calcium channels and post-synaptically to block glycinergic inhibition on dorsal horn neurons (Yaksh 2010, 2014). This glycinergic inhibition block can lead to further facilitation of dorsal horn excitability. COX inhibitors have been shown to reduce spinal prostaglandin release and diminish injury-induced hyperalgesia (Yaksh 2010).

NOS has also been shown to play a facilitatory role following spinal afferent activation through the formation of nitric oxide (NO) from arginine. NO acts presynaptically to increase transmitter release (Yaksh 2010, 2014). Therefore, spinal NOS inhibitors will reduce post–tissue injury hyperalgesia.

9.6 LOCAL INTERNEURONS

The excitatory input from large Aβ afferents normally does not lead to a pain state due to synaptic inhibition mediated by local interneurons containing amino acids such as γ-aminobutyric acid (GABA) and glycine (Figure 9.4). The dorsal horn GABAergic and glycinergic interneurons receive excitatory input from large low-threshold afferents and yield pre-synaptic and post-synaptic inhibition (Yaksh 2010, 2014; Todd 2010). The GABA and glycine receptors are chloride ionophores, thus resulting in increased chloride permeability with activation (Yaksh 2020). Increased chloride conductance at the post-synaptic membrane results in a mild hyperpolarization, thus stabilization, of the membrane (Yaksh 2010, 2020; Witschi et al. 2011). The release of products such as prostaglandins with peripheral tissue injury causes an alteration of chloride permeability, resulting in an increased chloride equilibrium potential and enhanced depolarization with increased chloride permeability (Yaksh 2020). Therefore, in the presence of tissue injury, a decrease in GABAergic and glycinergic inhibition leads to an exaggerated response to such tactile stimulation, resulting in tactile allodynia.

Many studies support the importance of GABA and glycine-mediated inhibition of spinal neurons. Yaksh demonstrated that intrathecal administration of glycine (strychnine) and GABA (bicuculline) antagonists produced a significantly enhanced response to light tactile stimulation (Figure 9.5) (Yaksh 1989; Ishikawa et al. 1999).

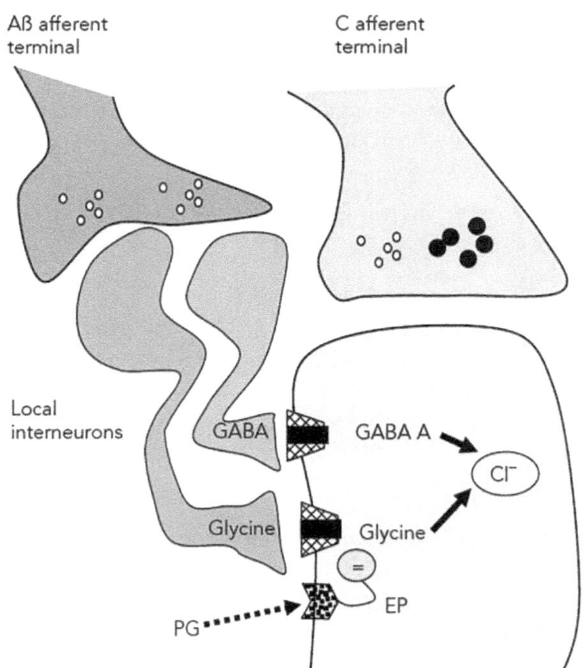

FIGURE 9.4 Regulation of dorsal horn excitability by GABA and glycine interneurons. Low-threshold primary afferents activate inhibitor GABA and glycine interneurons, which serve to reduce the excitatory drive produced by large afferent input. Loss of this inhibition would lead to a prominent increase in large afferent evoked excitation.

Source: Serhan, Ward, and Gilroy, *Fundamentals of Inflammation* (2010).

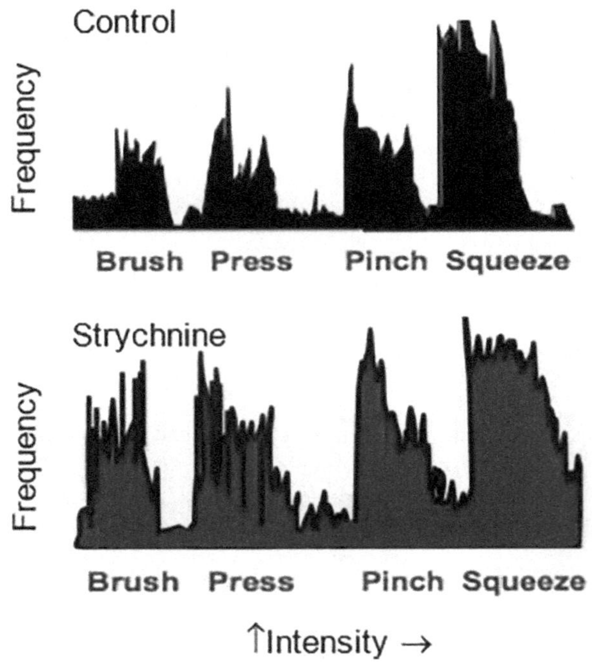

FIGURE 9.5 Effects of blockade on inhibitor interneuron receptors. Blocking the glycine receptor with an antagonist (strychnine) results in a prominent augmentation in the response of the WDR neuron to light touch.

Source: Modified from Yaksh, *Biology of Pain Processing* (2020).

This again emphasizes the role of intrinsic GABA and glycinergic interneurons—loss of interneuron regulation turns Aβ afferents into powerful drivers of WDR neuron activity.

9.7 BULBOSPINAL CIRCUITS

The bulbospinal pathways are descending serotonergic and noradrenergic projections from the brain stem to the dorsal horn that transmit excitatory and inhibitory signals to modulate the central sensitization at the dorsal horn level. Serotonergic pathways, activated by ascending projections into the medulla in response to small afferent input, originate from the nucleus raphe magnus of the medulla and project to the dorsal horn via bulbospinal-dorsolateral funiculus (DLF) (Figure 9.6) (Yaksh 2010, 2020; Yaksh and Luo 2011). The raphe spinal terminals in the deep dorsal horn excite WDR neurons by 5HT3 receptors, thus facilitating the windup (Yaksh and Luo 2011). In contrast, the noradrenergic pathways arising from the locus coeruleus mediate a local inhibition (Yaksh 2020). Norepinephrine (NE) reduces the

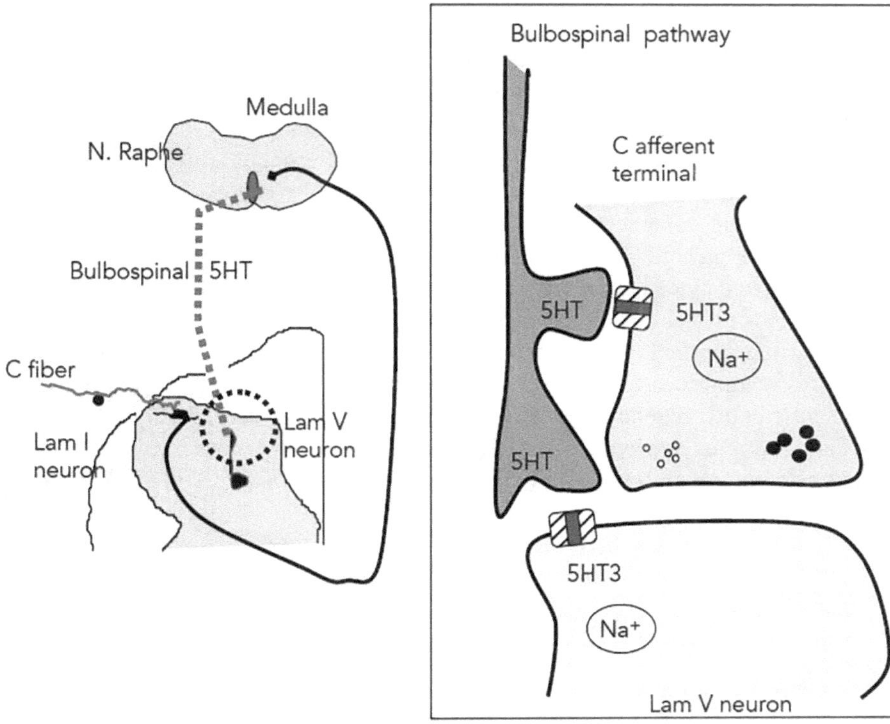

FIGURE 9.6 Ascending projections activated by small afferent input activate raphe spinal neurons that send serotonergic (5HT) projections to the dorsal horn. 5HT released from the bulbospinal pathway then activates WDR neurons through a $5HT_3$ receptor.

Source: Serhan, Ward, and Gilroy, *Fundamentals of Inflammation* (2010).

excitability of dorsal horn neurons through the inhibitory α2 adrenergic receptors on primary afferent and second-order neurons (Yaksh 2010, 2020).

The ascending activation of spinal circuits in response to high-frequency stimuli, in turn, results in enhanced pain states through the activation of spinal–bulbs–spinal (SBS) pathways (Yaksh 2020). This descending pathway may be activated by supraspinal systems, demonstrated by the light–shock pairing in a classical conditioning paradigm in rat models. The light–shock pairing leads to a blood pressure response that represents the activation of bulbospinal projections to spinal preganglionic neurons (Yaksh 2020). After such pairing, the subject will show the blood pressure response (and thus the activation of descending pathways) in response to the light alone (Yaksh 2020). This observation demonstrates that learned experiences can influence the spinal processing of nociceptive input and provide a link between the supraspinal affective component and facilitatory control of spinal sensory processing. This linkage suggests that concurrent stressors may enhance acute pain as well as the likelihood of pain chronification.

9.8 NONNEURONAL CELLS

At the spinal level, there are a variety of nonneuronal cells, including astrocytes and microglia, that play important trophic roles, such as blood–brain barrier integrity, extracellular water balance, glucose transport, and phagocytic functions (Yaksh 2010). It is also evident that these cells also regulate the excitability of local neuronal circuits. Astrocytes, microglia, and neurons form a complex tripartite network in which each can influence the excitability of synaptic transmission (Yaksh 2020). As shown in Figure 9.7, transmitters, such as glutamate, sP, adenosine triphosphate (ATP), and cytokines, at the synaptic cleft can overflow and directly activate adjacent nonneuronal cells (Yaksh 2010, 2014). Such activation leads to further secretion of active factors that mediate the excitability of neuronal transmission. Astrocytes communicate over a distance by the spread of excitation through local nonsynaptic contacts referred to as gap junctions (Yaksh 2010, 2020). Astrocytes may also communicate with other astrocytes and microglia by releasing several products, including glutamate and cytokines, such as TNF and IL1β (Yaksh 2010).

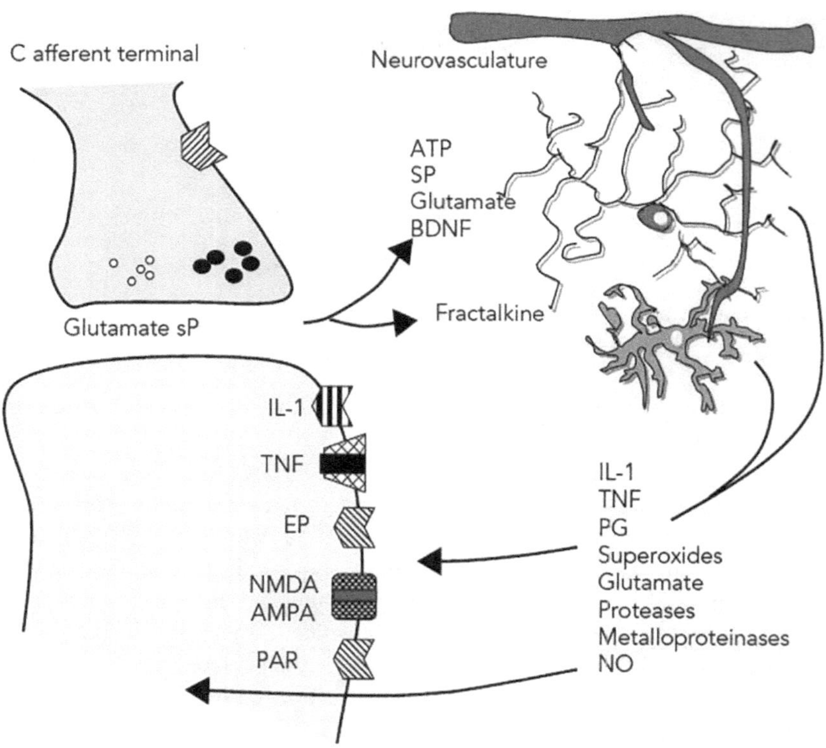

FIGURE 9.7 Nonneuronal cells, such as astrocytes and microglia, are activated by overflow from the synaptic cleft and through products in the cerebral vasculature. This activation leads to the secretion of inflammatory products that influence the excitability of neuronal transmission.

Source: Serhan, Ward, and Gilroy, *Fundamentals of Inflammation* (2010).

Similarly, microglia are activated by a variety of factors, such as membrane chemokine (fractalkine), which can act upon specific receptors on microglia (Yaksh 2010, 2020).

Nonneuronal cell activity is upregulated after peripheral injury and inflammation. The role of these cells is also supported by the use of spinal inhibitors of astrocytes (fluorocitrate) and microglia (minocycline and pentoxifylline). These agents have been shown to diminish hyperalgesic states by blocking the activation of astrocytes and microglia (Yaksh 2010, 2020; Milligan and Watkins 2009). After tissue injury, circulating cytokines can activate perivascular astrocytes and microglia to form parts of the blood–brain barrier. Therefore, these nonneuronal cells provide an avenue where circulating products can influence neuronal excitability.

9.9 ACUTE TO CHRONIC PAIN

Acute pain associated with tissue injury typically improves as a function of healing and resolution of the inflammation. There is an increased appreciation that a component of pain persists despite the resolution of the injury. This has been demonstrated in a variety of clinical conditions associated with post-surgical tissue trauma (Table 9.1) and chronic inflammatory changes. Studies performed using experimental pain models such as K/BxN and collagen antibody-induced arthritis (CAIA) have demonstrated that tactile allodynia persists long after resolution of visible swelling and inflammation (Polgár and Todd 2008; Lavand'homme 2017; Woller et al. 2017; Christianson et al. 2010; Gonçalves dos Santos et al. 2020; Yaksh 2020). This post-inflammatory phase tactile allodynia appears to involve phenotypically distinct mechanisms from acute inflammatory phase tactile allodynia. In the post-inflammatory phase, there is an increased expression of activating transcription factor 3 (ATF3) positive neurons in the DRG (Woller et al. 2017; Hunt, Raivich, and Anderson 2012). This marker is typically associated with satellite cell activation in

TABLE 9.1
Estimated Incidence of Chronic Post-Operative Pain after Surgical Procedures

Surgical Procedure	Estimated Incidence of Chronic Pain
Inguinal hernia repair	10%
Caesarean section	10%
Total knee replacement	15–20%
Breast surgery (lumpectomy and mastectomy)	20–30%
Thoracotomy	30–40%
Amputation	30–50%
Coronary artery bypass (sternotomy)	30–50%

Source: Adapted from Kehlet, Jensen, and Woolf (2006) and Lavand'homme and Thienpont (2015).

nerve injury and neuropathic pain. Moreover, in chronic inflammatory models, there is a sprouting of calcitonin gene–related peptide (CGRP), tyrosine hydroxylase (TH), and growth-associated protein (GAP 43) nerve fibers into the inflamed joint (Woller et al. 2017; Yaksh 2014; Jimenez-Andrade and Mantyh 2012). While CGRP reflects small afferent innervation, TH is associated with sympathetic post-ganglionic innervation (Woller et al. 2017). GAP 43 is a marker of axonal neurite formation and regeneration (Woller et al. 2017; Jimenez-Andrade and Mantyh 2012). The robust and inappropriate sprouting of afferents and post-ganglionic sympathetic fibers, along with the formation of neuroma-like structures, can lead to ectopic discharges. These observations suggest that the nociceptive processing underlying the chronic pain state reflects a neuropathic phenotype.

Additionally, studies have also demonstrated the role of the innate and adaptive immune systems in the development of chronic pain. The innate immune system detects damage and pathogens through toll-like receptors, such as TRL4, that are expressed in glia and primary afferent neurons (Woller et al. 2017; Yaksh and Luo 2011). TRL4 activation results in the release of pro-inflammatory cytokines, which evoke downstream events leading to increased synaptic transmission and nociceptive hypersensitivity. In mice models, the intrathecal administration of a TLR4 antagonist during the inflammatory phase showed no effect on inflammation but prevented the development of the persistent pain state (Yaksh, Ramachandran, and Woller 2020; Woller et al. 2017). This indicates that spinal TLR4 signaling plays a role in mediating the transition from acute to chronic pain.

The adaptive immune system also plays a role in the detection of invading pathogens and damage within the system through B and T cells. Chronic pain states have been linked to the activation of T-lymphocytes (Yaksh, Ramachandran, and Woller 2020). T cells have chemokine receptors involved in pain transmission and secrete a variety of pro-algesic cytokines (Yaksh, Ramachandran, and Woller 2020; Yaksh 2020). Animal models deficient in T cells showed less neuropathic after nerve injury (Yaksh, Ramachandran, and Woller 2020). There are also increasing studies on the role of antibodies in the induction of chronic pain states with chronic inflammation and nerve injury. This may also indicate a possible convergence between chronic inflammatory and neuropathic pain phenotypes.

9.10 CONCLUSION

Ongoing afferent traffic following tissue injury leads to a sensitization of the peripheral terminal, resulting in further generation of afferent input at the level of the dorsal horn, resulting in central sensitization, as exemplified by the windup phenomenon. This spinal facilitation, intricately mediated by complex facilitatory cascades involving local circuits, nonneuronal cells, and bulbospinal feedback loops, results in a series of events that change the way the system processes peripheral afferent input and the subsequent information. Although post–tissue injury pain mediated through acute spinal facilitation typically resolves with the resolution of the inflammation, pain may persist and transition into a chronic pain state. Many studies, as outlined earlier, have demonstrated that there is a convergence between chronic inflammatory and neuropathic pain states with signs of immune activation. It is important to understand the underlying mechanisms of pain processing and gain insight into the pharmacology and physiology of different aspects of the pain state to provide new tools for pain management.

REFERENCES

Christianson, Christina A., Maripat Corr, Gary S. Firestein, Anahita Mobargha, Tony L. Yaksh, and Camilla I. Svensson. 2010. Characterization of the Acute and Persistent Pain State Present in K/BxN Serum Transfer Arthritis. *Pain* 151 (2): 394–403. https://doi.org/10.1016/j.pain.2010.07.030.

Fisher, C.J., T.L. Yaksh, K. Bruno, and K.A. Eddinger. 2021. Basic Science of Pain. In *Pain Care Essentials and Innovations*, Ed S. Pangarkar, Q.G. Pham, and B.C. Eapen, 1-14. Elsevier. https://doi.org/10.1016/b978-0-323-72216-2.00001-6.

Gonçalves dos Santos, G., J.M. Jimenéz-Andrade, S.A. Woller, et al. 2020. The Neuropathic Phenotype of the K/BxN Transgenic Mouse with Spontaneous Arthritis: Pain, Nerve Sprouting and Joint Remodeling. *Scientific Reports* 10 (1). https://doi.org/10.1038/s41598-020-72441-5.

Hunt, D., G. Raivich, and P.N. Anderson. 2012. Activating Transcription Factor 3 (ATF3) and the Nervous System. *Frontiers in Molecular Neuroscience* 5 (7). https://doi.org/10.3389/fnmol.2012.00007.

Ishikawa, T., M. Marsala, T. Sakabe, and T.L. Yaksh. 1999. Characterization of spinal amino acid release and touch-evoked allodynia produced by spinal glycine or GABA receptor antagonist. *Neuroscience* 95 (3): 781–86

Jimenez-Andrade, J.M., and P.W. Mantyh. 2012. Sensory and Sympathetic Nerve Fibers Undergo Sprouting and Neuroma Formation in the Painful Arthritic Joint of Geriatric Mice. *Arthritis Research and Therapy* 14 (3). https://doi.org/10.1186/ar3826.

Jones, T.L., and L.S. Sorkin. 2005. Activated PKA and PKC, but Not CaMKIIα, Are Required for AMPA/Kainate-Mediated Pain Behavior in the Thermal Stimulus Model. *Pain* 117 (3): 259–70. https://doi.org/10.1016/j.pain.2005.06.003.

Kehlet, H., T.S. Jensen, C.J. Woolf. 2006. Persistent postsurgical pain: risk factors and prevention. *Lancet* 367: 1618–25.

Laird, J.M.A., V. Souslova, J.N. Wood, and F. Cervero. 2002. Deficits in Visceral Pain and Referred Hyperalgesia in Nav1.8 (SNS/PN3)-Null Mice. *Journal of Neuroscience* 22 (19): 8352–6. https://doi.org/10.1523/JNEUROSCI.22-19-08352.2002.

LaMotte, C.C. Organization of Dorsal Horn Neurotransmitter Systems. 1986. In *Spinal Afferent Processing,* Ed. T.L. Yaksh. 97–111. Springer Science+Business Media, LLC.

LaMotte, R.H., L.E.R Lundberg, and H.E. Torebjork. 1991. Pain, Hyperalgesia, and Activity in Nociceptive C Units in Humans After Intradermal Injection of Capsaicin. *Journal of Physiology* 448: 749–464.

Latremoliere, A. and C.J. Woolf. 2009. Central Sensitization: A Generator of Pain Hypersensitivity by Central Neural Plasticity. *Journal of Pain* 10(9): 895–926.

Lavand'homme, P. 2017. Transition from Acute to Chronic Pain after Surgery. *Pain* 158 (4): S50–54. https://doi.org/10.1097/j.pain.0000000000000809.

Lavand'homme, P. and E. Thienpont. 2015. Pain after Total Knee Arthroplasty. *The Bone and Joint Journal* 97-B (10): 45–48. https://doi.org/10.1302/0301–620X.97B10.

Li, J., D.A. Simone, and A.A. Larson. 1999. Windup Leads to Characteristics of Central Sensitization. *Pain* 79: 75–82.

Milligan, E.D. and L.R. Watkins. 2009. Pathological and Protective Roles of Glia in Chronic Pain. *Nature of Review Neuroscience* 10: 23–36.

Polgár, E., and A. J. Todd. 2008. Tactile Allodynia Can Occur in the Spared Nerve Injury Model in the Rat without Selective Loss of GABA or GABAA Receptors from Synapses in Laminae I-II of the Ipsilateral Spinal Dorsal Horn. *Neuroscience* 156 (1): 193–202. https://doi.org/10.1016/j.neuroscience.2008.07.009.

Sorkin, L.S., and M.S. Wallace. 1999. Acute Pain Mechanism. *Surgical Clinics of North America* 79 (2): 213–229.

Todd, A.J. 2010. Neuronal Circuitry for Pain Processing in the Dorsal Horn. *Nature Reviews Neuroscience* 11 (12): 823–36. https://doi.org/10.1038/nrn2947.

Westlund, K.N. 2006. The Dorsal Horn and Hyperalgesia. *Handbook of Clinical Neurology* 81: 103–215. doi:10.1016/S0072–9752(06)80013–8.

Willis, W.D. 2007. The Somatosensory System, With Emphasis on Structures Important for Pain. *Brain Research Reviews* 55: 297–313.

Witschi, R., P. Punnakkal, J.Paul, et al. 2011. Presynaptic A2-GABAA Receptors in Primary Afferent Depolarization and Spinal Pain Control. *Journal of Neuroscience* 31 (22): 8134–42. https://doi.org/10.1523/JNEUROSCI.6328–10.2011.

Woller, S.A., K.A. Eddinger, M. Corr, and T.L. Yaksh. 2017. An Overview of Pathways Encoding Nociception. *Clinical Experimental Rheumatology* 35: 40–46.

Yaksh, T.L. 1989. Behavioral and Autonomic Correlates of The Tactile Evoked Allodynia Produced by Spinal Glycine Inhibition: Effects of Modulatory Receptor Systems and Excitatory Amino Acid Antagonists. *Pain* 37: 111–23.

Yaksh, T.L. 2010. Mediators and Mechanisms of Inflammatory Pain. In *Fundamentals of Inflammation,* Ed. C.N. Serhan, P.A. Ward, and D.W. Gilroy, 217–233.

Yaksh, T.L. 2020. Biology of Pain Processing. Presentation at the University of California, San Diego.

Yaksh, T.L. and Z.D. Luo. 2011. Anatomy of the pain processing system. In *Pain Management,* Ed. S.D. Waldman. 2nd Edition. Elsevier, Philadelphia, PA.

Yaksh, T.L., R. Ramachandran, S.A. Woller. 2020. Molecular Biology of Pain. In *Principles and Practice of Pain Medicine,* Ed. Z.H. Bajwa, R.J. Wootton, and C.A. Warfield. 3rd edition. Chapter 1. McGraw Hill.

10 Post–Nerve Injury Pain States
Primary Afferent

Jasmin Villatoro-Lopez, Rany T. Abdallah, and Jennifer Tram

10.1 INTRODUCTION

Silas Weir-Mitchell (February 15, 1829–January 4, 1914) was an American neurologist and writer who was responsible for the discovery of causalgia (known as complex regional pain syndrome, or CRPS, today) and erythromelalgia (Mitchell, Morehouse, and Keen 2007). During the Civil War, Silas Weir-Mitchell discovered and treated causalgia while at Turners Lane Hospital, Philadelphia. In his book *Gunshot Wounds and Other Injuries of Nerves*, Weir-Mitchell describes the various symptoms associated with these kinds of injuries, including pain described as "mustard red-hot" or as a "red-hot file rasping the skin," known today as burning dysesthesia (Mitchell, Morehouse, and Keen 2007). Weir-Mitchell established that injury to the nerve would lead to complicated and debilitating states.

Peripheral nerve injury can occur due to a variety of events that lead to neuropathic pain states. If the injury impacts one nerve (i.e., a nerve transection, compression-carpal tunnel, or secondary to unilateral radiation), it is referred to as *mononeuropathy*. On the other hand, if the injury impacts all nerves (i.e., chemotherapy, diabetes, or immune disorders), it is referred to as *polyneuropathies* and may often be reflected in the distal extremities (Hanewinckel, Ikram, and Van Doorn 2016).

In the 1860s, Weir-Mitchell recognized that frequent components of this syndrome are (1) ongoing incidences of sharp, shooting sensations at the peripheral distribution of the injured nerve and (2) abnormal, painful sensations in response to light tactile stimulation of the peripheral body surface (*tactile allodynia*) (Mitchell, Morehouse, and Keen 2007).

10.2 EVENTS AFTER NERVE INJURY

After an acute focal injury of the peripheral afferent axon, there is an initial dying back, known as retrograde chromatolysis, that proceeds for some time, at which point the axon begins to sprout, sending growth cones forward. These growth cones will often fail to contact the original target and will display significant proliferation, which will then form what is known as neuromas (Stoll, Jander, and Myers 2002). Some of the barriers to recovery of the continuity between the proximal and distal sides of injury

DOI: 10.1201/9781003094302-10

are that the connections can be blocked by local debris and by the fact that the initial connections that were made in the embryo spanned a distance of less than a millimeter, while in the adult, the distances of the regenerating nerve could span up to a meter.

Peripheral axon injury induces substantial alterations in the dorsal root ganglion (DRG), despite the DRG itself remaining structurally intact. These alterations begin with the activation of immediate early genes. This is followed by an increase in the proliferation of activation transcription factor 3, or ATF3, as well as an increase in the activation of satellite cells (GFAP) (Chen and Sommer 2007; Znaor et al. 2007). Finally, there is a significant alteration in the DRG neuron protein expression in terms of receptors, channels, and enzymes (Baranowski, Priestley, and McMahon 1993) (Noguchi et al. 1990) (Cizkova et al. 2002).

In summary, in the early hours to days following nerve injury, acute axonal degeneration occurs. Fragmentation of axons and activation of Schwann cells are noticed as well. Moreover, a large release of growth factors and inflammatory mediators at the injury site, the dissociation of axonal Schwann cells, and Schwann cell proliferation happen. In the later phases, macrophage infiltration, myelin debris clearance, and growth cone formation occur (collections of sprouting axon terminals).

10.3 ORIGIN OF ONGOING DYSESTHESIA

Studies have revealed that in contrast to a normal afferent axon, an injured axon will display the development of ongoing afferent traffic. In normal conditions, primary afferent axons will show minimal to no spontaneous activity. However, following an acute injury, afferent axons display an initial burst of afferent firing following the injury, then silence for an interval of hours to days. Over time, this is then followed by the development of a measurable level of spontaneous afferent traffic in the axons (myelinated and unmyelinated) (Saade and Jabbur 2008). Thus, it is believed that this provides the source of the afferent activity, which leads to spontaneous ongoing sensation.

There is evidence that supports the claim that ectopic activity is partly responsible for the observed pain behavior. First, there is a parallel time course between the onset of ectopic activity in the neuroma/dorsal root ganglia (DRG) and the pain behavior. Second, the pain behavior can be blocked by the application of tetrodotoxin (TTX) or local anesthetics to the neuroma/DRG (Lyu et al. 2000). Third, a dorsal rhizotomy will reverse the pain behavior for a short term. Lastly, irritants applied to the DRG will initiate activity and yield pain behavior.

10.4 ORIGIN OF THE ECTOPIC AFFERENT ACTIVITY

There are two ways in which ectopic afferent activity occurs. One is from the neuroma, where terminal depolarization occurs and leads to orthodromic activity back to the spinal cord. The other is from the DRG, where cell bodies undergo depolarization after nerve injury. This input travels from the soma, down the glomerulus, to the main axon, which then generates an action potential in both directions (outside and to the spinal cord) (Burchiel 1984) (Devor, Wall, and Catalan 1992) (Kajander, Wakisaka, and Bennett 1992) (Han, Lee, and Chung 2000) (Abdulla and Smith 2001).

There are a few relative systems: (1) the afferent axon, which goes back and forth; (2) the glomerulus, which is the trafficking point between the cell body and the main axon; and (3) the afferent cell body itself (soma), which is surrounded by glial fibrillary acidic, protein-positive cells that invest in the DRG. Moreover, there is an increase in the activation of satellite cells and macrophages. Because the DRG lies outside the blood–brain barrier, it has a vasculature that is similar to the vasculature in the muscle. A peripheral vasculature is sympathetically innervated; thus, post-ganglionic sympathetic axons (which release norepinephrine, epinephrine, etc.) innervate those peripheral vessels. We then see post-ganglion sympathetic axons innervating the DRG, which can have a direct effect on satellite cells, macrophages, and the soma of the DRG.

We understand that the DRG can be a source of ectopic activity and can be complicated in terms of the type of information that they can process. Thus, it is not shocking to see the activation of toll receptors in the DRG by HSP, tenascin C, and other molecules that can be released from macrophages. There are also a variety of growth factor receptors activated by local products that are released: Satellite cells release BDNF, which can directly activate neurons (Yang et al. 2022). Schwann cells release a basic myelin protein at the local injury site, which initiates pain behavior through the generation of ectopic activity and sensory axons. Finally, the adrenergic input from post-ganglionic sympathetic innervating the DRG may also draw activity in the primary afferent.

10.5 DRG TRANSDUCTION

Two principal intrinsic cell types are within the DRG: DRG neurons and DRG *satellite cells* (SC). The satellite cells closely adhere to DRG neurons and often look like the thickening of the DRG cell wall (Konnova et al., 2023). There is evidence that SC and DRG cells may communicate with each other through GAP junctions, which allow the transfer of intracellular content from one cell to another (Spray et al., 2019) (Konnova et al., 2023). It is also known that SC and DRG cells may communicate with each other by the release of transmitters, such as cytokines, chemokines, purine, and a variety of lipids, that activate the DRG. Along with that, the DRG has significant sympathetic innervation that travels with the DRG vasculature. This means that the post-ganglionic sympathetic will often invest in the DRG neurons and enhance their excitability.

Inflammatory cells migrate into the DRG following nerve injury (Yu et al. 2020). DRG macrophage activation significantly increases staining intensity under microscopy. However, we see minimal macrophage movement from the outside of the DRG and only see an increase in activation, not in numbers. When this occurs, a variety of excitatory products are released.

10.6 SODIUM CHANNELS AND NERVE INJURY

After nerve injury, there is a significant increase in ectopic activity from the DRG, a significant portion of which may be related to the activation and increasing sensitivity of the injured axon (Suzuki and Dickenson, 2000). It was found that after nerve injury, DRG protein expression of sodium channels and calcium channels is significantly elevated, while potassium channels are reduced in expression. This phenomenon is referred to as "neonatal phenotype" and results in an instability of the DRG at the axon.

It was thought early on that this change in sodium channels was a possible source of the ongoing ectopic activity. However, in 1993, Marshal Devore demonstrated that when looking at the distribution of sodium channel binding by saxotoxin (a toxin that binds specifically to sodium channels), the ligated nerve was observed to express sodium channels in the sprouting neuroma in the area around the injury site itself. This suggests that increased sodium channel expression may occur after peripheral nerve injury (Devor et al. 1989). Along with this, it was observed that a block of sodium channels can alter the firing of these peripheral terminals (Devor, Wall, and Catalan 1992) (Chabal, Russell, and Burchiel 1989).

There are nine major classes of sodium channels, NaV1.1–NaV1.9 (differentially distributed in tissues). These are distributed in the DRG, CNS, muscle channels, cardiac channels, and some in small DRG. Each channel has a differential role in pain processing. For example, NaV1.7 was found to have its genetic manifestation in humans encoded in the SCN9A gene (Dormer et al. 2023). Individuals were found to have reduced sensitivity to pain or tissue-injuring stimuli, while others had severe episodic pain and erythromelalgia (Dormer et al., 2023). Both are associated with a significant increase in the functionality of NaV1.7 genes.

10.7 ORIGIN OF TACTILE ALLODYNIA

Tactile allodynia is a signal amplification by central sensitization which renders input arriving in the spinal cord along low-threshold mechanoreceptive Aβ fibers to produce pain behavior (Campbell et al. 1988; Torebjork, Lundberg, and LaMotte 1992). What causes Aβ afferent axons to initiate a "pain" message? This could be due to multiple reasons: (1) linkages between low- and high-threshold afferents, (2) increased dorsal horn excitability, (3) altered inhibitory control, (4) reorganization of dorsal horn connectivity, or (5) activation of nonneuronal cells (Devor and Wall 1990; Woolf, Shortland, and Coggeshall 1992; Wilson and Kitchener 1996; Suzuki and Dickenson 2000; Catheline et al. 1999).

After nerve injury, there is evidence that suggests that "cross-talk" between afferents in the DRG and the neuroma develops. This occurs when a depolarizing current in one axon generates depolarizing currents in an adjacent inactive axon (Fried, Govrin-Lippmann, and Devor 1993). The depolarization would allow the activity rising in one axon to drive the activity on the second axon. It is because of this that it is hypothesized that a large low-threshold axon can activate an adjacent high-threshold axon (Devor and Wall 1990). On the other hand, the DRG cells may release excitatory transmitters and have the respective receptors.

Many small interneurons that contain and release GABA and glycine are found in the spinal dorsal horn (Todd and Sullivan 1990; Todd 1996). GABA/glycinergic terminals are mostly pre-synaptic to the large central afferent terminal complexes and form reciprocal synapses (Carlton and Hayes 1990). Amino acids normally exert important evoked inhibitory control over the activity of Aβ primary afferent terminals and second-order neurons on the spinal dorsal horn (Rudomin 2002). This is relevant because it provides an observation that the simple intrathecal delivery of $GABA_A$ receptor or glycine receptor antagonists will lead to a strongly defined tactile allodynia (Yaksh 1989; Zhang, Hefferan, and Loomis 2001). This observation leads to the consideration that after nerve injury, there may be a loss of GABAergic neurons, albeit a minimal loss (Polgar et al. 2003; Ibuki et al. 1997).

An alternative observation that has recently arisen is that following nerve injury, spinal neurons regress to a neonatal phenotype where $GABA_A$ activation becomes excitatory (Ben-Ari 2002; Rudomin and Schmidt 1999). This effect is secondary to reduced activity of the membrane Cl^- transporter, which then changes the reversal current for the Cl^- conductance. The increasing membrane Cl^- conductance results in membrane depolarization, while under normal conditions, transmembrane (Cl^-) are at equilibrium. Increasing Cl permeability by $GABA_A$ or glycine-r yields hyperpolarization and inhibition.

In the neuronal tissues, cation–chloride cotransporters regulate Cl^- homeostasis, and the activity/expression of said transporters has an important implication for the direction/magnitude of anion flow through $GABA_A$ channels (Price, Cervero, and de Koninck 2005). The targeting of these cation–chloride cotransporters to restore normal GABA1/glycinergic transmission in the spinal cord represents an entirely new approach to the development of analgesics.

10.8 CONCLUSION

In conclusion, nerve injury is an ongoing afferent activity and is a result of neuroma/DRG activity (ectopic activity). This ectopic activity arises from the inflammatory milieu of the terminal proliferation of Schwann cells and invasion of macrophages and neutrophils into the nerve injury site. There is also a significant increase in channel (NaV) expression and a decrease in potassium channels to enhance the excitability of the sensory axon. Sympathetic sprouting into the DRG can contribute to the increased drive in pain states. Finally, Aβ cross-talk in the neuroma and into the DRG, which may lead to activation of small afferents that signal pain inflammation.

REFERENCES

Abdulla, F. A., and P. A. Smith. 2001. "Axotomy- and autotomy-induced changes in Ca2+ and K+ channel currents of rat dorsal root ganglion neurons." *J Neurophysiol* 85 (2):644–58. doi: 10.1152/jn.2001.85.2.644.

Baranowski, A. P., J. V. Priestley, and S. McMahon. 1993. "Substance P in cutaneous primary sensory neurons—a comparison of models of nerve injury that allow varying degrees of regeneration." *Neuroscience* 55 (4):1025–36. doi: 10.1016/0306–4522(93)90316–8.

Ben-Ari, Y. 2002. "Excitatory actions of GABA during development: the nature of the nurture." *Nat Rev Neurosci* 3 (9):728–39. doi: 10.1038/nrn920.

Burchiel, K. J. 1984. "Spontaneous impulse generation in normal and denervated dorsal root ganglia: sensitivity to alpha-adrenergic stimulation and hypoxia." *Exp Neurol* 85 (2):257–72. doi: 10.1016/0014–4886(84)90139–0.

Campbell, J. N., S. N. Raja, R. A. Meyer, and S. E. Mackinnon. 1988. "Myelinated afferents signal the hyperalgesia associated with nerve injury." *Pain* 32 (1):89–94. doi: 10.1016/0304–3959(88)90027–9.

Carlton, S. M., and E. S. Hayes. 1990. "Light microscopic and ultrastructural analysis of GABA-immunoreactive profiles in the monkey spinal cord." *J Comp Neurol* 300 (2):162–82. doi: 10.1002/cne.903000203.

Catheline, G., S. Le Guen, P. Honore, and J. M. Besson. 1999. "Are there long-term changes in the basal or evoked Fos expression in the dorsal horn of the spinal cord of the mononeuropathic rat?" *Pain* 80 (1–2):347–57. doi: 10.1016/s0304–3959(98)00234–6.

Chabal, C., L. C. Russell, and K. J. Burchiel. 1989. "The effect of intravenous lidocaine, tocainide, and mexiletine on spontaneously active fibers originating in rat sciatic neuromas." *Pain* 38 (3):333–8. doi: 10.1016/0304–3959(89)90220–0.

Chen, Y., and C. Sommer. 2007. "Activation of the nociceptin opioid system in rat sensory neurons produces antinociceptive effects in inflammatory pain: involvement of inflammatory mediators." *J Neurosci Res* 85 (7):1478–88. doi: 10.1002/jnr.21272.

Cizkova, D., J. Marsala, N. Lukacova, M. Marsala, S. Jergova, J. Orendacova, and T. L. Yaksh. 2002. "Localization of N-type Ca2+ channels in the rat spinal cord following chronic constrictive nerve injury." *Exp Brain Res* 147 (4):456–63. doi: 10.1007/s00221-002-1217-3.

Devor, M., C. H. Keller, T. J. Deerinck, S. R. Levinson, and M. H. Ellisman. 1989. "Na^+ channel accumulation on axolemma of afferent endings in nerve end neuromas in Apteronotus." *Neurosci Lett* 102 (2–3):149–54. doi: 10.1016/0304–3940(89)90070–0.

Devor, M., and P. D. Wall. 1990. "Cross-excitation in dorsal root ganglia of nerve-injured and intact rats." *J Neurophysiol* 64 (6):1733–46. doi: 10.1152/jn.1990.64.6.1733.

Devor, M., P. D. Wall, and N. Catalan. 1992. "Systemic lidocaine silences ectopic neuroma and DRG discharge without blocking nerve conduction." *Pain* 48 (2):261–8. doi: 10.1016/0304–3959(92)90067-L.

Dormer, A., M. Narayanan, J. Schentag, D. Achinko, E. Norman, J. Kerrigan, G. Jay, and W. Heydorn. 2023. "A Review of the Therapeutic Targeting of SCN9A and Nav1.7 for Pain Relief in Current Human Clinical Trials." *J Pain Res* 16:1487–98. doi: 10.2147/JPR.S388896.

Fried, K., R. Govrin-Lippmann, and M. Devor. 1993. "Close apposition among neighboring axonal endings in a neuroma." *J Neurocytol* 22 (8):663–81. doi: 10.1007/BF01181491.

Han, H. C., D. H. Lee, and J. M. Chung. 2000. "Characteristics of ectopic discharges in a rat neuropathic pain model." *Pain* 84 (2–3):253–61. doi: 10.1016/s0304–3959(99)00219–5.

Hanewinckel, R., M. A. Ikram, and P. A. Van Doorn. 2016. "Peripheral neuropathies." *Handb Clin Neurol* 138:263–82. doi: 10.1016/B978-0-12-802973-2.00015-X.

Ibuki, T., A. T. Hama, X. T. Wang, G. D. Pappas, and J. Sagen. 1997. "Loss of GABA-immunoreactivity in the spinal dorsal horn of rats with peripheral nerve injury and promotion of recovery by adrenal medullary grafts." *Neuroscience* 76 (3):845–58. doi: 10.1016/s0306–4522(96)00341–7.

Kajander, K. C., S. Wakisaka, and G. J. Bennett. 1992. "Spontaneous discharge originates in the dorsal root ganglion at the onset of a painful peripheral neuropathy in the rat." *Neurosci Lett* 138 (2):225–8. doi: 10.1016/0304–3940(92)90920–3.

Konnova, E. A., A. F. Deftu, P. Chu Sin Chung, M. Pertin, G. Kirschmann, I. Decosterd, and M. R. Suter. 2023. "Characterisation of GFAP-Expressing Glial Cells in the Dorsal Root Ganglion after Spared Nerve Injury." *Int J Mol Sci* 24 (21). doi: 10.3390/ijms242115559.

Lyu, Y. S., S. K. Park, K. Chung, and J. M. Chung. 2000. "Low dose of tetrodotoxin reduces neuropathic pain behaviors in an animal model." *Brain Res* 871 (1):98–103. doi: 10.1016/s0006–8993(00)02451–3.

Mitchell, S. W., G. R. Morehouse, and W. W. Keen. 2007. "Gunshot wounds and other injuries of nerves. 1864." *Clin Orthop Relat Res* 458:35–9. doi: 10.1097/BLO.0b013e31803df02c.

Noguchi, K., E. Senba, Y. Morita, M. Sato, and M. Tohyama. 1990. "Alpha-CGRP and beta-CGRP mRNAs are differentially regulated in the rat spinal cord and dorsal root ganglion." *Brain Res Mol Brain Res* 7 (4):299–304. doi: 10.1016/0169–328x (90)90080-w.

Polgar, E., D. I. Hughes, J. S. Riddell, D. J. Maxwell, Z. Puskar, and A. J. Todd. 2003. "Selective loss of spinal GABAergic or glycinergic neurons is not necessary for development of thermal hyperalgesia in the chronic constriction injury model of neuropathic pain." *Pain* 104 (1–2):229–39. doi: 10.1016/s0304–3959(03)00011–3.

Price, T. J., F. Cervero, and Y. de Koninck. 2005. "Role of cation-chloride-cotransporters (CCC) in pain and hyperalgesia." *Curr Top Med Chem* 5 (6):547–55. doi: 10.2174/1568026054367629.

Rudomin, P. 2002. "Selectivity of the central control of sensory information in the mammalian spinal cord." *Adv Exp Med Biol* 508:157–70. doi: 10.1007/978-1-4615-0713-0_19.

Rudomin, P., and R. F. Schmidt. 1999. "Presynaptic inhibition in the vertebrate spinal cord revisited." *Exp Brain Res* 129 (1):1–37. doi: 10.1007/s002210050933.

Saade, N. E., and S. J. Jabbur. 2008. "Nociceptive behavior in animal models for peripheral neuropathy: spinal and supraspinal mechanisms." *Prog Neurobiol* 86 (1):22–47. doi: 10.1016/j.pneurobio.2008.06.002.

Spray, D. C., R. Iglesias, N. Shraer, S. O. Suadicani, V. Belzer, R. Hanstein, and M. Hanani. 2019. "Gap junction mediated signaling between satellite glia and neurons in trigeminal ganglia." *Glia* 67 (5):791–801. doi: 10.1002/glia.23554.

Stoll, G., S. Jander, and R. R. Myers. 2002. "Degeneration and regeneration of the peripheral nervous system: from Augustus Waller's observations to neuroinflammation." *J Peripher Nerv Syst* 7 (1):13–27. doi: 10.1046/j.1529–8027.2002.02002. x.

Suzuki, R., and A. H. Dickenson. 2000. "Neuropathic pain: nerves bursting with excitement." *Neuroreport* 11 (12): R17–21. doi: 10.1097/00001756-200008210-00001.

Todd, A. J. 1996. "GABA and glycine in synaptic glomeruli of the rat spinal dorsal horn." *Eur J Neurosci* 8 (12):2492–8. doi: 10.1111/j.1460–9568. 1996.tb01543.x.

Todd, A. J., and A. C. Sullivan. 1990. "Light microscope study of the coexistence of GABA-like and glycine-like immunoreactivities in the spinal cord of the rat." *J Comp Neurol* 296 (3):496–505. doi: 10.1002/cne.902960312.

Torebjork, H. E., L. E. Lundberg, and R. H. LaMotte. 1992. "Central changes in processing of mechanoreceptive input in capsaicin-induced secondary hyperalgesia in humans." *J Physiol* 448:765–80. doi: 10.1113/jphysiol.992.sp019069.

Wilson, P., and P. D. Kitchener. 1996. "Plasticity of cutaneous primary afferent projections to the spinal dorsal horn." *Prog Neurobiol* 48 (2):105–29. doi: 10.1016/0301–0082(95)00040–2.

Woolf, C. J., P. Shortland, and R. E. Coggeshall. 1992. "Peripheral nerve injury triggers central sprouting of myelinated afferents." *Nature* 355 (6355):75–8. doi: 10.1038/355075a0.

Yaksh, T. L. 1989. "Behavioral and autonomic correlates of the tactile evoked allodynia produced by spinal glycine inhibition: effects of modulatory receptor systems and excitatory amino acid antagonists." *Pain* 37 (1):111–23. doi: 10.1016/0304–3959(89)90160–7.

Yang, J. X., H. F. Wang, J. Z. Chen, H. Y. Li, J. C. Hu, A. A. Yu, J. J. Wen, S. J. Chen, W. D. Lai, S. Wang, Y. Jin, and J. Yu. 2022. "Potential Neuroimmune Interaction in Chronic Pain: A Review on Immune Cells in Peripheral and Central Sensitization." *Front Pain Res (Lausanne)* 3:946846. doi: 10.3389/fpain.2022.946846.

Yu, X., H. Liu, K. A. Hamel, M. G. Morvan, S. Yu, J. Leff, Z. Guan, J. M. Braz, and A. I. Basbaum. 2020. "Dorsal root ganglion macrophages contribute to both the initiation and persistence of neuropathic pain." *Nat Commun* 11 (1):264. doi: 10.1038/s41467-019-13839-2.

Zhang, Z., M. P. Hefferan, and C. W. Loomis. 2001. "Topical bicuculline to the rat spinal cord induces highly localized allodynia that is mediated by spinal prostaglandins." *Pain* 92 (3):351–61. doi: 10.1016/S0304–3959(01)00276–7.

Znaor, L., S. Lovric, Q. Hogan, and D. Sapunar. 2007. "Association of neural inflammation with hyperalgesia following spinal nerve ligation." *Croat Med J* 48 (1):35–42.

11 Post–Nerve Injury Pain States
Spinal Cord

Jasmin Villatoro-Lopez, Rany T. Abdallah, and Jennifer Tram

11.1 INTRODUCTION

In the early nineties, it was believed that after nerve injury, *sprouting* occurred. Since sprouting does occur in the peripheral nerve, this led to the belief that this could also occur within the central nervous system. However, this hypothesis was refuted.

After peripheral nerve injury, an increase in innervation of the peripheral neuroma by post-ganglionic sympathetic terminals is seen (Ramer et al. 1998). In more recent studies, however, it has been observed that there is an ingrowth of post-ganglionic sympathetic terminals into the dorsal root ganglion (DRG) of the injured axons (Chung et al. 1996).

This innervation involves all sizes of ganglion cells, particularly type A (large ganglion cells). It occurs mainly in the DRG, ipsilateral to the lesion. However, there is also an innervation of the contralateral ganglion cell (Chen et al. 1996). The stimulation of the ventral roots which contain the pre-ganglionic efferent neurons will produce activity in the sensory axon by an interaction at the peripheral terminal at the site of the injury or by an interaction at the level of the DRG.

11.2 "SYMPATHETICS" IN NEUROPATHIC PAIN

Rene Leriche (1879–1955) worked on *causalgia* and phantom limbs in the early thirties. Leriche's work suggested the importance of vasomotor changes and was able to show alleviation of nerve injury pain through periarterial sympathectomy, in which he would use lidocaine and novocaine injections into sympathetic ganglia, which would reduce the pain state due to a block of sympathetic input from the injured nerve.

11.3 ASTROCYTES AND MICROGLIA FOLLOWING NERVE INJURY

Nerve injury leads to a persistent appearance on the ipsilateral dorsal horn of active spinal astrocytes and microglia (Ma and Quirion 2002). These glia secrete a variety of products that can sensitize dorsal horn function, and nerve injury–induced sensory neuropathies as well. Many treatments leading to hyperpathic states yield similar changes in the axon, DRG, and dorsal horn protein expression.

11.4 TISSUE INJURY: EVOLUTION OF PERSISTENT PAIN STATE

Tissue injury pain will normally improve as a function of "healing" and resolution of inflammation. However, in some instances, the inflammatory/injury state may

 DOI: 10.1201/9781003094302-11

resolve but the pain persists. Individuals with chronic inflammatory conditions can experience intense pain that will persist even after remission of inflammatory signs. At this point, the pain is pathologic, maladaptive, and debilitating. Why does this occur? Is there something else that occurs secondary to significant and persistent inflammation/tissue injury?

Despite the persistent inflammation conditions, there could be an evolution of a neuropathic phenotype with signs of immune activation. This has been experimentally demonstrated in an antibody-generated murine models of joint inflammation, such as K/BxN and collagen antibody-induced arthritis (CAIA) (Christianson et al. 2010). Even after the resolution of inflammation, it was observed that tactile allodynia was persistent (Kim and Moalem-Taylor 2011). In the periphery, robust sprouting of small sensory (CFRP) and sympathetic nerve fibers in the joint, along with the formation of neuroma-like structures, was observed after inflammation (Jimenez-Andrade and Mantyh 2012); in the DRG, an increased expression of activating transcription factor 3 (ATF3) was observed (Kim and Moalem-Taylor 2011); while in the dorsal horn, activation of astrocytes and microglia was observed, along with increased expression of many pro-algogenic enzymes and channels (Kim and Moalem-Taylor 2011).

It should be noted that in the early stages, anti-inflammatory agents and anti-hyperalgesic (gabapentin) would reverse the allodynia; however, during the later stages, only gabapentin was effective (Christianson et al. 2010). This resembles a neuropathic phenotype.

11.5 CONCLUSION

In summary, after peripheral nerve injury, an increase in innervation of the peripheral neuroma by post-ganglionic sympathetic terminal is observed. More so, an ingrowth of post-ganglionic sympathetic terminals into the dorsal root ganglion (DRG) of the injured axons is seen (Chung et al. 1996). The stimulation of the ventral roots containing the pre-ganglionic efferents produces activity in the sensory axon by an interaction at the peripheral terminal at the site of the injury or by an interaction at the level of the DRG (Chen et al. 1996). It was also found that the alleviation of nerve injury pain through periarterial sympathectomy was found by blocking the sympathetic input from the injured nerve.

In terms of tissue injury, individuals with chronic inflammatory conditions can continue to experience persistent intense pain even after remission of inflammatory signs. Research, however, has noted that anti-inflammatory agents and anti-hyperalgesic (gabapentin) can reverse the allodynia, resembling a neuropathic phenotype (Christianson et al. 2010).

REFERENCES

Chen, Y., M. Michaelis, W. Janig, and M. Devor. 1996. "Adrenoreceptor subtype mediating sympathetic-sensory coupling in injured sensory neurons." *J Neurophysiol* 76 (6):3721–30. doi: 10.1152/jn.1996.76.6.3721.

Christianson, C. A., M. Corr, G. S. Firestein, A. Mobargha, T. L. Yaksh, and C. I. Svensson. 2010. "Characterization of the acute and persistent pain state present in K/BxN serum transfer arthritis." *Pain* 151 (2):394–403. doi: 10.1016/j.pain.2010.07.030.

Chung, K., B. H. Lee, Y. W. Yoon, and J. M. Chung. 1996. "Sympathetic sprouting in the dorsal root ganglia of the injured peripheral nerve in a rat neuropathic pain model." *J Comp Neurol* 376 (2):241–52. doi: 10.1002/(SICI)1096-9861(19961209)376:2<241::AID-CNE6>3.0.CO;2-3.

Jimenez-Andrade, J. M., and P. W. Mantyh. 2012. "Sensory and sympathetic nerve fibers undergo sprouting and neuroma formation in the painful arthritic joint of geriatric mice." *Arthritis Res Ther* 14 (3):R101. doi: 10.1186/ar3826.

Kim, C. F., and G. Moalem-Taylor. 2011. "Detailed characterization of neuro-immune responses following neuropathic injury in mice." *Brain Res* 1405:95–108. doi: 10.1016/j.brainres.2011.06.022.

Ma, W., and R. Quirion. 2002. "Partial sciatic nerve ligation induces an increase in the phosphorylation of extracellular signal-regulated kinase (ERK) and c-Jun N-terminal kinase (JNK) in astrocytes in the lumbar spinal dorsal horn and the gracile nucleus." *Pain* 99 (1–2):175–84. doi: 10.1016/s0304-3959(02)00097-0.

Ramer, M. S., P. G. Murphy, P. M. Richardson, and M. A. Bisby. 1998. "Spinal nerve lesion-induced mechanoallodynia and adrenergic sprouting in sensory ganglia are attenuated in interleukin-6 knockout mice." *Pain* 78 (2):115–21. doi: 10.1016/S0304-3959(98)00121-3.

12 Visceral Pain System/ Neuro-Immune Interaction

Laura Case

12.1 INTRODUCTION: ORIGINS OF VISCERAL SENSATION

Visceral sensations originate from sensory afferents in the organs of the thoracic and abdominal cavities, including blood vessels and connective tissues. As seen in Figure 12.1, these organs include the heart, lung, great vessels, lower airway, esophagus, stomach, gallbladder, small bowel, liver, spleen, pancreas, kidney, colon, rectum, uterus, prostate, bladder, anus, and genitalia. While these structures are all believed to be capable of producing painful sensations, the vast majority of this afferent information never reaches the level of conscious perception.

Despite their lower sensory innervation density, the viscera can transmit intense pain. Visceral pain is one of the most common types of pain caused by disease and one of the most frequent reasons patients seek medical care. Yet visceral pain has received little research compared with somatic pain, based on an outdated assumption that visceral pain is simply a variant of somatic pain. Though visceral pain and somatic pain have much in common, we now recognize many important differences between them, as well as the critical role that visceral sensation plays in the transmission of pain.

12.2 VISCERAL INNERVATION

Visceral innervation differs in several important ways from somatic innervation. The viscera have significantly fewer afferents than the skin, comprising only about 5% of the number of somatic afferents [1]. In addition, the viscera contain very few Aβ afferents [2, 3] and are predominantly innervated by slow-conducting unmyelinated C fibers and thinly myelinated Aδ fibers. Another distinguishing characteristic of visceral innervation is that visceral afferents are polymodal, responding to mechanical, chemical, and thermal stimuli.

Visceral information is transmitted by somatic afferent fibers, sympathetic afferents from the spine, and parasympathetic afferents from the vagus nerve (cranial nerve X) and pelvic nerves. As seen in Figure 12.1, each visceral structure receives dual innervation from at least two distinct nerve supplies, the sympathetic and parasympathetic. These are named based on their efferent (outgoing) functions, but they also contain afferent fibers that relay distinct types of information, including pain,

DOI: 10.1201/9781003094302-12

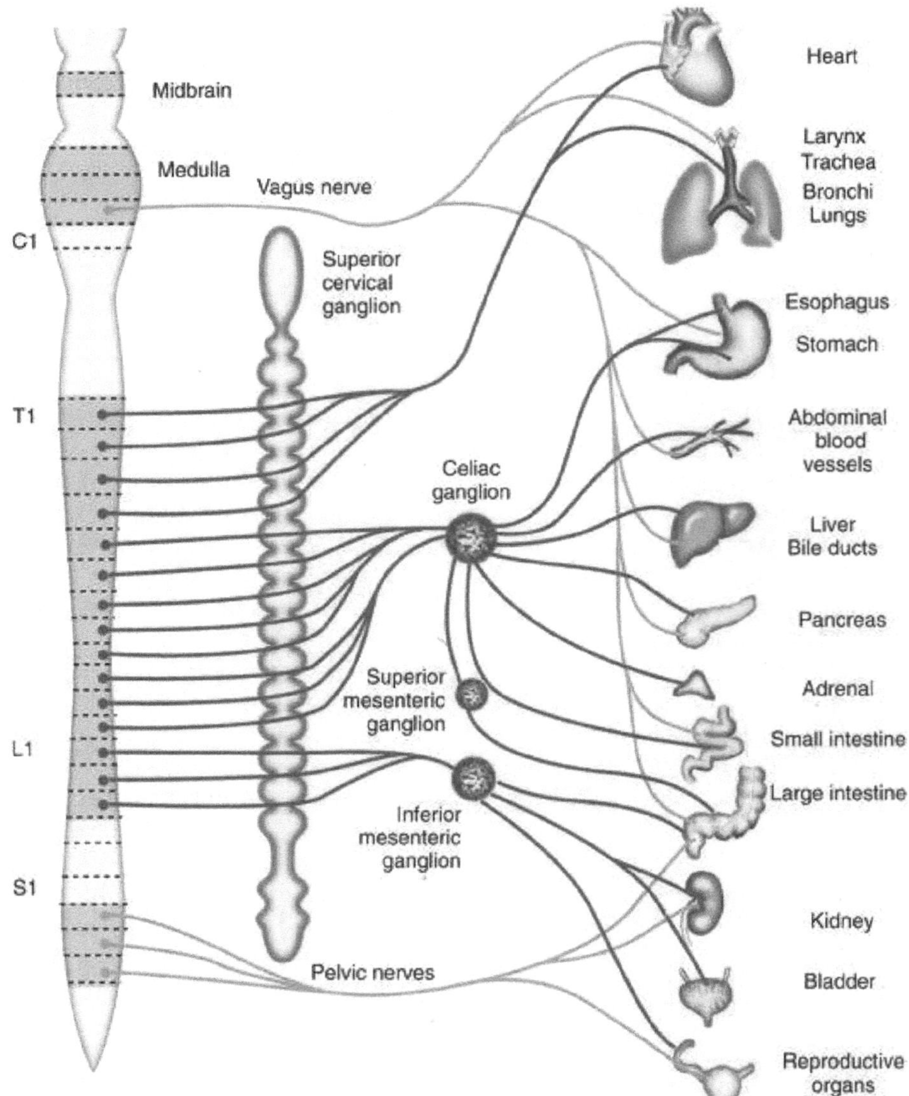

FIGURE 12.1 Dual innervation of visceral organs by the sympathetic nervous system and parasympathetic nervous system.

Source: https://www.us.elsevierhealth.com/sleisenger-and-fordtrans-gastrointestinal-and-liver-disease-review-and-assessment-9780323636599.html

to the central nervous system. Thoracic and upper abdominal viscera are predominantly innervated by the vagus nerve and spinal sympathetic nerves. In contrast, the lower abdominal viscera, including intestines and urogenital organs, are innervated by spinal sympathetic and sacral nerves.

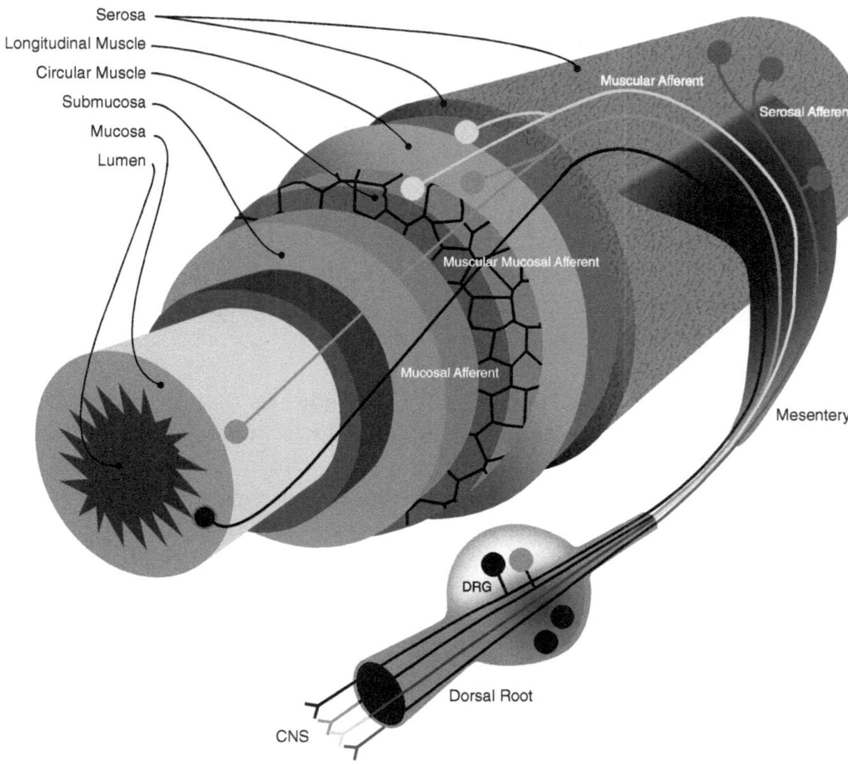

FIGURE 12.2 Visceral sensations originate from sensory afferents in the organs of the thoracic and abdominal cavities, and blood vessels and connective tissues, including mesentery, organ capsules, and lining of the peritoneal cavity.

Source: https://www.ncbi.nlm.nih.gov/pmc/articles/PMC2732716/.

Solid visceral organs, like the pancreas, liver, lung, and spleen, have minimal sensory innervation [4], leading to injuries and damage often going unnoticed, as seen in conditions like liver cirrhosis [5]. Instead, most visceral pain originates from hollow visceral organs, elicited by strong contraction, stretch, tension, or ischemia of the walls of the organ [6]. As pictured in Figure 12.2, in hollow organs such as the GI tract, all tissue layers receive innervation from distinct types of sensory afferent fibers. For example, the mucosa, muscle, and serosa layers of the gastrointestinal tract are innervated by different populations of sensory afferents that respond to distinct types of mechanical stimuli, such as mechanical stroking or stretch.

In the past, researchers debated whether the viscera were innervated by separate classes of sensory receptors for autonomic regulation versus sensation, or whether a single class of receptors signaled regulatory information at low levels of stimulation and pain at high levels of stimulation. It is now understood that there are two categories of receptors, one encoding low-threshold stimuli that span the natural stimulus range from innocuous to noxious, and another with a high threshold, responding mostly to mechanical stimuli and transmitting pain. This first class is comprised of the **parasympathetic afferents**, which produce intensity-encoded responses throughout the physiologic stimulus range, exhibiting characteristics of a wide dynamic range (WDR) response. These afferents are believed to transmit pain under normal conditions. Intensity-encoding receptors have been demonstrated in the heart, esophagus, colon, urinary bladder, and testes [7, 8]. In contrast, the second class is comprised of the **sympathetic afferents,** which in the viscera, are specific for high-intensity stimuli and are believed to maintain pain under pathologic conditions. High-threshold receptors have been identified in the heart, vein, lung and airways, esophagus, biliary system, small intestine, colon, ureter, urinary bladder, and uterus [7, 8].

Figure 12.3, which follows, shows data from a study examining the mechanosensitivity of visceral afferents to the colon. Parasympathetic afferents exhibited greater sensitivity to graded intensities of stretch stimuli, whereas sympathetic afferents responded only to high-intensity stimuli. These differences have led to the hypothesis that parasympathetic afferents likely relay sensory information under normal conditions, while sympathetic afferents play a role in pain transmission, particularly in pathologic conditions.

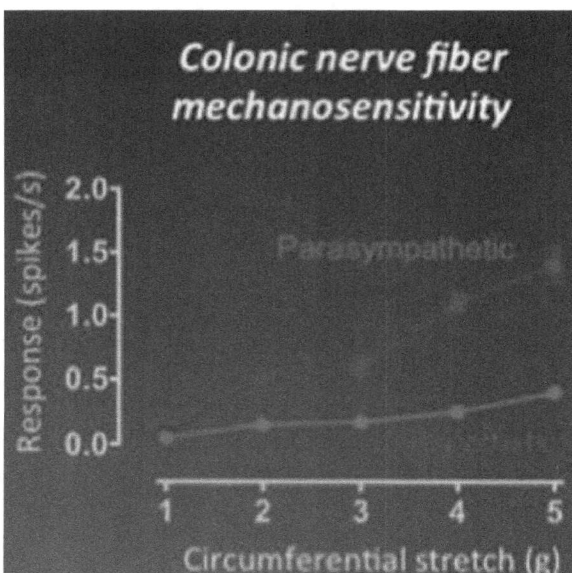

FIGURE 12.3 Colonic nerve fiber mechanosensitivity. Parasympathetic afferents were much more sensitive to different intensities of a stretch stimulus (1–5 g) applied to their receptive fields, whereas sympathetic afferents responded only to high-intensity stimuli.

Source: Adapted from Brierly et al., *Gastroenterol* 127:166.

12.3 CENTRAL PROJECTIONS AND CONVERGENCE

Visceral information is encoded by neurons in the dorsal horn of the spinal cord in laminae V, VI, and X. Visceral afferents exhibit a unique feature of extensive arborization of afferents in their central projections. In contrast to sensory afferents from the skin, which enter the spinal cord, ascend a few spinal levels, and form a discrete synapse, Figure 12.4 will show that afferents ascend and descend the cord at multiple levels and form multiple synapses with second-order neurons. This unique organization contributes to the diffuse nature of visceral sensations and poor spatial discriminability of visceral pain.

Another unique feature of visceral innervation is the phenomenon of **cross-organ sensitization** between visceral organs. For example, Figure 12.5b illustrates visceral–visceral convergence between the bladder and the colon. Convergence occurs in the dorsal root ganglion (DRG) as well as in the laminar structures throughout the spinal cord; when afferents from distinct organs project to a single spinal neuron, activity in one organ may stimulate the distal organ. An additional, unique feature of visceral innervation pictured in Figure 12.5a is the occurrence of direct organ-to-organ transmission of action potentials that bypass the spinal cord. This is due to the branching of afferent fibers to multiple organs, such as the colon and the bladder (also called "axonal dichotomy"). Convergence further contributes to the highly diffuse nature of visceral pain perception.

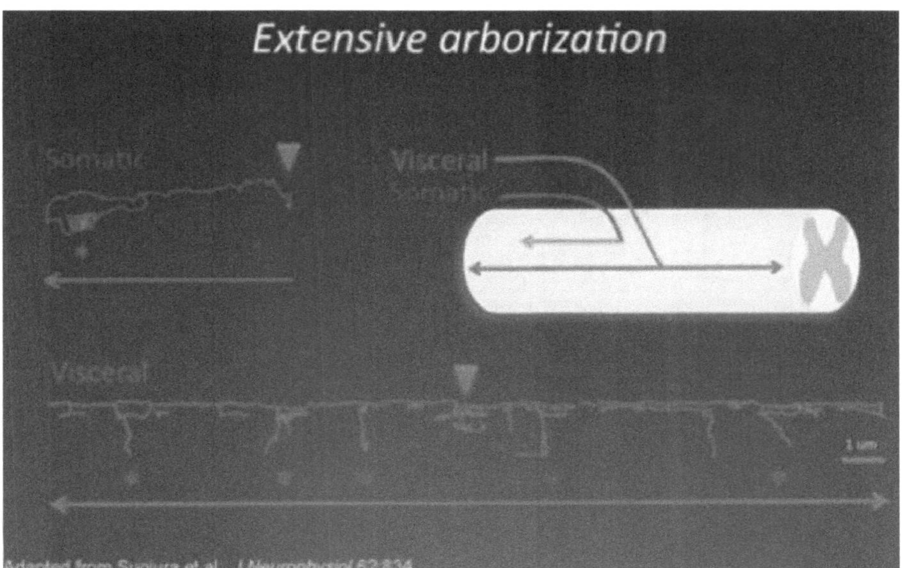

FIGURE 12.4 Visceral afferents exhibit extensive arborization in the spinal cord, contributing to poor spatial discriminability and referred pain sensations.

Source: Adapted from Sugiura et al., *J Neurophysiol* 315–325 [9].

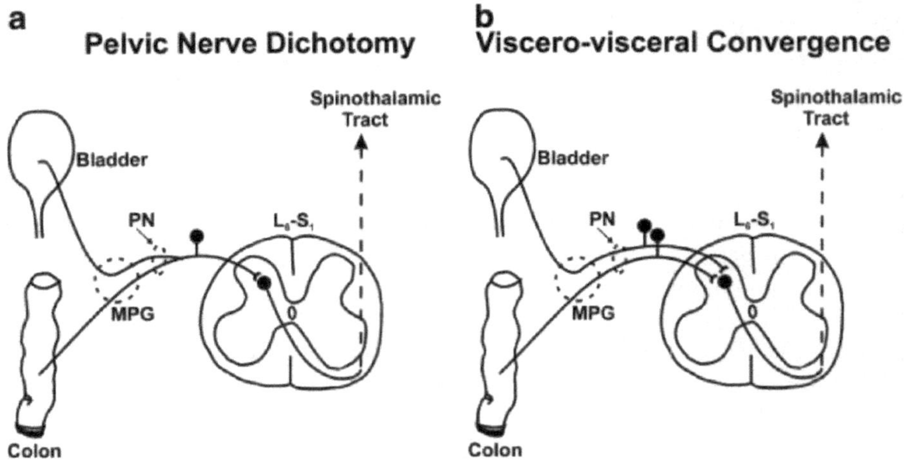

FIGURE 12.5 Cross-organ convergence and branching [10].

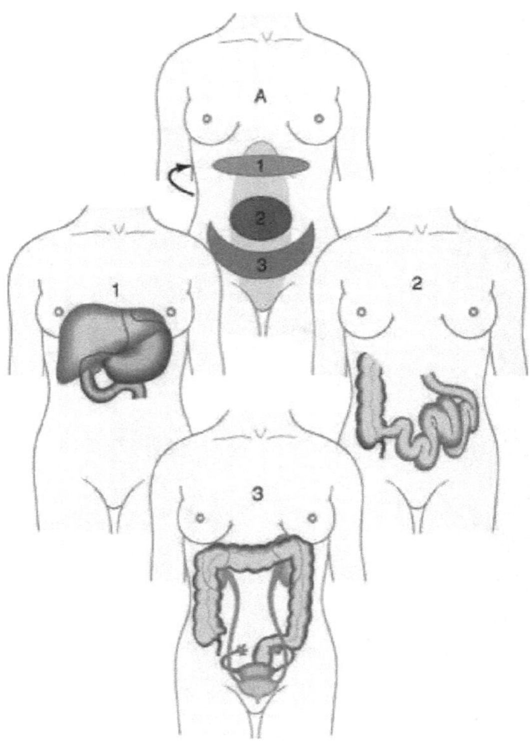

FIGURE 12.6 Localization of visceral pain. Pain arising from organ areas depicted in 1, 2, 3 is felt in the epigastrium, midabdomen, and hypogastrium, respectively as shown in A. The arrow in A indicates biliary pain that is referred to the right scapular area.

Source: https://www.us.elsevierhealth.com/sleisenger-and-fordtrans-gastrointestinal-and-liver-disease-review-and-assessment-9780323636599.html

One of the most unique features of visceral pain is **referred pain**, a phenomenon depicted in Figure 12.6, wherein visceral pain is perceived in distant skin and muscle of the same spinal segments. An early explanation for referred pain was MacKenzie's 1909 "convergence-facilitation" theory, which postulated that nociceptive activity could induce an "irritable focus" in the spinal cord (referenced in [11]), activating somatic afferents in the same spinal segment. This explanation foreshadows the concept of central sensitization and explains the lingering effect of hyperalgesia after referred pain but does not explain the immediate nature of referred sensations.

A contemporary explanation for the cutaneous referral pattern of visceral pain is the convergence of primary sensory afferent neurons from the skin and viscera onto individual second-order neurons in the dorsal horn of the spinal cord. If the second-order neuron is responsible for relaying sensations to the brain stem and brain, stimulation of our organs can be sensed as emanating from not just the organ itself but also areas of the skin that converge onto those same second-order neurons. Pain referral also occurs between visceral organs. For example, about 35% of patients with chronic pelvic pain improve substantially when treated for functional bowel disorders, suggesting referral of colorectal pain to the pelvis [12].

12.4 SENSITIZATION OF VISCERAL AFFERENTS

Peripheral neurons innervating the viscera can be sensitized by thermal and chemical stimuli. When a visceral organ is inflamed, reflex responses are initiated, leading to changes in blood flow and muscle contraction. An additional insult on top of the first elicits **visceral afferent sensitization** that produces a greater response than if not sensitized. Figure 12.7 shows data from a study demonstrating the sensitization of afferent fibers in the stomach by application of acid to experimentally induce ulcers in rats, as would occur in human patients with stomach ulcers and gastric acid secretion sensitization [13]. Acute gastric thermal and chemical stimuli sensitized mechanosensitive gastric vagal afferents. Notably, this exposure also activated the afferents, causing increases in spontaneous activity.

A minority of visceral afferents, dubbed "**silent afferents**," are unresponsive to mechanical stimuli until inflammation occurs [3, 14]. Afferent activity unmasked by inflammation may contribute to central sensitization, such as in maintained excitation of central neurons after inflammation of the bladder [15]. Many visceral pain models exhibit inflammation-driven hyperalgesia.

Due to the previously discussed principle of convergence, visceral sensitization can also induce somatic sensitization. Laird and colleagues injected capsaicin into the colon of a mouse, evoking visceral C fiber activity [16]. As seen in Figure 12.8, repeated touch to the abdomen, hind paw, and tail revealed an agitation response, demonstrating the convergence of visceral to somatic sensitization. Similarly, in patients with irritable bowel syndrome (IBS), the referred pain of bowel distention is increased by colonic distention (see Figure 12.9) [17]. Pain referral was not localized to the site of distention and was instead referred to larger segments of the abdominal cavity, demonstrating increases in pain referral in patients with chronic pain. IBS patients also experience pain referral to a greater number of abdominal and lower thoracic locations [18].

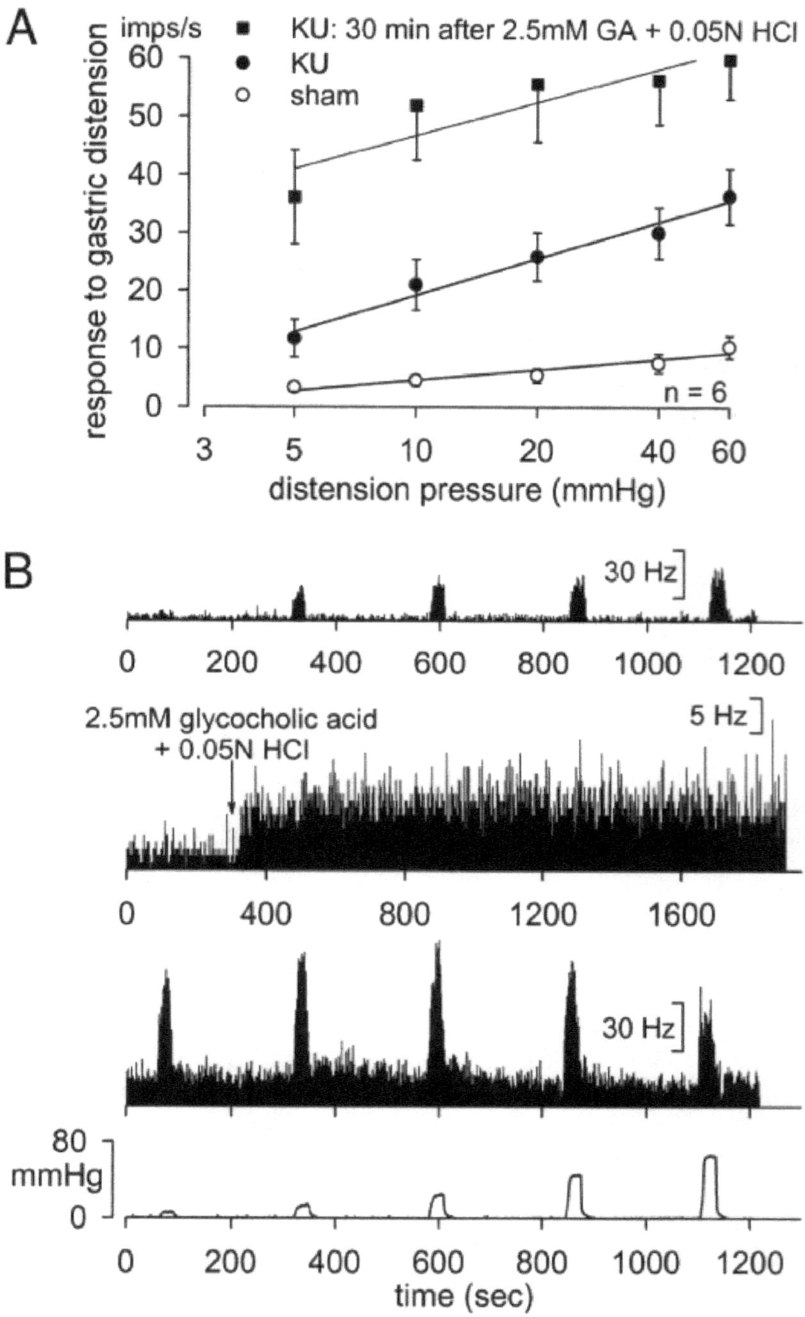

FIGURE 12.7 Cutaneous referral pattern of visceral pain.

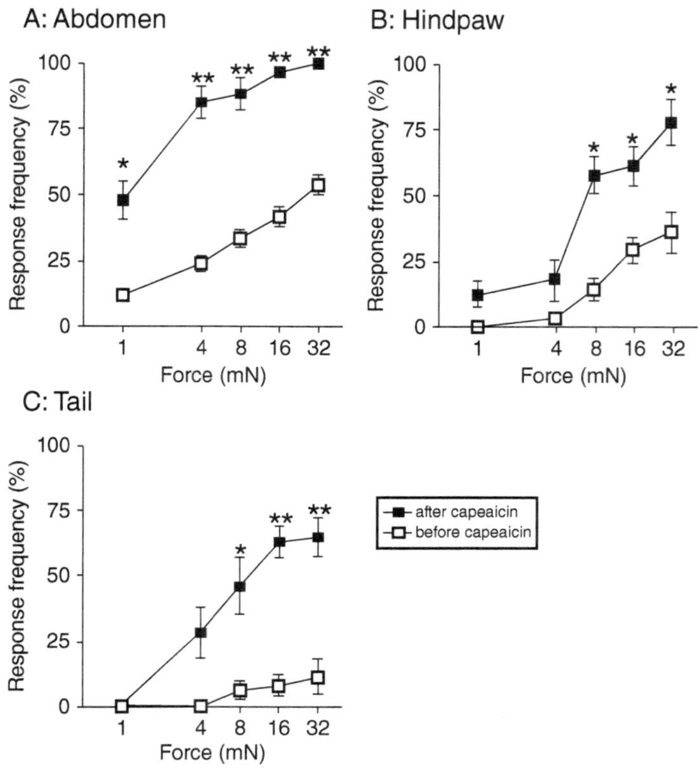

FIGURE 12.8 (a) Afferent fiber response to distension of the stomach at different pressures (5–60 mmHg). The stimulus response function is shifted to the left in rats after induction of ulcers, and then leftward again when acid is applied to animals with ulcers. (b) Traces from representative afferent vagal nerve fibers and action potentials generated by distension alone (*top*), application of acid (*middle*), and response to distension after acid application (*bottom*).

Source: Kang et al. (2004).

Convergence of visceral and somatic sensitization. Laird et al. injected capsaicin into the colon, evoking visceral C fiber input. Repeated touch stimuli applied to areas of the body surface revealed an enhanced response to somatic stimuli applied to various body surfaces [16].

12.5 CENTRAL PATHWAYS FOR VISCERAL PAIN

From the spinal cord, visceral sensory information travels to the brain stem and cerebral cortex primarily via the spinothalamic tract, as with cutaneous nociceptive sensory pathways. Pain signals are also conveyed by the spinoreticular pathway, dorsal column pathway, spino(trigeminal)-parabrachial-amygdaloid pathway, and spinohypothalamic pathway; the contributions of these pathways to the perception of visceral pain are an active area of research. An additional pathway for visceral pain is afferent

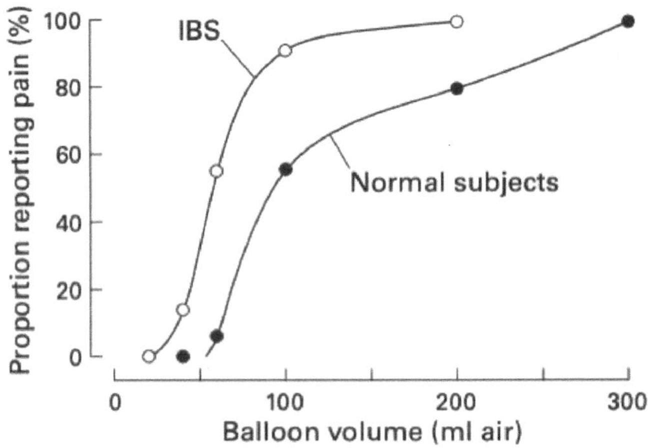

FIGURE 12.9 Patients with chronic abdominal pain from irritable bowel syndrome (IBS) experience pain at lower volumes of colonic balloon distention than healthy participants. This shift in the psychophysical function demonstrates hyperalgesia in IBS.

Source: [17].

parasympathetic information traveling through the vagus nerve, which travels to the nucleus tractus solitarius (NTS) in the brain stem, then crosses the midline and joins the spinothalamic tract to the thalamus. However, some nociceptive signals are also transmitted in a post-synaptic dorsal column pathway. In particular, visceral pain signals originating from cell bodies in lamina X ascend the dorsal columns to the dorsal column nuclei and onto the ventral posterolateral (VPL) nucleus of the thalamus [19].

The dorsal column–medial lemniscal pathway was traditionally believed to contain low-threshold primary afferent A fibers that, when stimulated, released GABA—and potentially other neurotransmitters—into the spinal cord. This organization was the foundation for applying transcutaneous electrical nerve stimulation (TENS) to the dorsal column, which reduces acute pain perception [20]; indeed, GABA has been found to mediate the effects of TENS in rats [21]. However, it is now also understood that stimulation of the dorsal column also activates ascending A delta and C fiber pathways that recruit the brain's descending pain modulation system [20]. TENS has demonstrated some ability to decrease visceral pain, including post-operative pain after uterine tube ligation [22], rectal hypersensitivity [23], and uterine contractions during labor [24], but its clinical efficacy remains debated [25, 26].

Visceral pain processing in the brain has been investigated using several methods, including gastric and rectal distention. A recent meta-analysis of fMRI studies compared visceral and somatic pain and identified high overlap in distributed brain areas specific to pain perception. One difference observed was the relatively higher activation of the somatomotor network for cutaneous pain versus the frontoparietal network for visceral (rectal) pain [27]. Additional research is needed to determine the significance of this difference.

12.6 PSYCHOPHYSICS/PERCEPTION OF VISCERAL PAIN

As previously discussed, visceral pain is diffuse and difficult to localize and is frequently referred to other visceral and/or cutaneous locations. Visceral pain is not evoked from all viscera and is not always caused by visceral injury. For example, cutting the intestines causes no pain, while a stretch of the bladder evokes pain in the absence of injury. Visceral afferents are therefore not always considered "sensory" [2]. Visceral pain is also different in the quality of sensation, with visceral pain more likely to elicit dull and cramping sensations in response to muscle contraction, distention, or chemical processes, while cutaneous pain is sharp, in response to mechanical, thermal, or chemical triggers (see Table 12.1).

Another distinguishing difference between visceral and somatic stimuli is the lack of withdrawal reflex to visceral stimuli that is ubiquitous for cutaneous pain [4]. Visceral stimuli may instead provoke motor and autonomic reflexes, such as sweating, nausea, hunched posture, or vomiting, though these responses typically onset at a delay. These reactions may serve as the visceral equivalent of protective reflexes, warning the sufferer to rest [2]. Visceral pain is also characterized by heightened emotional responses due to the strong involvement of the autonomic nervous system in detecting visceral pain [28].

Visceral pain sensation exhibits spatial summation; pain threshold and perceived intensity are determined by the area of tissue stimulated. A strong but localized pain stimulus will not reach the threshold necessary for pain transmission and perception. This contrasts with cutaneous stimuli, for which changes in the size of the area stimulated have little effect on perception [1].

In the viscera, repeated noxious stimulation increases the excitability of viscerosomatic neurons in the spinal cord [29]. However, in contrast to the somatic pain

TABLE 12.1
Comparison of Features of Visceral and Somatic Pain

Feature	Visceral	Somatic
Effective stimuli	Ischemia Contraction Distention Chemical	Noxious mechanical Noxious thermal Noxious chemical
Character	Dull Cramping	Sharp
Autonomic symptoms	Frequent	Rare
Localization	Poor	Good
Referral of pain	Yes	No
Spatial summation	Yes	Minimal
Windup	No	Yes

Source: Adapted from [32].

system, these spinal nociceptive neurons do not exhibit **windup**—the term used in somatic pain for frequency-dependent increases in excitability [30]. Instead, their excitability may be induced by neuronal networks activated by the stimuli or the release of certain transmitters. Strong positive feedback loops between spinal and supraspinal structures which are prominent on visceral nociceptive neurons [31] may underlie the heightened motor and autonomic reflexes triggered by visceral pain. In addition, afferent discharges after injury or inflammation may be stronger and longer-lasting than discharges provoked by acute injury, potentially enhancing these central effects. The post-synaptic activity of neurotransmitters released by noxious stimuli may also contribute to the increased excitability of visceral pain pathways after prolonged stimulation [2]. Cumulatively, these changes can make visceral pain persist long after an initial injury is sustained.

12.7 BIOCHEMISTRY OF VISCERAL PAIN

In contrast to somatic afferents, visceral afferents are peptidergic, expressing calcitonin gene–related peptide (CGRP), NF200, and TRPV1 [33]. As with somatic afferents, these peptidergic visceral afferents terminate in laminae I and V of the spinal cord. Visceral afferents display pro- and antinociceptive ion channels and receptors that determine afferent sensitivity, which can be strongly altered by inflammation [33]. Most visceral afferents are of the nerve growth factor (NGF)–dependent peptidergic class [32, 34]. NGF is implicated in inflammatory responses leading to pain [35–37]. Administration of NGF can upregulate and sensitize bladder afferents and recruit the involvement of silent afferents [38]. Tachykinins, ATP, and the tetrodotoxin-resistant sodium channel Na(v)1.8 have also been implicated in visceral hyperalgesia and inflammation-induced activation of visceral afferents [32].

Piezo2 is a mechanically activated ion channel that transduces mechanosensation in various populations of sensory neurons [39, 40]. A growing body of studies has begun to also implicate Piezo2 in visceral sensation. In the skin, Piezo2 has generally been associated with myelinated A fiber sensory functions [41]. However, Piezo2 has been implicated in several visceral sensory functions, including sensory neurons that sense airway stretch [42], colorectal mechanotransduction and mechano-nociception [43], and bladder stretch and micturition reflexes [44]. In rats, it may play a role in visceral sensation [45]. Expression of Piezo2 in the colon correlates with visceral sensitivity, making Piezo2 a potential marker for visceral hypersensitivity in IBS [45]. Piezo proteins also appear to play an important role in endothelial pain [46].

12.8 VISCERAL HYPERSENSITIVITY AND NEURO-IMMUNE INTERACTION

Visceral hypersensitivity can be caused at multiple levels, including sensitization of primary visceral afferents, central sensitization of spinal neurons, and changes in descending pain modulatory pathways [10]. For example, early life stress or trauma can lead to chronic pain via dysregulation of the hypothalamic–pituitary–adrenal axis, and inflammatory conditions can alter the descending opioidergic pain system, resulting in heightened pain perception [10].

Leaky gut, characterized by the disruption of the barrier between luminal contents and the underlying interstitium, increases intestinal epithelial permeability, allowing luminal substances to directly interact with underlying tissues. This exposure heightens afferent pain signaling, intensifying nociceptive input. Inflammatory responses, driven by the infiltration of immune cells and the release of pro-inflammatory mediators, further activate sensory afferents, amplifying pain perception. Persistent visceral inflammation induces long-term neuroplastic changes in both peripheral and central pain processing pathways. Dysregulated immune signaling and the release of pro-inflammatory cytokines contribute to the pathophysiology of IBS [33]. Neurogenic inflammation, driven by efferent nerve activation and immune cell infiltration, plays a key role in maintaining visceral hypersensitivity. Additionally, stress-mediated alterations in gut–brain and bladder–brain axis communication exacerbate pain sensitivity and immune dysregulation [33]. Local immune responses to food antigens further perpetuate mucosal inflammation, reinforcing the cycle of pain, immune activation, and visceral dysfunction [47].

Epithelial cells also play a recently discovered role in visceral afferent activation. For example, activation of colon epithelial cells can initiate the firing of colon afferents and pain responses. Given common alterations in the colon epithelium in inflammatory bowel disease and irritable bowel disorders, epithelial changes may play a significant role in visceral pain in these conditions [48].

12.9 CONCLUSION

Visceral pain feels different than cutaneous pain, and its unique mechanisms reflect this difference. Visceral pain is internal, originating from sympathetic and parasympathetic afferents innervating the thoracic and abdominal organs. These afferents are predominantly peptidergic, polymodal A delta and C fibers. Visceral pain is difficult to localize due to the extensive arborization and convergence of visceral afferents. Visceral nociception is conveyed primarily by the spinothalamic tract and vagus nerve and invokes different responses than cutaneous pain. Thermal and chemical stimuli can also sensitize visceral afferents and can induce somatic sensitization. Finally, visceral afferents are strongly altered by inflammation and can be hypersensitized by peripheral or central sensitization or changes in descending pain modulatory pathways. This may explain the frequent co-occurrence of psychological and visceral symptoms. Recurring visceral inflammation can lead to long-term plastic changes in the nervous system, an active area of ongoing research.

REFERENCES

1. McMahon, S.B., *Are there fundamental differences in the peripheral mechanisms of visceral and somatic pain*? Behavioral and Brain Sciences, 1997. **20**(3): p. 381–391.
2. Cervero, F. and J.M. Laird, *Visceral pain*. The Lancet, 1999. **353**(9170): p. 2145–2148.
3. Sengupta, J. and G. Gebhart, *Mechanosensitive properties of pelvic nerve afferent fibers innervating the urinary bladder of the rat*. Journal of Neurophysiology, 1994. **72**(5): p. 2420–2430.
4. Cervero, F. and J.M. Laird, *Understanding the signaling and transmission of visceral nociceptive events*. Journal of Neurobiology, 2004. **61**(1): p. 45–54.

5. Marotta, P.J., I.W. Graziadei, and C.N. Ghent, *Muscle Cramps: A 'Complication 'of Cirrhosis.* Canadian Journal of Gastroenterology, 2000. **14**(Suppl D): p. 21D-25D.
6. Miranda, A., *Abdominal pain*, in *Nelson Pediatric Symptom-Based Diagnosis*. 2018, Elsevier. p. 161–181. e2.
7. Cervero, F., *Visceral nociceptors*, in *Neurobiology of nociceptors.*, B.C.C. F, Editor. 1996, Oxford University Press: Oxford. p. 220–40.
8. JN, G.G.S., *On visceral nociceptors*, in *Peripheral neurons in nociception: physiopharmacological aspects*, G.G. Besson JM, & Ollat H, Editor. 1994, John Libbey Eurotext: Paris. p. 23–37.
9. Sugiura, Y., et al., *Quantitative Analysis of Central Terminal Projections of Visceral and Somatic Unmyelinated (C) Primary Afferent Fibers in the Guinea Pig*. The Journal of Comparative Neurology, 1993. 332: p. 315–325. https://doi.org/10.1002/cne.903320305.
10. Sengupta, J.N., *Visceral pain: the neurophysiological mechanism.* Sensory Nerves, 2009: p. 31–74.
11. McMahon, S., N. Dmitrieva, and M. Koltzenburg, *Visceral pain.* British journal of anaesthesia, 1995. **75**(2): p. 132–144.
12. Williams, R.E., et al., *Recognition and treatment of irritable bowel syndrome among women with chronic pelvic pain.* American journal of obstetrics and gynecology, 2005. **192**(3): p. 761–767.
13. Kang, Y.-M., K. Bielefeldt, and G. Gebhart, *Sensitization of mechanosensitive gastric vagal afferent fibers in the rat by thermal and chemical stimuli and gastric ulcers.* Journal of Neurophysiology, 2004. **91**(5): pp. 1981–1989.
14. Koltzenburg, M. and S. McMahon, *Mechanically insensitive primary afferents supplying the bladder.* 1995, Visceral pain. Seattle: IASP Press.
15. Coderre, T.J., et al., *Contribution of central neuroplasticity to pathological pain: review of clinical and experimental evidence.* Pain, 1993. **52**(3): p. 259–285.
16. Laird, J., et al., *A new model of visceral pain and referred hyperalgesia in the mouse.* PAIN®, 2001. **92**(3): p. 335–342.
17. Ritchie, J., *Pain from distension of the pelvic colon by inflating a balloon in the irritable colon syndrome.* Gut, 1973. **14**(2): p. 125–132.
18. Mayer, E.A. and G.F. Gebhart, *Basic and clinical aspects of visceral hyperalgesia.* Gastroenterology, 1994. **107**(1): p. 271–293.
19. Al-Chaer, E.D., et al., *Visceral nociceptive input into the ventral posterolateral nucleus of the thalamus: a new function for the dorsal column pathway.* Journal of Neurophysiology, 1996. **76**(4): p. 2661–2674.
20. Sluka, K.A., and D. Walsh, *Transcutaneous electrical nerve stimulation: basic science mechanisms and clinical effectiveness.* The Journal of Pain, 2003. **4**(3): p. 109–121.
21. Maeda, Y., et al., *Release of GABA and activation of GABAA in the spinal cord mediates the effects of TENS in rats.* Brain research, 2007. **1136**: p. 43–50.
22. DeSantana, J.M., K.A. Sluka, and G.R. Lauretti, *High and low-frequency TENS reduce postoperative pain intensity after laparoscopic tubal ligation: a randomized controlled trial.* The Clinical journal of pain, 2009. **25**(1): p. 12–19.
23. Xiao, W.-B. and Y.-L. Liu, *Rectal hypersensitivity reduced by acupoint TENS in patients with diarrhea-predominant irritable bowel syndrome: a pilot study.* Digestive diseases and sciences, 2004. **49**(2): p. 312–319.
24. Chao, A.-S., et al., *Pain relief by applying transcutaneous electrical nerve stimulation (TENS) on acupuncture points during the first stage of labor: a randomized double-blind placebo-controlled trial.* Pain, 2007. **127**(3): p. 214–220.
25. Bergeron-Vézina, K., et al., *High-and low-frequency transcutaneous electrical nerve stimulation does not reduce experimental pain in elderly individuals.* Pain, 2015. **156**(10): p. 2093.
26. Rakel, B.A., et al., *Transcutaneous electrical nerve stimulation for the control of pain during rehabilitation after total knee arthroplasty: a randomized, blinded, placebo-controlled trial.* PAIN®, 2014. **155**(12): p. 2599–2611.

27. Van Oudenhove, L., et al., *Common and distinct neural representations of aversive somatic and visceral stimulation in healthy individuals.* Nature Communications, 2020. **11**(1): p. 1–11.
28. Cueva, J.G., A. Mulholland, and M.B. Goodman, *Nanoscale organization of the MEC-4 DEG/ENaC sensory mechanotransduction channel in Caenorhabditis elegans touch receptor neurons.* Journal of Neuroscience, 2007. **27**(51): p. 14089–14098.
29. Roza, C., J.M. Laird, and F. Cervero, *Spinal mechanisms underlying persistent pain and referred hyperalgesia in rats with an experimental ureteric stone.* Journal of Neurophysiology, 1998. **79**(4): p. 1603–1612.
30. Laird, J., P.G. De La Rubia, and F. Cervero, *Excitability changes of somatic and viscero-somatic nociceptive reflexes in the decerebrate-spinal rabbit: role of NMDA receptors.* The Journal of Physiology, 1995. **489**(2): p. 545–555.
31. Tattersall, J., F. Cervero, and B. Lumb, *Viscerosomatic neurons in the lower thoracic spinal cord of the cat: excitations and inhibitions evoked by splanchnic and somatic nerve volleys and by stimulation of brain stem nuclei.* Journal of Neurophysiology, 1986. **56**(5): p. 1411–1423.
32. Farquhar-Smith, W.P. and S. Jaggar, *Visceral pain mechanisms*, in *Urogenital pain in clinical practice.* 2008, Informa Healthcare Inc New York. p. 61–69.
33. Grundy, L., A. Erickson, and S.M. Brierley, *Visceral pain.* Annual review of physiology, 2019.
34. Bennett, D.L., et al., *trkA, CGRP and IB4 expression in retrogradely labeled cutaneous and visceral primary sensory neurons in the rat.* Neuroscience letters, 1996. **206**(1): p. 33–36.
35. McMahon, S.B., *NGF as a mediator of inflammatory pain.* Philosophical Transactions of the Royal Society of London. Series B: Biological Sciences, 1996. **351**(1338): p. 431–440.
36. Lewin, G.R., A. Rueff, and L.M. Mendell, *Peripheral and central mechanisms of NGF-induced hyperalgesia.* European Journal of Neuroscience, 1994. **6**(12): p. 1903–1912.
37. Levi-Montalcini, R., et al., *Nerve growth factor: from neurotrophin to neurokinin.* Trends in neurosciences, 1996. **19**(11): p. 514–520.
38. Dmitrieva, N., et al., *The role of nerve growth factor in a model of visceral inflammation.* Neuroscience, 1997. **78**(2): p. 449–459.
39. Ranade, S.S., et al., *Piezo2 is the major transducer of mechanical forces for touch sensation in mice.* Nature, 2014. **516**(7529): p. 121.
40. Schrenk-Siemens, K., et al., *PIEZO2 is required for mechanotransduction in human stem cell-derived touch receptors.* Nature Neuroscience, 2015. **18**(1): p. 10–16.
41. Chesler, A.T., et al., *The role of PIEZO2 in human mechanosensation.* The New England Journal of Medicine, 2016. **2016**(375): p. 1355–1364.
42. Nonomura, K., et al., *Piezo2 senses airway stretch and mediates lung inflation-induced apnoea.* Nature, 2017. **541**(7636): p. 176–181.
43. Feng, B. and T. Guo, *Visceral pain from colon and rectum: the mechanotransduction and biomechanics.* Journal of Neural Transmission, 2020. **127**(4): p. 415–429.
44. Marshall, K.L., et al., *PIEZO2 in sensory neurons and urothelial cells coordinates urination.* Nature, 2020: p. 1–6.
45. Yang, J., et al., *The potential role of Piezo2 in the mediation of visceral sensation.* Neuroscience letters, 2016. **630**: p. 158–163.
46. Ferrari, L.F., et al., *Contribution of Piezo2 to endothelium-dependent pain.* Molecular pain, 2015. **11**: p. s12990-015-0068-4.
47. Aguilera-Lizarraga, J., et al., *Local immune response to food antigens drives meal-induced abdominal pain.* Nature, 2021. **590**(7844): p. 151–156.
48. Najjar, S.A., B.M. Davis, and K.M. Albers, *Epithelial–Neuronal Communication in the Colon: Implications for Visceral Pain.* Trends in neurosciences, 2020. **43**(3): p. 170–181.

13 Preclinical Models of Pain

Danielle Zheng

13.1 INTRODUCTION

Preclinical models of pain help researchers and clinicians develop an understanding of the mechanisms involved in pain processing and can help facilitate the development of human medications. Through the use of animal models, such as mice and rats, researchers can validate the mechanisms, pharmacology, and functional phenotype of various pain types. Remember, however, that while single cells, receptors, and brain slices can reflect mechanisms and target engagement, it is behavior that defines pain.

In this chapter, you will learn about the preclinical models used as a surrogate for the various pain states, including acute pain states, tissue injury and inflammation, visceral pain, nerve injury, and spontaneous pain. Additionally, we will briefly cover the genetics of pain and ethical guidelines for pain research in animals.

13.2 ACUTE PAIN STATES

Acute pain is a product of a complex physiological cascade of events in response to an adverse stimulus, often due to tissue injury [1]. As one of the most important biological instincts for survival, the response to acute pain is proportional to the degree of the adverse stimulus and tissue injury.

A classic and pedagogic example to illustrate this is the reaction to touching a hot object, such as a stovetop. If an extremely hot stovetop is inadvertently touched by an individual, that person would remove their hand from the stovetop as quickly as possible, in a matter of milliseconds. However, if the stovetop is warm, or even cold, the reaction to touching the stovetop would be drastically different than in the previous example. The former is a normal response to an acute, painful stimulus, commonly referred to as the nociceptive flexion reflex, which is a paradigm that has been used for decades in pain research to study the threshold of pain [2]. There can certainly be abnormal reactions, such as in neurodegenerative disorders, where the circuitry for the nociceptive flexion reflex is damaged and a painful stimulus to a limb, for example, does not produce flexion withdrawal of that limb. However, in normal reflexive physiology of pain, the area of referred pain should coincide with the location of the painful stimulus, with a proportional response to that stimulus if a certain threshold for pain is reached.

This section examines classic models used to study acute pain states.

DOI: 10.1201/9781003094302-13

13.2.1 Transient High-Intensity Stimuli

The molecular basis of the physiological response to high-intensity stimuli involves the following steps: first, a painful stimulus (e.g., thermal or mechanical pressure) is applied to an area of an organism. Nociceptors are mostly polymodal, thereby responsive to any pressure, thermal, or chemical stimuli. Signals, via action potentials, travel along the afferent A delta fibers and C nociceptors. The rate of these action potentials is proportional to stimulus intensity. This leads to the release of neurotransmitters that act on their respective receptors (e.g., glutamate on the AMPA receptor, substance P on the neurokinin 1 receptor) [3–5]. There is then a proportional response in the discharge of the dorsal horn of the spinal cord that will be relayed to the brain for both the sensory-discriminative and affective aspects of perception of pain, resulting in a behavioral response, usually an acute escape behavior from the stimulus [4, 6, 7]. Observation and study of these behaviors can help delineate the physiology of the pain response. It is also crucial that these responses do not generate damage, as once a permanent insult has been done, it is then subject to a different state or mechanism of pain response. Therefore, utilizing models that do not necessarily cause tissue injury while pain is being elicited is important.

13.2.2 Acute Non-Injurious Models

13.2.2.1 Thermally Evoked Escape to the Hind Paw

This is a classic test, also known as the **hot plate test**, first described by Woolf and Macdonald in 1944 and later modified by Eddy and Leimbach [8, 9]. In this experiment, an animal (e.g., a rodent) is placed on top of the hot plate and enclosed in a transparent cylinder (Figure 13.1). The hot plate is heated to a certain temperature that is hot enough to provide a noxious thermal stimulus, and the latency to an initial response is measured, such as the hind paw lick. The hind paw lick was initially presumed to be an acute escape behavior, later validated by Yeomen et al. [8, 10, 11].

More recently, in 1988, the Hargreaves method began to be utilized, which directly applies a thermal stimulus with heat (radiant or infrared) to the individual hind paw of an unrestrained animal, and observations were made for the withdrawal of the hind paw. Again, the latency between the onset of the thermal stimulus and the withdrawal of the hind paw was measured as an outcome in seconds. This revised method minimized handling and allowed for individual assessment of the hind paw separately [13].

This is complex behavior that requires the rodent to stop moving around on the hot plate, shift its weight, and remove or lick the hind paw, indicating that it is a supraspinally organized behavior. Similar behavior with the withdrawal of the tail upon thermal stimulation of the tail (known as tail flick) has been observed by D'Amour and Smith. In the **tail flick test**, the animal's tail is exposed to a thermal stimulus and time is measured until the animal flicks its tail forward, indicating latency to pain threshold (Figure 13.2) [14, 15]. The tail flick response has been replicated in rodents with tail immersion in heated water baths, as well as in primates [16–19].

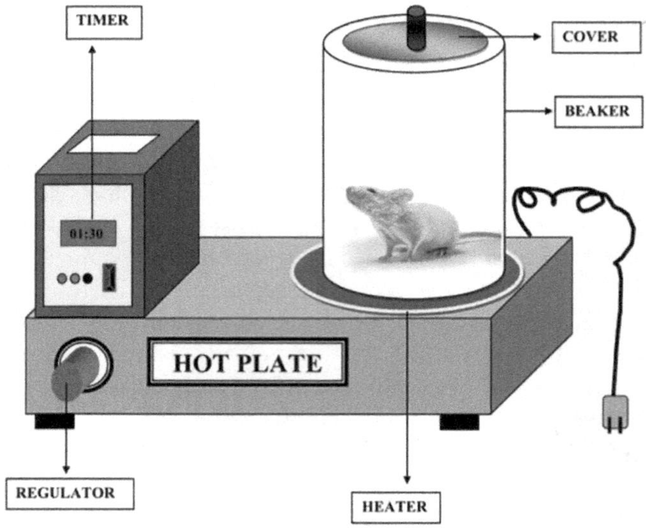

FIGURE 13.1 Illustration of the hot plate test apparatus and set-up.

Source: [12]. Open-access, free to re-use (https://www.sciencepublishinggroup.com/information/open-access).

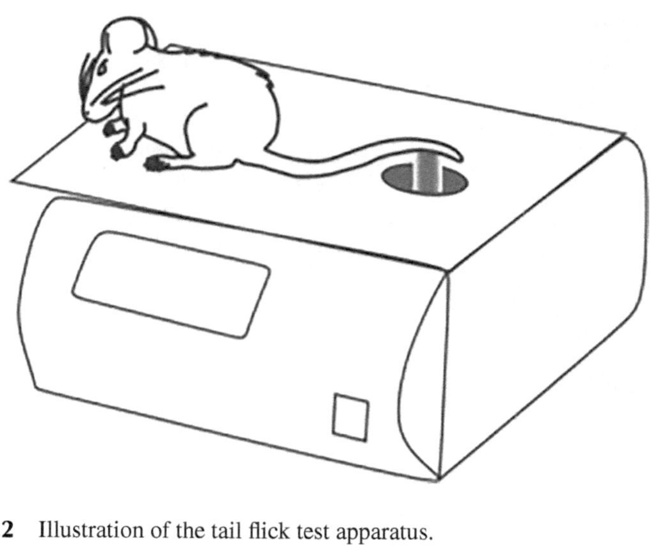

FIGURE 13.2 Illustration of the tail flick test apparatus.

Source: [20]. Open-access, free to re-use (https://creativecommons.org/licenses/by/4.0/).

13.2.2.2 Mechanically Evoked Escape to Hind Paw

In addition to a thermal stimulus to evoke pain and an escape response, mechanical stimuli can be applied as well to observe the behavior in animals. The **Randall–Selitto test** is one method that has been used in pain research since the 1950s. The rodent is restrained in a handheld device clenched to a hind paw, and progressively increasing pressure is applied on the body part. The pressure is measured and recorded until it leads to withdrawal or vocalization of the mice and rats, thereby serving as a useful tool for assessing pain thresholds [21, 22]. Mechanically evoked pain has been observed in dogs as well by Martin et al., where intestinal Doyen forceps were used to apply pressure to toes [23].

13.2.3 Common Properties of Acute Nociception Models

There are many properties shared by the various models of nociception. First, stimulus evokes an unconditioned escape. For example, if an animal is shown a red light before a pain stimulus is applied in its setting, it would be conditioned to associate the red light with the pain and attempt an escape before the onset of the painful stimulus. Thus, it is important and common that certain non-aversive cues (lights, sounds) are avoided that trigger the animal to anticipate the pain and an escape response.

Additionally, the stimuli applied to the animals do not cause side effects or adverse events that may alter the physiology and confound the animal's natural response. Some side effects from certain stimuli may include motor weakness, incoordination, sedation, hyperactivity, or loss of organized behavior. Any of these adverse events can impact our ability to assert that a specific reaction is indeed the behavioral pain response.

The presence of adverse events in an animal model can be discerned using a "tier system" of assays, which often consists of tier 1 via Irwin test/functional observational battery (Table 13.1), mainly to screen for neurotoxicity evaluations. The question here is, "Does a chemical act on the neurons?" [24] Behaviors evaluated include activity or excitability, discerned by an animal's arousal, gait, responses, reflexes, grip strength, etc. [25]

Tier 2 testing is a more specific series of complex tests to further assess cognition as well as dose-dependent responses of the subjects being tested. This can be done by testing learning, attention, and memory, as well as motor and sensory function, by utilizing gait analyses, rotarod, grip strength, acoustic startle response, etc., all of which may represent neuronal loss, if present [25].

The consideration to have a cutoff for the stimulus duration and intensity to prevent tissue injury is important not just with the study of acute pain in non-injurious models but also because it may affect the methods of the study (e.g., repetitive exposures with low-intensity stimulus vs. single exposure with high-intensity stimulus). It is important to be reminded that the more intense the stimulus, the shorter the response latency. In addition, the inter-animal variation will be smaller with higher-intensity stimuli, but the response will be less sensitive to a given treatment. A similar pattern of inter-animal variability is observed in a drug dose–response curve, where higher

TABLE 13.1
Types of Behavioral Tests Often Used at the First and Second Tier of Neurotoxicity Evaluations

Type of Test	Behaviors Evaluated	Specific Test/End Point
Tier 1: Screening, Hazard Identification		
FOB, Irwin screen	Activity, excitability, sensorimotor, neuromuscular	Arousal, rearing, reactivity, gait, posture, responses, reflexes, landing foot splay, grip strength, excretions
Tier 2: Hazard Characterization		
Cognition	Learning, conditioning, memory, attention	Passive/active avoidance, water maze, T-maze, operant schedules of reinforcement
Motor	Quantitative measures: coordination, equilibrium, strength	Gait analysis, rotarod, grip strength, landing foot splay, motor activity
Sensory	Quantitative measures: stimuli-specific response	Acoustic startle response, prepulse inhibition

Source: [25] (https://us.sagepub.com/en-us/nam/pre-approved-permission-requests-journals).

analgesic dosage leads to an increase in the response latency to painful stimuli, but at very high doses, the slope of the dose–response curve is smaller, where the analgesic may become a partial agonist.

Lastly, analgesics can be used in these models to modulate an animal's response to pain. *Analgesics* can be defined as drugs that reduce the nociceptive stimulus–response relationship without altering motor function or other aspects of sensory integration. For example, a well-known analgesic is morphine, a μ-opioid agonist, which can be used to demonstrate its analgesic properties by increasing the response latency to thermal escape. Morphine can be used in conjunction with an antagonist, such as naloxone, or other opioid agonists, such as fentanyl or meperidine, for structural activity relationship.

13.3 TISSUE INJURY AND INFLAMMATION

Inflammatory pain states often follow an acute local tissue injury. Inflammation is classically characterized by the constellation of symptoms of rubor (redness), tumor (swelling), calor (warmth), and dolor (pain). This is mediated by a complex physiologic response involving an increase in the serum concentration of proteins collectively referred to as acute phase reactants [26]. This phenomenon, termed the acute phase response, was first noted by the discovery of an increase in the concentration of C-reactive protein in the serum of patients with pneumococcal pneumonia [27]. Since then, numerous acute phase reactants have been identified as contributing to the classic cardinal signs of inflammation. These signs of inflammation often persist after the acute painful stimuli have been withdrawn and oftentimes follow a complicated tissue referral pattern.

This section will cover some of the important studies that have contributed to our current understanding of tissue injury and inflammation.

13.3.1 Physiology of Pain Response Secondary to Local Tissue Injury

When a tissue sustains a local injury, there is typically an associated local area of primary hyperalgesia. Less intuitively, there is often an area of secondary tactile allodynia, characterized by an enhanced pain response secondary to otherwise-innocuous stimuli in an area that was not involved in the initial tissue injury [28]. In the case of primary hyperalgesia, the area of initial inflammation gives rise to increased spontaneous Aδ/C fiber activity. This afferent signal drives increased spinal neuron activity and activates the spinal facilitatory cascade that results in exaggerated outflow from the dorsal horn, which can then cause secondary tactile allodynia [29]. Numerous models have been developed to further characterize this physiologic response to tissue injury.

13.3.1.1 Carrageenan-Evoked Inflammation

Post-injury pain states have been studied using **carrageenan-evoked inflammation** as a model for the acute inflammatory response (Figure 13.3). Carrageenan is extracted from seaweed and serves as an irritant that evokes innate immune signaling. It is a natural polysaccharide, cheap and readily available. Furthermore, it produces an acute, highly reproducible inflammation, which has led to its use in numerous research studies for characterizing the inflammatory response. In these

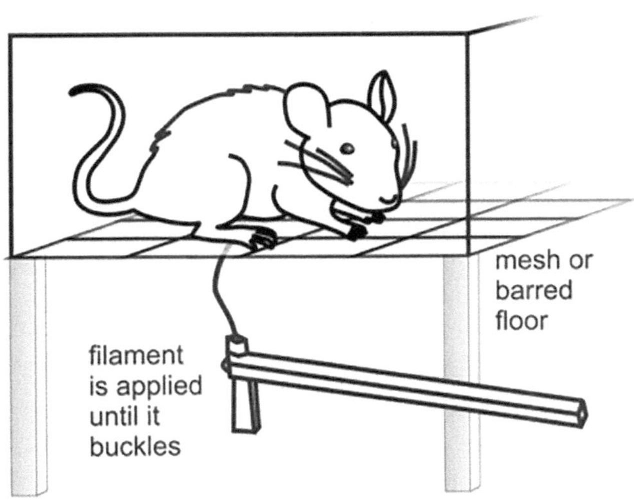

FIGURE 13.3 Application of von Frey hair testing to deliver uniform, repeatable stimulus.

Source: [20] Open-source, free to re-use (https://www.frontiersin.org/journals/molecular-neuroscience/about#about-open).

studies, carrageenan is injected into the paw of a rodent model, and the inflammatory response is measured using various metrics. The thickness of the paw (tumor) shows increased swelling for several hours post-injection, then gradually returns to baseline over 24–48 hours. Other measures of inflammation can be measured in this model as well. Measuring the thermal escape latency is achieved by placing the rodent's paw in contact with a hot surface and then recording the time elapsed until the rodent displays withdrawal behavior. Using this model for inflammation, many studies have been able to characterize the efficacy of medications and interventions for treating inflammatory states. One such study demonstrated that anti-inflammatory agents such as indomethacin predictably lowered the level of acute paw swelling observed as a result of carrageenan injection [30].

13.3.1.2 Hind Paw Formalin-Evoked Flinching (Rodent)

Formalin-induced flinching studies have proven useful to characterize the time course and mechanism of the inflammatory response. In this study, 20–50 μl of 1–5% formalin were injected into the hind paw of rodent models, and the flinching behavior of the rodent was documented. The flinching behavior follows a biphasic distribution with an initial high number of flinching responses immediately following injection, followed by a phase II of elevated flinching responses approximately 20 minutes post-injection. The flinching behavior in phase I is thought to be due to the acute high-frequency firing of peripheral afferents. However, in phase II, low-level firing of peripheral afferents is noted. It is believed this second phase is caused by sensitization of the second-order neuron in the spinal dorsal horn secondary to high-frequency C fiber input during phase I. This sensitization increases flinching behavior from the low level of continued peripheral afferent activity. Furthermore, at 5–7 days, a phase III of flinching behavior is noted, thought to be due to microglial activation [31].

13.3.1.3 Von Frey Hair Testing

Applying a consistent stimulus to animal models is difficult to achieve consistently by hand but is an important component of many studies. Thus, **von Frey hair testing** was developed to address this common obstacle. This technique utilizes a thin, deformable hair as a mechanism to apply consistent pressure to the paw of the rodent model. The amount of pressure applied can be varied by changing the thickness of the hair. An innocuous threshold of <15 g of pressure typically does not induce a response; however, with sensitization, the threshold of pressure necessary to induce a withdrawal response from the rodent decreases. Further advances in von Frey hair testing have allowed measuring the timing of the response accurately down to thousands of a seconds, as well as allowing for the precise application of a stimulus for a particular duration [32].

13.3.1.4 Post-Surgical Incision/Brennan Model (Rodent) (Post-Surgical Allodynia)

The **Brennan model** characterizes post-surgical allodynia in rodents, wherein a plantar paw incision is used as the source of inflammation. The incision is spread and then closed. Post-operatively, the withdrawal threshold is measured, which shows an onset of tactile allodynia within minutes that persists for several days. This has been used to test methods for the management of post-operative allodynia. Intrathecal bupivacaine and intrathecal morphine were administered preoperatively in one group and post-operatively in another group. Neither group showed a reduction in hyperalgesia, suggesting that incisional pain may be maintained differently than pain in other models [33].

13.3.1.5 KBxN Arthritis (Mouse) (Acute to Chronic)

K/BxN arthritis serves as a model of the acute-to-chronic transition of inflammatory pain states. This model utilizes the serum of rodents with a type of congenital inflammation. Mice transgenetic for a T cell receptor that recognized bovine RNase are then bred into NOD (non-obese diabetic) mice. These mice were found to develop severe destructive inflammatory arthritis. Importantly, this inflammatory state was found to be serum-transferrable [34]. When this serum was injected into otherwise-healthy mice, their ankle width was found to increase for 12–15 days. The threshold of tactile pressure necessary to induce a brisk withdrawal of their paw (tactile allodynia) was also measured. The mechanical allodynia in these mice persisted long after the initial inflammation had resolved, demonstrating a transition to a chronic pain state. Thus, this model has proven useful wherein arthritic pain and other chronic pain states can be studied [35].

13.4 VISCERAL PAIN

Viscera is a highly innervated part of the body, and much of the innervation is communicated by sympathetic afferents, whose cell bodies are in the dorsal root ganglia, which travel with the parasympathetic afferents to deliver sensory input regarding distension of hollow organs as well as chemosensitivity (secondary to inflammatory products).

Visceral pain is often described as sharp and diffuse and can have referred pain areas in specific body surfaces, a concept known as **somatic referral**. For example, if one suffers a myocardial infarction, the heart muscle will release substances such as ATP that can activate the C fiber terminals that innervate the heart. Since the cell bodies of nerves innervating the visceral organs are located in the dorsal root ganglia, as previously mentioned, the pain signal in this example will be sent to the T3/T4 level of the spinal cord on the left side. The nociceptive afferents converge in the area of the dorsal root ganglia that also pertains to a certain area of skin or muscle, thereby generating somatic referred pain (Figure 13.4) [36]. Therefore, the referred pain is increased in the setting of visceral inflammation. There have been several models to study the nature of visceral pain.

The classic study by Hendershot et al. was performed by delivering solutions such as hypertonic saline or dilute acetic acid that **irritated peritoneal space** and visceral organs like colon and bladder [38]. When a rat experiences irritation to the viscera, it exhibits writhing, also known as abdominal visceral distention, rubbing its abdomen on the floor. This finding is corroborated by increased abdominal tone on electromyography (EMG), which is akin to guarding in humans in a setting of peritonitis. An increase in blood pressure and heart rate also occurs, as signs of autonomic drive in response to noxious stimuli [39].

Similar sequelae arise with **visceral distension**, which can occur in the absence of, or in conjunction with, visceral irritation. Kamp et al. subjected rats to colorectal

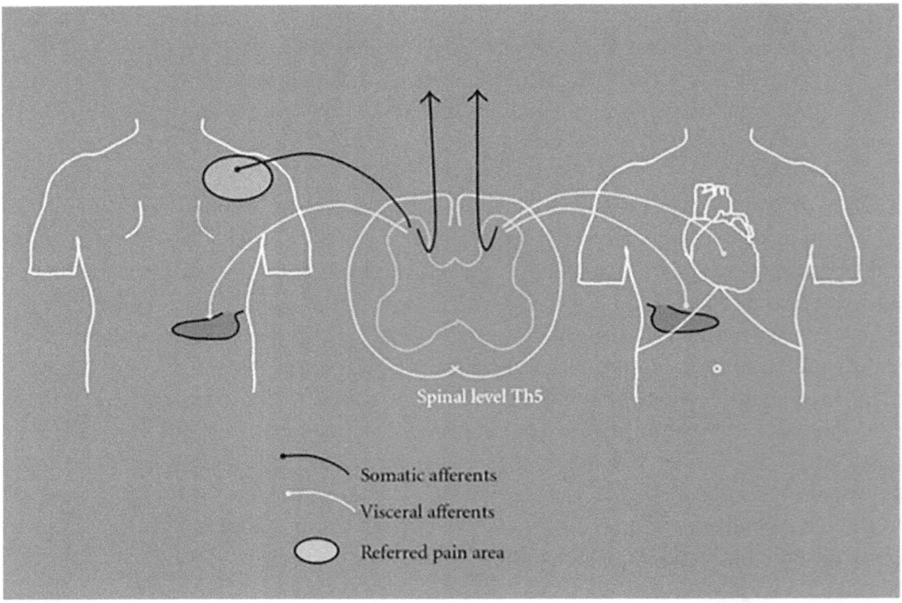

FIGURE 13.4 Convergence of afferent inputs from the skin (black), liver, and heart (white) onto the dorsal root ganglion. Two tracts (DCML: dorsal column medial lemniscal; STT: spinothalamic tract) convey the afferent signals via the medial spinal cord.

Source: [37]. Open-source.

distension by inflating a balloon and measuring the distension pressure with an abdominal EMG, and the evoked contractions were proportional to the degree of colorectal distension. Results revealed that low distension pressure did not cause signs and symptoms, such as an increase in heart rate, blood pressure, and writhing, but as the distension pressure increased, these responses became evident, suggesting visceral distension as a cause for pain [40].

The concept of somatic referral applies to visceral pain as well. Tactile thresholds (i.e., number of times an animal would vocalize in response to a painful stimulus) were measured by Laird et al. in mice with and without **intracolonic capsaicin** administration, and it was found that visceral irritation synergistically increased the animal's response to pain, suggesting that activation of visceral afferents evokes referred somatic sensitization [41].

13.5 NERVE INJURY

13.5.1 Physiology of Nerve Injury

Nerve injuries occur via a variety of mechanisms that can influence the symptoms experienced. Insults can affect one nerve (mononeuropathy) or multiple nerves (polyneuropathy). Numerous models exist to characterize the underlying physiology of these often-encountered pain states. Although the mechanism of injury varies, many of the resultant symptoms are quite similar [42].

13.5.2 Mononeuropathy Models

13.5.2.1 Chronic Constrictive Injury Model

The **chronic constrictive injury model** is one of the first widely used models for studying nerve injuries. In this model, four ligatures are placed around a nerve while the rodent is under anesthesia. The wound is then closed, and the animal is allowed to recover for 24 hours after the procedure. The pain threshold can then be measured utilizing any number of techniques. For example, von Frey hair testing can be used to measure the withdrawal threshold, which demonstrates the sensitizing effects produced by chronic constrictive injury [43].

13.5.2.2 Spinal Nerve Ligation Model

The **spinal nerve ligation model** is another commonly used model to study neuropathic pain. In this model, one or two spinal nerves are tightly ligated in the rat, typically L5/L6. This procedure results in a chronic pain state with measurable behavioral changes, such as mechanical allodynia and heat hyperalgesia, that typically have an onset within 3–4 days. In some studies, this allodynia has been noted to extend to 60–90 days with no recovery. This model has seen widespread usage in characterizing neuropathic pain, as well as in drug research for new analgesic pharmacologic agents [44].

13.5.2.3 Spared Nerve Injury Model

The **spared nerve injury model** in rodents is a partial denervation model in which the common peroneal and tibial nerves are injured and, importantly, the sural nerve is left intact. However, when force is applied to the lateral hindfoot (distribution of the sural nerve), there is marked tactile allodynia. This model has been important to help characterize the mechanisms of neuropathic pain (Figure 13.5) [45].

13.5.3 Polyneuropathy

Polyneuropathy refers to damage to multiple peripheral nerves and can be caused by a wide variety of insults. For example, diabetic neuropathy is an exceedingly common cause of polyneuropathy and can be studied using mutant mice. The db gene is an autosomal recessive mutation on mouse chromosome 4. These db mice have been used as a model to further characterize diabetic peripheral polyneuropathy [46]. Chemotherapeutic agents such as cisplatin and paclitaxel are other well-known culprit for tactile allodynia. When administered to mice, this tactile allodynia develops within a few days. This has been used as a model to study analgesic efficacy in chemotherapy-induced polyneuropathy [47]. To study viral neuropathy, mice can be infected with HSV-1 or HIV, which results in these mice developing polyneuropathy, much like humans. In addition to these models, many other models have been developed to help further characterize these polyneuropathies, as detailed in Table 13.2.

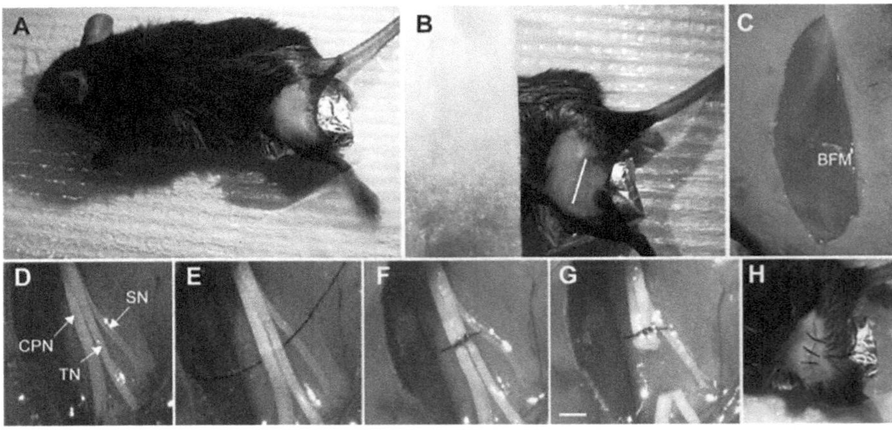

FIGURE 13.5 Surgical ligation of common peroneal and tibial nerves. A 2 cm section of these nerves was removed to prevent nerve regeneration. Contact with the sural nerve was carefully avoided. Steps E to G were omitted for the sham operation control group.

Source: [45]. Open-source (https://bio-protocol.org/en/about?type=policy). Also published by a colleague of Dr. Zheng's.

TABLE 13.2
Methods of Studying Various Polyneuropathy Models

Chemotherapy-Induced Neuropathy	Vincristine, Taxol, Cisplatin
Viral neuropathy	HSV-1, HIV injection
Trigeminal neuropathy	Infraorbital constriction, formalin injection
Inflammatory neuritis	Perisciatic zymosan injection
Neuroma	Nerve transection, cryo-neurolysis of the sciatic nerve
Spinal cord injury	Contusion, hemisection of T3, excitotoxic, quisqualic acid
Spinal stenosis	Silicone rubber, steel rod
Gout	Urate crystals in joint spaces
Fibromyalgia	Acidic saline injection, gastrocnemius muscle
Cystitis	Cyclophosphamide
Charcot–Marie–Tooth	Chr17p11.2, PMP22 transgenic
Guillain–Barre syndrome	Experimental autoimmune neuritis (EAN)
Demyelinating polyneuropathy (CIDP)	Peripheral myelin in Freund's Adjuvant

Source: Dr. Yaksh.

13.6 SPONTANEOUS PAIN ASSESSMENT STRATEGIES

Some argue that what we are measuring in rodent models is some kind of spinal threshold regulation. However, we know that pain is more than a spinal threshold. In the 1960s, Melzack and Casey [48] formalized the notion that pain has

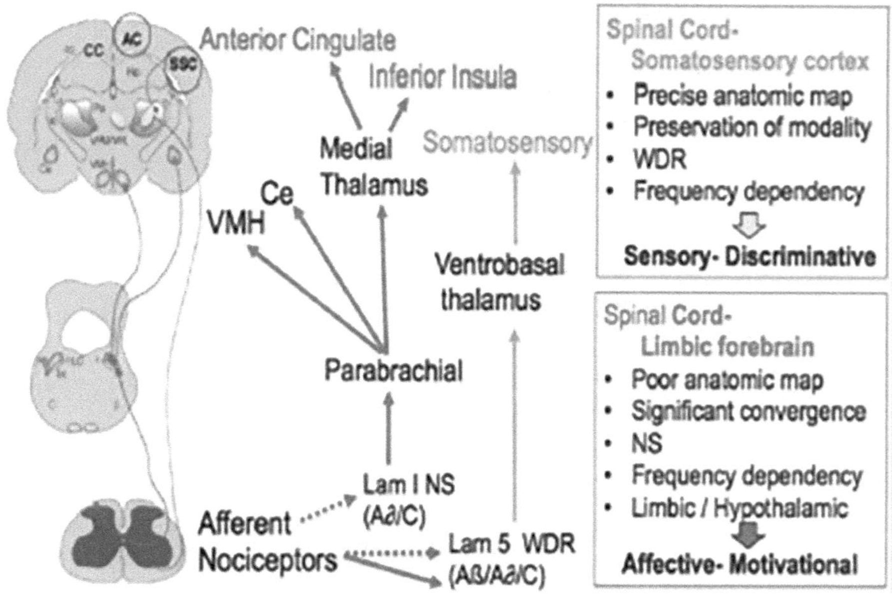

FIGURE 13.6 Duality of ascending projections.

Source: Dr. Yaksh.

two orthogonal components: (1) sensory-discriminative and (2) affective-motivational. These components are organized into separate pathways in the brain and spinal cord (Figure 13.6). In the sensory-discriminative pathway, the afferent nociceptors activate the dorsal horn neurons, which project to the ventrobasal thalamus. These fibers are organized in a precise anatomical map, with preservation of modality, and are highly psychophysically organized. However, the output from the dorsal horn may also go to areas of the brain stem and diencephalon, including the hypothalamus, amygdala, and medial thalamus, which then refers to the limbic forebrain (anterior cingulate and inferior insula). These pathways have poor anatomical mapping and significant convergence between various modalities. Given the areas this pathway targets, it has been argued that this pathway underlies the affective-motivational component of pain. There has been much interest in developing models that will allow us to determine how aversive a pain state is perceived to be.

13.6.1 Spontaneous Activity

Measurement of spontaneous activity has been used to determine the effect of pain on function. In mice, measurement of a **24-hour activity cycle** will reveal disruption in the cycle with a pain generator [49]. Similarly, the function can be measured by **weight-bearing**, in which an animal stands on two strain gauges

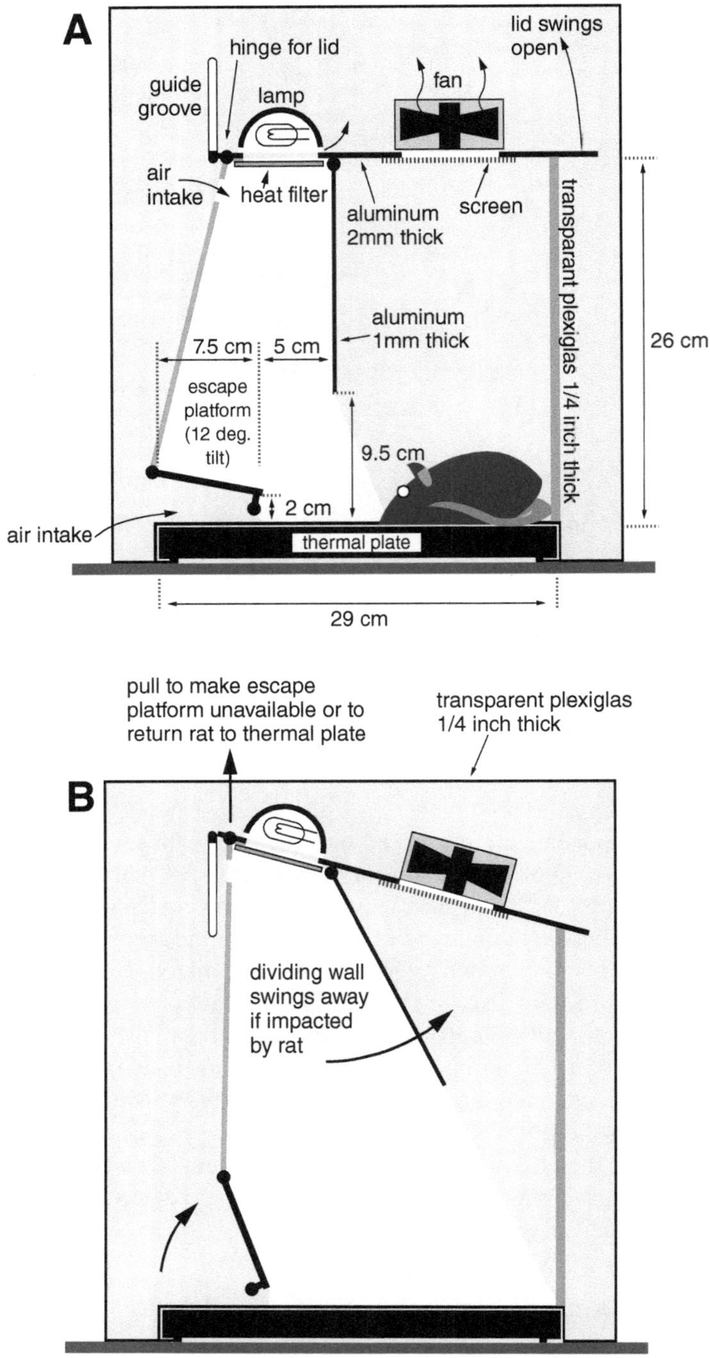

FIGURE 13.7 Measurement of spontaneous activity: (a) Measurement of activity over 24 24-hour activity cycle; the activity of a mouse in an arthritis model (*middle*) is altered compared to normal sleep/wake activity (*top*), and administration of ketorolac allows for recovery of activity (*bottom*). (b) Measurement of weight-bearing.

Source: [49].

and the researcher can measure whether the left or right paw is bearing more weight [50]. There are also many devices to measure **ambulatory patterns** in normal and pain states [20]. What is common about all these models is that there is typically a recovery of function with the administration of an analgesic (Figure 13.7).

13.6.2 Conditioned Place Preference

Another commonly used test is the **conditioned place preference** paradigm [50–52]. In this classical conditioning paradigm, two distinct chambers are connected by a middle "neutral" chamber. During conditioning, a specific state (e.g., administration of medication or placebo) is associated with first chamber, while another state is linked to the second chamber. On test day, the animal is placed in the neutral chamber without administration of medication and allowed to freely move between the chambers, and the amount of time that the animal spends in each chamber is assessed. The animal is said to show a "preference" for the chamber that it spends more time in, and that chamber (and its associated medication) is said to be positively reinforcing (or that the other chamber is negatively reinforcing). In pain states, the assumption is made that pain is a negatively reinforcing experience (i.e., it is associated with a negative affective motivation), and therefore, if a drug alters the input associated with driving the aversive state, then it should be positively reinforcing. However, some medications, such as morphine, are intrinsically positively reinforcing even in the absence of pain; these medications could not be assessed for analgesia in the conditioned place preference model (Figure 13.8).

13.6.3 Operant Escape Models

Operant conditioning pairs a behavior with a consequence. Unlike classical conditioning, in which the behavior is involuntary, in operant conditioning, the consequence of a behavior drives the strength of that behavior. In pain research, animals are assessed by the **escape test**, in which animals are placed in a device that provides a painful thermal stimulus that forces the animal to escape to a different environment to avoid the painful experience. Latency and duration of escape from the painful compartment are measured. Unlike reflex responses, which occur within 100 ms, the minimum reaction time for sensory perception and then a conscious response to somatosensory stimulation is longer (250 ms), and pain is only extinguished after the operant response (escape) (Figure 13.9) [53, 54].

13.6.4 Veterinary Pain Drug Trials

In the laboratory, large animals are not commonly employed in preclinical models of pain behavior. However, companion animals such as cats and dogs can also suffer from painful diseases, such as osteosarcoma, and are brought to the veterinarian to be euthanized due to the inability to improve their quality of life. Some veterinary clinics now offer experimental pain medication/treatment in studies that are often randomized and double-blinded, with protocols similar to those for human studies. Many behavioral inventories have been created for the assessment

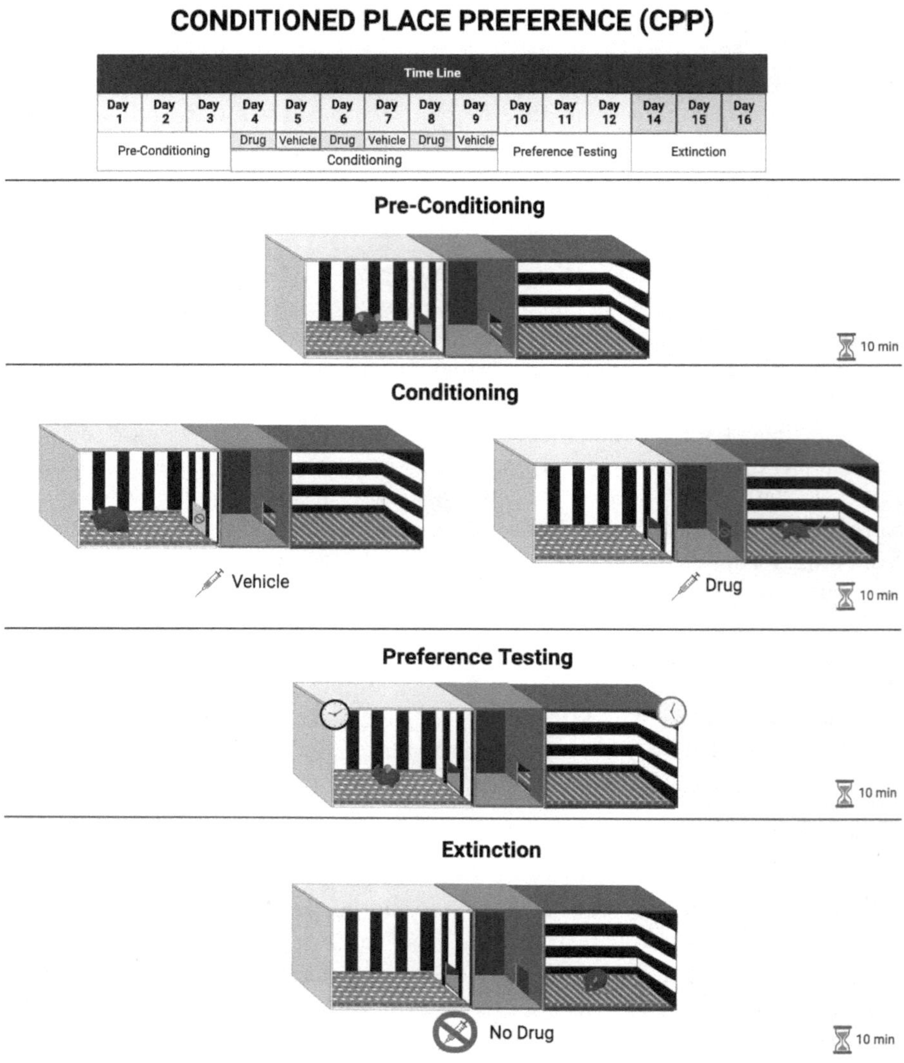

FIGURE 13.8 Conditioned place preference.

of pain in animals. There is increased interest in enrolling companion animals in studies that may benefit not only the companion animals but also potentially the human population [55].

13.7 GENETICS OF PAIN

13.7.1 Knockout/Transgenic Strains

There is a broad range of reported knockouts/transgenic mice strains in pain studies (Table 13.3). While these strains are helpful in the elucidation of specific genes on

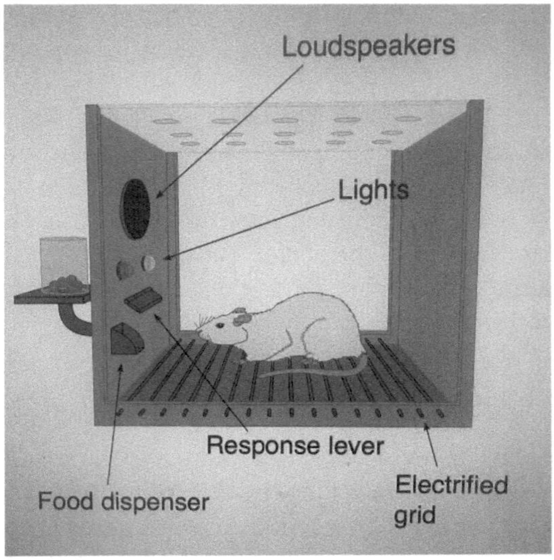

FIGURE 13.9 Operant escape test.

Source: [54] (https://www.sciencedirect.com/science/article/abs/pii/S0165027000001606?via%3Dihub).

TABLE 13.3
Published Knockout/Transgenic Mouse Strains with Phenotypes

Genotype	Phenotype
β-endorphin KO	Abolished opioid analgesia induced by stress
Galanin OE	Elevation of nociceptive threshold to thermal stimulation
G protein Go-αo KO	Thermal hyperalgesia and motor control impairment
IFN-γ KO	Abolished pain behavior after sciatic section
IL-6 KO	Reduced analgesic effects of morphine
κ-opioid R KO	Enhanced sensitivity to visceral pain; no effect of κ-opioid
NET KO	Enhanced opioid analgesia
NGF KO	Mediate inflammation-induced peripheral/central sensitization
NGF OE	Hyperalgesic to mechanical and thermal stimulation
NK-1 R	Attenuation in response to heat hyperalgesia
NMDA-NR2B, OE	Enhanced responsiveness to formalin/CFA
NPY KO	Increased autotomy behavior after sciatic transection
PKA Riβ KO	Reduction in tissue injury–induced persistent pain
PKC-γ KO	Blocked neuropathic syndrome after sciatic injury
Prodynorphin KO	Accelerated recovery after nerve ligation
ppENK KO	Reduced supraspinal, but not spinal, pain threshold
μ-opioid R KO	Shortened latencies on thermal escape
Δ-opioid R KO	Abolished spinal δ-opioid analgesia
Substance P OE	Facilitation of opioid-mediated antinociceptive mechanism
TNF OE	Enhanced allodynia after spinal nerve transection

Source: Courtesy of Z David Luo, MD.

pain and pain behaviors, it is important to remember that in these studies, all pain end points were not the same, and background strains for appropriate controls were not the same.

Additionally, pain behavior varies with the strain of the animal being studied. In a study of licking behavior after intraplantar formalin administration, for example, there was a wide range of behaviors in various mouse strains [56]. This indicates that pain and analgesic mechanisms may vary by strain. Also, analgesic effects are impacted by the characteristics of the model. The drug may have the same effect, but via different mechanisms, in different models. It is important to select a model based on hypothesized mechanisms.

13.8 ETHICAL GUIDELINES FOR PAIN RESEARCH IN ANIMALS

The charge of the individual who works with animals is to treat animals as well as they can. In the study of pain, unfortunately, cell culture can elucidate mechanisms but cannot tell us what nociception is—animals must experience pain as part of pain research. While the use of preclinical models in understanding the biology of nociception has led to important advances that have benefited both animal and human patients, researchers must also follow guidelines to conduct research humanely and ethically.

Research in animals is governed by the mandate "**reduce, refine, and replace**" [57]. It is important to make the experimental groups robust and to calculate how many animals are necessary to adequately power an experiment, and to use as few animals as possible. Refining an experiment allows for minimizing animal suffering and improving welfare. And when possible, consider replacing a higher-order animal with a lower-order one (e.g., replace a dog with a guinea pig model).

In chronic studies, consideration must also be given to the overall condition of the animal. One can **minimize stressors** by singly housing animals and ensuring accessibility to food and water. It is also important to **minimize stimulus exposure/consequences** by utilizing soft bedding and strict attention to euthanasia criteria (e.g., weight loss, loss of mobility, overall appearance of animal, piloerection). **Minimizing study duration and defining criteria for earliest sacrifice** is also important to ensure the well-being of the research animal.

The **Ethics Committee of the International Association for the Study of Pain** (IASP) has also formulated recommendations on this subject. In a preamble, the committee stated that experiments are indispensable if we are to gain a better understanding of the mechanism of pain. The committee, while acknowledging that some experiments have the aim of trying to reproduce chronic syndromes in animals, stated clearly that experimental protocols have to minimize or avoid unnecessary pain. The practical consequences of those recommendations include [58]:

- Experiments involving the study of pain on conscious animals must be reviewed by scientists and laypersons, and the potential benefit of these experiments must be demonstrated.
- As far as possible, the scientists must test the painful stimuli on themselves.
- Investigators should assess all behavioral and physiological changes in the animal and report them in resulting manuscripts.

TABLE 13.4
USDA Pain and Distress Categories for Vertebrate Animals

Pain Category	Description	Examples
B	Breeding or holding colony	Bred but not yet used
C	Produce minimal, transient pain or distress	Injections, blood sampling; observational study of animal behavior; acute escape; intraplantar irritants
D	Produce pain or distress, but employ anesthetics and post-procedure analgesics	Non-survival physiological studies; surgical protocol with perioperative analgesia
E	Pain states not accompanied by treatment to alleviate pain or are not amenable to such therapies	Nerve injury; cancer; chronic inflammation; lethal dosing studies

Source: Made by Dr. Yaksh based on [60].

- There must be no question of using animals paralyzed with a neuromuscular blocking agent without a general anesthetic or an appropriate surgical procedure that eliminates sensory awareness.
- The experiment duration must be as short as possible, and the number of animals involved kept to a minimum.

Before performing research on animals, the study protocol must be approved by an institution's **institutional animal care and use committee** (IACUC). This committee is responsible for reviewing all animal use protocols, ensuring compliance with federal regulations, inspecting animal facilities and laboratories, and overseeing training and educational programs. All vertebrate animals used in research, teaching, or testing must also be assigned a **pain category** (B to E; there is no USDA Pain Category A) (Table 13.4) [59, 60].

REFERENCES

1. Carr, D.B. and L.C. Goudas, *Acute pain*. Lancet, 1999. **353**(9169): p. 2051–8.
2. Rhudy, J.L. and C.R. France, *Defining the nociceptive flexion reflex (NFR) threshold in human participants: a comparison of different scoring criteria*. Pain, 2007. **128**(3): p. 244–253.
3. Mense, S., *Nociception from skeletal muscle in relation to clinical muscle pain*. Pain, 1993. **54**(3): p. 241–289.
4. Hoheisel, U. and S. Mense, *Long-term changes in discharge behavior of cat dorsal horn neurons following noxious stimulation of deep tissues*. Pain, 1989. **36**(2): p. 239–247.
5. Schaible, H.G. and F. Richter, *Pathophysiology of pain*. Langenbecks Arch Surg, 2004. **389**(4): p. 237–43.
6. Ikeda, H., et al., *Synaptic amplifier of inflammatory pain in the spinal dorsal horn*. Science, 2006. **312**(5780): p. 1659–62.
7. Amir, S. and Z. Amit, *Endogenous opioid ligands may mediate stress-induced changes in the affective properties of pain-related behavior in rats*. Life Sci, 1978. **23**(11): p. 1143–51.

8. Woolf, G. and MacDonald, *The evaluation of the analgesic action of pethidine hydrochloride (Demerol)*. Journal of Pharmacology and Experimental Therapeutics, 1944. **80**(3): p. 300–7.
9. Eddy, N.B. and D. Leimbach, *Synthetic analgesics. II. Dithienylbutenyl- and dithienylbutylamines*. J Pharmacol Exp Ther, 1953. **107**(3): p. 385–93.
10. O'Callaghan, J.P. and S.G. Holtzman, *Quantification of the analgesic activity of narcotic antagonists by a modified hot-plate procedure*. J Pharmacol Exp Ther, 1975. **192**(3): p. 497–505.
11. Yeomen, D.C. and H.K. Proudfit, *Characterization of the foot withdrawal response to noxious radiant heat in the rat*. Pain, 1994. **59**(1): p. 85–94.
12. Patel, P., J. Sahu, and S. Chandel, *A detailed review on nociceptive models for the screening of analgesic activity in experimental Animals*. Int J Neurol Phys Ther, 2016. **2**(6): p. 44–50.
13. Dirig, D.M., et al., *Characterization of variables defining hindpaw withdrawal latency evoked by radiant thermal stimuli*. J Neurosci Methods, 1997. **76**(2): p. 183–91.
14. D'Amour, F. and D. Smith, *A method for determining loss of pain sensation*. J Pharmacol Exp Ther, 1941. **72**(1): p. 74–79.
15. Bannon, A.W. and A.B. Malmberg, *Models of nociception: hot-plate, tail-flick, and formalin tests in rodents*. Curr Protoc Neurosci, 2007. Chapter 8: p. Unit 8 9.
16. Luttinger, D., *Determination of antinociceptive efficacy of drugs in mice using different water temperatures in a tail-immersion test*. J Pharmacol Methods, 1985. **13**(4): p. 351–7.
17. Saeki, S. and T.L. Yaksh, *Suppression of nociceptive responses by spinal mu opioid agonists: effects of stimulus intensity and agonist efficacy*. Anesth Analg, 1993. **77**(2): p. 265–74.
18. Dykstra, L.A., and J.H. Woods, *A tail withdrawal procedure for assessing analgesic activity in rhesus monkeys*. J Pharmacol Methods, 1986. **15**(3): p. 263–9.
19. Gatch, M.B., et al., *Antinociceptive effects of cocaine/opioid combinations in rhesus monkeys*. J Pharmacol Exp Ther, 1995. **275**(3): p. 1346–54.
20. Deuis, J.R., L.S. Dvorakova, and I. Vetter, *Methods Used to Evaluate Pain Behaviors in Rodents*. Front Mol Neurosci, 2017. **10**: p. 284.
21. Randall, L.O. and J.J. Selitto, *A method for measurement of analgesic activity on inflamed tissue*. Arch Int Pharmacodyn Ther, 1957. **111**(4): p. 409–19.
22. Green, A.F. and P.A. Young, *A comparison of heat and pressure analgesiometric methods in rats*. Br J Pharmacol Chemother, 1951. **6**(4): p. 572–85.
23. Martin, W.R., et al., *Use of hindlimb reflexes of the chronic spinal dog for comparing analgesics*. J Pharmacol Exp Ther, 1964. **144**: p. 8–11.
24. Mathiasen, J.R. and V.C. Moser, *The Irwin test and functional observational battery (FOB) for assessing the effects of compounds on behavior, physiology, and safety pharmacology in rodents*. Curr Protoc Pharmacol, 2018. **83**(1): p. e43.
25. Moser, V.C., *Functional assays for neurotoxicity testing*. Toxicol Pathol, 2011. **39**(1): p. 36–45.
26. Gabay, C. and I. Kushner, *Acute-phase proteins and other systemic responses to inflammation*. N Engl J Med, 1999. **340**(6): p. 448–54.
27. Kushner, I., *The phenomenon of the acute phase response*. Ann N Y Acad Sci, 1982. **389**: p. 39–48.
28. La, J.H., et al., *Differential involvement of reactive oxygen species in a mouse model of capsaicin-induced secondary mechanical hyperalgesia and allodynia*. Mol Pain, 2017. **13**: p. 1744806917713907.
29. Kimura, S. and H. Kontani, *Separate recording of A-delta and C fiber-mediated nociceptive flexor reflex responses of mouse hindlimb using electromyography and the characteristics of wind-up appearing in the responses*. J Pharmacol Sci, 2008. **108**(2): p. 172–8.

30. Morris, C.J., *Carrageenan-induced paw edema in the rat and mouse.* Methods Mol Biol, 2003. **225**: p. 115–21.
31. Dubuisson, D. and S.G. Dennis, *The formalin test: a quantitative study of the analgesic effects of morphine, meperidine, and brain stem stimulation in rats and cats.* Pain, 1977. **4**(2): p. 161–174.
32. Lambert, G.A., G. Mallos, and A.S. Zagami, *Von Frey's hairs—a review of their technology and use—a novel automated von Frey device for improved testing for hyperalgesia.* J Neurosci Methods, 2009. **177**(2): p. 420–6.
33. Brennan, T.J., E.F. Umali, and P.K. Zahn, *Comparison of pre- versus post-incision administration of intrathecal bupivacaine and intrathecal morphine in a rat model of postoperative pain.* Anesthesiology, 1997. **87**(6): p. 1517–28.
34. Monach, P.A., D. Mathis, and C. Benoist, *The K/BxN arthritis model.* Curr Protoc Immunol, 2008. Chapter 15: p. 15 22 1–15 22 12.
35. Christensen, A.D., et al., *K/BxN serum-transfer arthritis as a model for human inflammatory arthritis.* Front Immunol, 2016. **7**: p. 213.
36. Merskey, H., *Classification of chronic pain. Descriptions of chronic pain syndromes and definitions of pain terms. Prepared by the International Association for the Study of Pain, Subcommittee on Taxonomy.* Pain Suppl, 1986. **3**: p. S1–226.
37. Lottrup, C., S.S. Olesen, and A.M. Drewes, *The pain system in oesophageal disorders: mechanisms, clinical characteristics, and treatment.* Gastroenterol Res Pract, 2011. **2011**: p. 910420.
38. Hendershot, L.C. and J. Forsaith, *Antagonism of the frequency of phenylquinone-induced writhing in the mouse by weak analgesics and nonanalgesics.* J Pharmacol Exp Ther, 1959. **125**(3): p. 237–40.
39. Schwartz, E.S. and G.F. Gebhart, *Visceral pain.* Curr Top Behav Neurosci, 2014. **20**: p. 171–97.
40. Kamp, E.H., et al., *Quantitative assessment and characterization of visceral nociception and hyperalgesia in mice.* Am J Physiol Gastrointest Liver Physiol, 2003. **284**(3): p. G434–44.
41. Laird, J.M.A., et al., *A new model of visceral pain and referred hyperalgesia in the mouse.* Pain, 2001. **92**(3): p. 335–342.
42. Burnett, M.G. and E.L. Zager, *Pathophysiology of peripheral nerve injury: a brief review.* Neurosurg Focus, 2004. **16**(5): p. E1.
43. Austin, P.J., A. Wu, and G. Moalem-Taylor, *Chronic constriction of the sciatic nerve and pain hypersensitivity testing in rats.* J Vis Exp, 2012(61).
44. Chung, J.M., H.K. Kim, and K. Chung, *Segmental spinal nerve ligation model of neuropathic pain.* Methods Mol Med, 2004. **99**: p. 35–45.
45. Cichon, J., L. Sun, and G. Yang, *Spared nerve injury model of neuropathic pain in mice.* Bio Protoc, 2018. **8**(6).
46. Bahary, N., et al., *Molecular mapping of the mouse db mutation.* Proc Natl Acad Sci U S A, 1990. **87**(21): p. 8642–6.
47. Park, H.J., et al., *Persistent hyperalgesia in the cisplatin-treated mouse as defined by threshold measures, the conditioned place preference paradigm, and changes in dorsal root ganglia activated transcription factor 3: the effects of gabapentin, ketorolac, and etanercept.* Anesth Analg, 2013. **116**(1): p. 224–31.
48. Melzack, R. and K. Casey, *Sensory, motivational and central control determinants of pain,* in *The Skin Senses*, D. Kenshalo, Editor. 1968, Thomas: Springfield, IL. p. 423–443.
49. Suhail, M.S., et al., *Effects of long-term polyarthritis and subsequent NSAID treatment on activity with disassociation of tactile allodynia in the mouse.* Neurocomputing (Amst), 2012. **84**: p. 47–52.
50. Liu, P., et al., *Ongoing pain in the MIA model of osteoarthritis.* Neurosci Lett, 2011. **493**(3): p. 72–5.

51. King, T., et al., *Unmasking the tonic-aversive state in neuropathic pain.* Nat Neurosci, 2009. **12**(11): p. 1364–6.
52. Okun, A., et al., *Transient inflammation-induced ongoing pain is driven by TRPV1 sensitive afferents.* Mol Pain, 2011. **7**: p. 4.
53. Vierck, C.J. and R.P. Yezierski, *Comparison of operant escape and reflex tests of nociceptive sensitivity.* Neurosci Biobehav Rev, 2015. **51**: p. 223–42.
54. Mauderli, A.P., A. Acosta-Rua, and C.J. Vierck, *An operant assay of thermal pain in conscious, unrestrained rats.* J Neurosci Methods, 2000. **97**(1): p. 19–29.
55. Hansen, B.D., *Assessment of pain in dogs: veterinary clinical studies.* ILAR J, 2003. **44**(3): p. 197–205.
56. Bon, K., et al., *Genetic evidence for the correlation of deep dorsal horn Fos protein immunoreactivity with tonic formalin pain behavior.* J Pain, 2002. **3**(3): p. 181–9.
57. Daneshian, M., et al., *A framework program for the teaching of alternative methods (replacement, reduction, refinement) to animal experimentation.* ALTEX, 2011. **28**(4): p. 341–52.
58. Zimmermann, M., *Ethical guidelines for investigations of experimental pain in conscious animals.* Pain, 1983. **16**(2): p. 109–110.
59. DeHaven, W. *Pain and Distress: USDA Perspective.* in *Definition of Pain and Distress and Reporting Requirements for Laboratory Animals: Proceedings of the Workshop Held June 22, 2000.* 2000. Washington, DC: National Academies Press.
60. Kentucky, U.o. *USDA Pain & Distress Categories.* 2024; Available from: https://www.research.uky.edu/division-laboratory-animal-resources/usda-pain-distress-categories.

14 Human Experimental Pain Models

Clinical Applications and Molecular Mechanisms in Drug Development

Maja Green, Mustafa Broachwala, and Amna Hassan

14.1 INTRODUCTION

The life cycle of a pharmaceutical agent can be divided into four key phases: preclinical research, clinical trials, regulatory approval, and post-marketing surveillance. This progression reflects the balance between scientific innovation and commercial feasibility that defines the pharmaceutical industry [1]. During preclinical research, *in vitro* studies of biological products or synthetic compounds help identify lead candidates, laying the foundation for drug discovery. These leads are then tested in *in vivo* animal models to evaluate their mechanisms of action, efficacy, and safety, creating an essential bridge from the laboratory to clinical application [2, 3]. The transition from preclinical to clinical research marks a pivotal moment in drug development, shifting from theoretical evaluation to real-world application (Figure 14.1).

Clinical trials follow a well-structured, three-phase progression. Phase I trials focus on safety and pharmacokinetics, typically involving a small cohort of healthy volunteers or patients to identify adverse events and establish the maximum tolerated dose. Once safety is confirmed, phase II trials assess the drug's efficacy and dose response in a population relevant to the therapeutic indication. These trials are crucial in determining whether the drug achieves the intended therapeutic effect. Phase III trials, the final stage before regulatory approval, are large-scale, multi-center studies designed to confirm efficacy, monitor adverse effects, and gather comprehensive data required for regulatory submission. After completing phase III, the drug undergoes review by authorities, such as the FDA, for potential market approval.

The process of drug development is outlined across four major stages: research and development (3–6 years), preclinical studies (1 year), clinical trials (4–7 years), and review and approval (1–2 years). During the research and development phase, target identification, compound screening, and lead identification are performed. Preclinical studies involve *in vitro* and *in vivo* studies, along with toxicity testing,

DOI: 10.1201/9781003094302-14

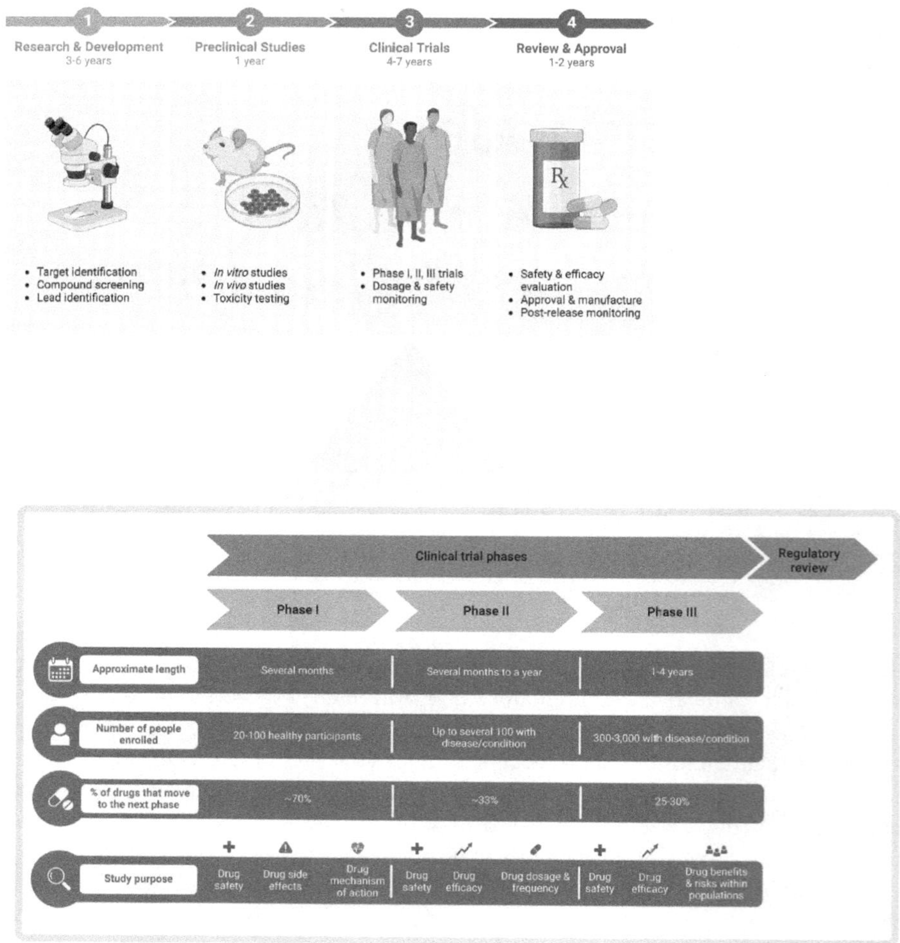

FIGURE 14.1 Overview of drug development stages and clinical trial phases.

to ensure the safety of the compound before advancing to human trials. Clinical trials progress through three phases: Phase I trials evaluate drug safety and side effects in 20–100 healthy participants, with approximately 70% of drugs advancing to the next phase. Phase II assesses efficacy in 100–300 participants with the condition being studied, with about 33% of drugs progressing to phase III. Phase III involves 300–3,000 participants, assessing drug efficacy, dosage, safety, and long-term effects, with 25–30% of drugs advancing to approval. Review and approval ensures regulatory evaluation of safety and efficacy data, approval, manufacturing, and post-release monitoring. The second panel illustrates the distinct characteristics of clinical trial phases, highlighting the number of participants, duration, and study focus for each phase.

Despite significant financial investment, often hundreds of millions of dollars, many drugs, particularly pain therapeutics, fail in phase II or III trials. Pain, as a complex and multifaceted condition, presents unique challenges due to variability in patient populations, subjective outcome measures, and the intricate nature of pain pathways. The failure of pain medications in late-stage trials represents both a scientific setback and a substantial financial loss for companies that have invested years in development [1, 4, 5]. In this context, human experimental pain models (HEPMs) provide a valuable tool for early-stage drug development, offering critical "go/no-go" signals during phase I trials. These models allow researchers to assess a drug's ability to modulate pain responses in real time, reducing the risk of costly failures in later phases. By simulating pain conditions, such as thermal or mechanical stimuli, HEPMs evaluate how drugs affect nociceptive pathways. Advanced models, including capsaicin-induced hyperalgesia or neuropathic pain paradigms, are used to assess drug effects on more complex, chronic pain conditions [6–9].

The clinical and commercial implications of HEPMs are substantial. Clinically, these models provide early insights into a drug's interaction with pain pathways, informing dosing strategies, identifying target populations, and predicting potential adverse effects. From a commercial perspective, early data on pain modulation helps mitigate the financial risks associated with late-stage failures due to unanticipated side effects or inadequate efficacy. By offering a controlled, reproducible framework to evaluate drug effects, HEPMs can shorten development timelines, increase the likelihood of regulatory approval, and more efficiently bring effective pain therapies to market. Preclinical research plays an integral role in shaping these models. Animal pain studies using thermal, mechanical, or chemical stimuli (e.g., hot plate tests or von Frey filaments) provide foundational data that inform human experimental pain paradigms. This translational approach improves the chances that preclinical efficacy will translate into clinical success, as similar stimuli are applied to human volunteers in a controlled setting to test pharmacological interventions [10, 11].

HEPMs also enable the investigation of pharmacodynamic effects over time, aligned with a drug's pharmacokinetic profile. For example, assessing a drug's effect at peak plasma concentrations post-administration provides valuable information on both onset and duration of action [12–15]. This is especially important in pain management, where rapid onset and sustained pain relief are key therapeutic goals. Additionally, these models help clarify dose–response relationships, which are essential for optimizing dosing strategies in later trials. However, a challenge in utilizing HEPMs is ensuring precise experimental design and subject selection. Participants often undergo multiple test sessions, particularly when evaluating different pain models, requiring careful scheduling to avoid carryover effects. Adequate recovery time between sessions is critical, especially for models that induce persistent hyperalgesia, such as capsaicin or ultraviolet radiation models, where prolonged sensitization may affect subsequent tests. Ensuring proper recovery is crucial for data reliability and model validity [11, 16, 17].

Ultimately, HEPMs represent a promising strategy for improving the clinical and commercial success of new pain therapies. By providing early insights into efficacy, safety, and mechanisms of action, these models help inform critical go/no-go decisions, reducing the financial burden of late-stage failures. As pharmaceutical companies continue to invest in developing novel pain treatments, integrating HEPMs into early-stage research may prove pivotal for enhancing outcomes and accelerating the development of effective pain therapies [18, 19].

The following sections will elucidate the cold pressor (CP) test, brief thermal sensitization model, UV-B hyperalgesia model, heat/capsaicin sensitization model, and intradermal capsaicin pain model, which are commonly used to assess analgesic efficacy across a range of pain mechanisms, from nociceptive to neuropathic. These models offer controlled and reproducible insights into both peripheral and central pain pathways, supporting the development of targeted pain treatments.

14.2 COLD PRESSOR TEST: A REPRODUCIBLE MODEL FOR ASSESSING ANALGESIC EFFICACY AND PAIN MECHANISMS

The CP test is a well-established experimental pain model frequently used in both clinical and research settings to study pain mechanisms and evaluate the efficacy of analgesics. In this model, participants submerge their hand and forearm into ice-cold water (typically maintained at 1.0°C ± 0.3°C), with key outcomes such as time to onset of pain, pain intensity, and pain tolerance (measured as time to hand withdrawal) being recorded. The CP test induces a reproducible, tonic noxious cold pain stimulus, activating both peripheral nociceptors (Aδ and C fibers) and central thalamic pain processing systems. This is often accompanied by autonomic responses, such as changes in heart rate and blood pressure [20].

At the molecular level, the cold stimulus triggers the release of inflammatory mediators and modulates ion channels, such as transient receptor potential melastatin (TRPM8) and transient receptor potential vanilloid (TRPV1), which are critical to nociception. TRPM8 responds to cold temperatures, while TRPV1 plays a role in pain sensitization and the central modulation of pain. Further, the cold stimulus induces glutamate release in the dorsal horn of the spinal cord, activating NMDA receptors, which contribute to central sensitization and prolonged pain responses [21–24].

From a clinical perspective, the CP test is invaluable for assessing the analgesic effects of various drug classes. Opioids, such as morphine and fentanyl, significantly reduce pain intensity and prolong pain tolerance in the CP test by binding to μ-opioid receptors and inhibiting ascending pain pathways. Meta-analyses confirm that opioids enhance pain tolerance in CP trials, with effects comparable to those observed in clinical pain management. Gabapentin, when combined with opioids, augments analgesia through its action on calcium channels, highlighting its potential for combination therapy in reducing opioid doses and minimizing side effects.

In contrast, non-opioid analgesics, such as acetaminophen, demonstrate modest effects in the CP test, likely through modulation of serotonergic pathways and weak inhibition of COX enzymes. Results for nonsteroidal anti-inflammatory drugs (NSAIDs), like ibuprofen, have been inconsistent, possibly due to variations in methodology and differences in COX inhibition among individuals. Furthermore, serotonin-norepinephrine reuptake inhibitors (SNRIs), such as venlafaxine and amitriptyline, have shown limited efficacy in this model, suggesting a complex role for descending inhibitory pathways in cold-induced pain [25–31].

The CP test's reproducibility also makes it a valuable model for evaluating non-pharmacological therapies. Acupuncture and transcutaneous electrical nerve stimulation (TENS) have demonstrated analgesic effects, possibly by modulating endogenous opioid release and inhibiting nociceptive signals via Aβ fibers, as supported by recent clinical trials [32–34].

Variability in CP test results can stem from differences in water temperature, circulation, and participant characteristics. Even a variation as small as 2°C can significantly impact pain perception and tolerance, highlighting the need for standardized conditions. Gender differences have also been observed, with women generally reporting higher pain intensity and shorter tolerance times than men, potentially due to differences in pain processing, hormonal influences, and nociceptive thresholds [35–37].

14.2.1 Methodology

To ensure consistency, participants with extreme tolerance (those who can endure the ice bath for the maximum time) are excluded from the study. The dominant arm is preconditioned in a 35°C warm bath for 2 minutes, followed by submersion of at least 16 cm into the cold-water tank, maintained at 1.0°C ± 0.3°C with continuous circulation. The test duration is capped at 120 seconds to prevent prolonged exposure, and participants provide continuous pain intensity ratings, while pain tolerance time is measured (Figure 14.2).

In this figure, the subject's dominant hand and forearm are preconditioned in a warm bath at 35°C for 2 minutes to normalize skin temperature. The participant's hand is then submerged in a 1°C ice water bath, with continuous circulation to maintain a constant temperature. Pain intensity and tolerance are recorded throughout the

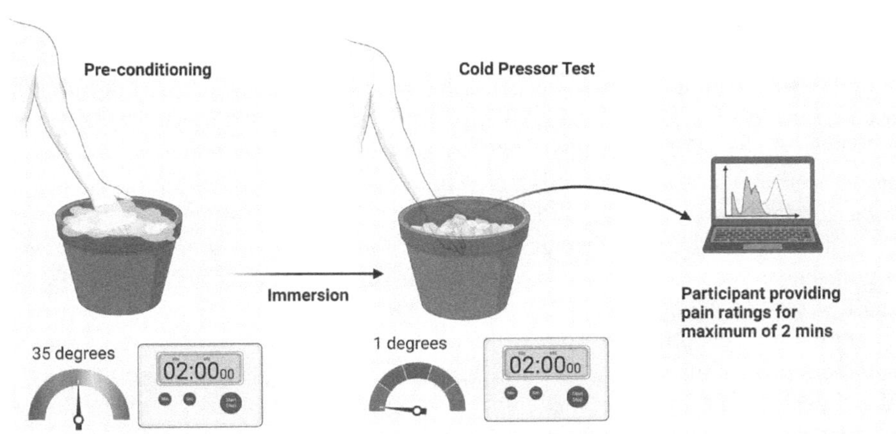

FIGURE 14.2 Methodology of the cold pressor (CP) test for pain assessment.

immersion, with the subject providing continuous pain ratings while submerged for a maximum duration of 2 minutes. Data is captured in real time, showing the subject's pain response over time.

The CP test's simplicity, reproducibility, and ability to activate both peripheral and central pain pathways make it an ideal model for studying pain mechanisms, assessing analgesic efficacy, and understanding variability in pain tolerance across different populations.

14.3 BRIEF THERMAL SENSITIZATION MODEL: A NONINVASIVE TOOL FOR ASSESSING CENTRAL SENSITIZATION AND ANALGESIC EFFICACY

The brief thermal sensitization model is a widely utilized, noninvasive paradigm for inducing secondary hyperalgesia, providing a practical and efficient alternative to more intense models, such as intradermal capsaicin injection or the time-consuming UV-B and heat/capsaicin sensitization models. This model reliably mimics the mechanisms underlying central sensitization and secondary hyperalgesia, making it a valuable tool in pain research. It is frequently used in the assessment of analgesic efficacy and to explore the development of opioid tolerance [38, 39].

In this model, heat application sensitizes peripheral nociceptors and induces a central sensitization process characterized by increased excitability of dorsal horn neurons. This sensitization is mediated by the activation of key molecular pathways, including NMDA receptor upregulation and the release of excitatory neurotransmitters, such as glutamate and substance P. The transition from acute thermal pain to secondary hyperalgesia involves the amplification of pain signals via windup phenomena and long-term potentiation, resulting in allodynia.

The brief thermal sensitization model has proven to be sensitive to both opioid and gabapentin-mediated analgesia. Gabapentin, which acts by inhibiting voltage-gated calcium channels and reducing excitatory neurotransmitter release, has demonstrated efficacy in attenuating thermal-induced hyperalgesia, further supporting its use in clinical settings for conditions involving neuropathic pain. Additionally, opioids have shown efficacy in this model by activating μ-opioid receptors and dampening nociceptive signal transmission (Figure 14.3). However, the model has also been employed to investigate the development of opioid tolerance, a critical issue in chronic opioid therapy. Repeated opioid administration has been associated with diminished efficacy in reducing hyperalgesia in this model, underscoring the clinical challenge of managing opioid tolerance [40–43].

On the pre-synaptic side, opioids, such as fentanyl and morphine, bind to opioid receptors and inhibit the release of glutamate. This is mediated by G protein–coupled receptor (GPCR) activation, which decreases GIRK channel activity and lowers SNARE complex formation, reducing neurotransmitter release.

Recent clinical trials have validated the model's utility in distinguishing between different analgesic mechanisms. Studies evaluating gabapentin's role in reducing central sensitization have reported a significant reduction in the area of secondary hyperalgesia, reinforcing the model's translational value. Opioid studies have also

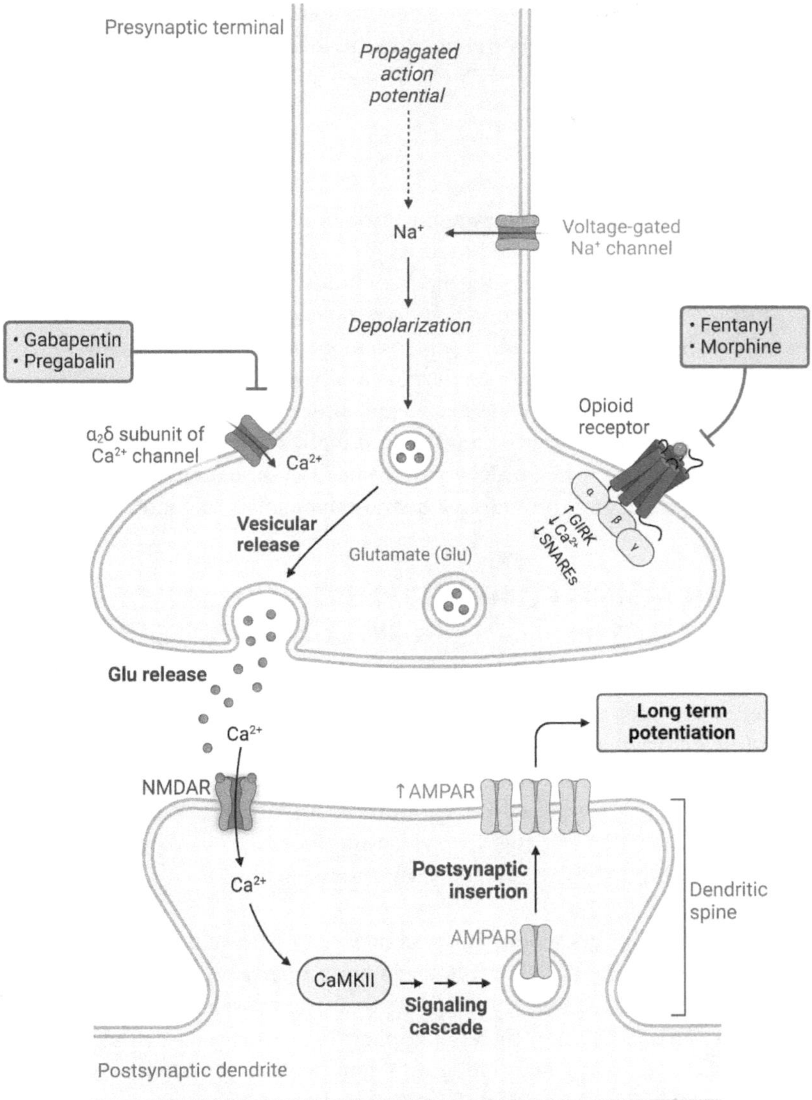

FIGURE 14.3 Mechanisms of synaptic transmission and modulation by pharmacological agents in pain pathways. The pre-synaptic terminal is activated by a propagated action potential, leading to Na^+ influx through voltage-gated sodium channels, followed by membrane depolarization. Depolarization triggers Ca^{2+} influx through voltage-gated calcium channels containing the $\alpha_2\delta$ subunit, the target of gabapentin and pregabalin. Calcium influx facilitates vesicular release of glutamate (Glu) into the synaptic cleft. In the synaptic cleft, glutamate binds to NMDARs on the post-synaptic membrane, leading to Ca^{2+} influx and the activation of the Ca^{2+}/calmodulin-dependent protein kinase II (CaMKII) signaling cascade. This promotes the insertion of α-amino-3-hydroxy-5-methyl-4-isoxazolepropionic acid receptors (AMPARs) into the post-synaptic membrane, contributing to long-term potentiation at the synapse, which is associated with enhanced synaptic strength and pain signal transmission.

highlighted the model's sensitivity in detecting early signs of tolerance, with data indicating reduced efficacy in both hyperalgesia area size and pain thresholds after prolonged opioid use [44].

14.3.1 Methodology

Brief thermal sensitization involves application of a 2 × 4 cm thermal probe to the anterior thigh. This probe is heated to 45°C for 5 minutes, inducing a localized area of sensitization. After removing the heat stimulus, a 26-gauge von Frey filament is used to map the region of secondary hyperalgesia. The assessment begins at a non-painful peripheral region and progresses tangentially toward the thermal application site. Subjects report pain or tenderness as the filament moves closer to the sensitized area, allowing researchers to define the borders of the hyperalgesia zone. This process is repeated from different angles until eight points around the perimeter of the area are determined. The borders are outlined, and the area of secondary hyperalgesia is measured in cm^2, providing a quantifiable metric of central sensitization.

14.4 CLINICAL AND COMMERCIAL SIGNIFICANCE OF UV-B HYPERALGESIA MODEL IN PRECLINICAL RESEARCH

The use of ultraviolet radiation (UV-B) to induce hyperalgesia is a well-established and reproducible model for studying peripheral pain mechanisms. Unlike models that induce continuous, spontaneous pain, the UV-B model enables localized hyperalgesic inflammation, allowing for precise assessment of both mechanical and thermal pain thresholds without the confounding influence of central sensitization. This model is especially valuable for evaluating the efficacy of peripherally acting analgesics, including NSAIDs, selective cyclooxygenase-2 (COX-2) inhibitors, and opioids [23].

The UV-B model offers unique insights into early pain sensitization mechanisms by specifically activating peripheral nociceptors. In particular, it targets silent nociceptors, normally inactive sensory receptors that become sensitized in the context of inflammation. This activation triggers peripheral sensitization, mediated by inflammatory mediators, such as histamine, prostaglandins, and cytokines, like TNF-α and IL–6. These molecules act on ion channels, such as TRPV1, TRPA1, and ASIC3, which modulate nociceptive signaling. Additionally, studies on ultraviolet erythema formation have demonstrated that mast cells play a critical role. Mast cell degranulation, triggered by UV-C radiation, releases histamine and other pro-inflammatory mediators, contributing to both erythema and hyperalgesia observed following UV exposure [21, 23, 45–47].

The controlled nature of UV-B-induced hyperalgesia allows for the isolation and precise examination of pharmacological interventions' effects on peripheral pain pathways. This targeted approach is particularly useful for studying agents that modulate peripheral pain mechanisms, avoiding the complexity introduced by central sensitization. Compared to models like capsaicin-induced hyperalgesia which involve both peripheral and central pain pathways, the UV-B model provides a more focused evaluation of peripherally acting analgesics. This distinction is crucial for determining their efficacy in treating conditions associated with peripheral sensitization, such as osteoarthritis and post-surgical pain [48, 49].

Pharmacological studies using the UV-B model have provided valuable, though sometimes variable, results. For example, morphine has been shown to increase pain thresholds in UV-B-treated areas, but it does not affect mechanical pain thresholds. Remifentanil increases heat pain tolerance but has a limited effect on secondary hyperalgesia. COX-2 inhibitors, such as rofecoxib, have demonstrated efficacy by increasing heat pain tolerance and reducing the area of secondary hyperalgesia. Ibuprofen has also been found to reduce mechanical hyperalgesia. Interestingly, gabapentin, which is effective in some neuropathic pain models, has shown no significant effect on UV-B-induced hyperalgesia or on enhancing the effects of remifentanil. These mixed outcomes underscore the importance of matching pharmacological interventions to specific pain mechanisms, with the UV-B model being especially suitable for testing agents targeting peripheral sensitization [48, 50].

From a commercial perspective, the UV-B model holds great promise for reducing the risks associated with drug development for pain therapies. It provides early-stage, mechanistic insights into how compounds modulate peripheral pain pathways, offering pharmaceutical companies a strategic advantage in conducting proof-of-concept studies. Given the high cost of developing analgesics, especially for chronic pain, where many drugs fail in phase II or III trials due to inadequate efficacy or safety concerns, integrating the UV-B model into preclinical research can inform critical go/no-go decisions before advancing to expensive clinical trials. By focusing on primary hyperalgesia, the model enables a more targeted approach to developing treatments for conditions driven by peripheral sensitization, such as inflammatory pain disorders.

Aligning drug testing with the pharmacokinetics and pharmacodynamics of UV-B-induced pain allows researchers to assess the temporal relationship between drug administration and pain modulation. This provides valuable data on both the onset and the duration of analgesic effects, with important implications for the commercial development of pain medications. Compounds that demonstrate rapid onset and sustained efficacy in preclinical models are more likely to succeed in clinical trials, meeting market demands for fast-acting, long-lasting pain relief therapies.

14.4.1 Methodology

Determining the minimum effective dose (MED) of UV-B irradiation is crucial before initiating hyperalgesia studies, due to interindividual variability in UV-B sensitivity. Testing is typically conducted on areas with minimal sun exposure, such as the inner thigh or volar forearm, to ensure consistent UV-B absorption. The chosen site is cleaned with an antiseptic solution to remove any contaminants that might interfere with absorption.

Five distinct skin spots are irradiated using a UV-B multi-tester, which delivers graded doses of UV-B light through specific filters. The starting doses range from 100 to 400 mJ/cm^2, with the highest dose passing through an unfiltered aperture and progressively lower doses attenuated by up to 60%. The exposure time is kept

TABLE 14.1
Erythema Formation Scores

	Erythema Formation Score
0	No erythema
1	Very slight erythema (barely perceptible, equivalent to the MED)
2	Well-defined erythema
3	Moderate to severe erythema
4	Severe erythema (beet redness) to eschar formation preventing erythema grading

Note: This table provides a standardized method for grading erythema in response to UV-B irradiation, ensuring consistency in determining the MED for subsequent hyperalgesia testing.

under 60 seconds to avoid tissue damage while ensuring an effective inflammatory response. The MED is determined 24 hours after irradiation, coinciding with the peak of inflammation and hyperalgesia [20].

The erythema formation score (Table 14.1) is used to assess the MED, with a score of 1 (very slight erythema) considered the MED. Subjects who do not develop a MED are excluded from further study [51–53].

For the testing phase, a different site is irradiated with 3× the MED. Assessments are conducted 24 hours after irradiation and repeated approximately 6 hours after administering the experimental medication. Inflammation and flare responses are measured using color Doppler imaging to quantify localized blood flow changes. Heat pain thresholds and heat pain tolerance are assessed using a thermal sensory testing device. A computer-assisted Peltier device is applied to the irradiated area, and the temperature is increased by 1°C per second until the subject perceives heat (heat threshold) or pain (heat pain threshold). For heat pain tolerance, the subject terminates the test when the heat becomes intolerable. A maximum temperature of 50°C is set to avoid burn injury. This methodology ensures reliable, valid assessments of both inflammatory responses and pain thresholds in the context of UV-B-induced hyperalgesia.

14.5 HEAT/CAPSAICIN SENSITIZATION PAIN MODEL: METHODOLOGY AND CLINICAL UTILITY

The heat/capsaicin sensitization model is a well-established, noninvasive paradigm that induces areas of both primary and secondary hyperalgesia, which can be periodically reactivated with heat application. This model allows for the induction of cutaneous hyperalgesia without causing tissue injury, making it a suitable method for testing the efficacy of oral analgesic agents. Unlike the intradermal capsaicin injection model, which is associated with significant pain, or the burn injury model, which carries a risk of tissue damage, the heat/capsaicin model is a safer and more patient-friendly alternative for pain research [54]. Reactivation of hyperalgesia is achieved by reheating the sensitized skin to 40°C for 5 minutes at 40-minute intervals throughout the study day. This rekindling maintains central sensitization by sustaining peripheral nociceptive input. Studies have demonstrated that secondary hyperalgesia to von Frey filament stimulation is more consistent and reproducible compared to brush stimulation, making it a preferred assessment tool in this model.

Pharmacologically, this model has shown sensitivity to opioids, such as remifentanil, oral hydromorphone, and morphine, demonstrating its utility in evaluating opioid analgesics. However, the combination of dextromethorphan and morphine was not found to be superior to morphine alone. Additionally, lamotrigine, an anticonvulsant with sodium channel–blocking properties, had no significant effect on pain modulation in this model, highlighting the specificity of the heat/capsaicin model for certain analgesic classes.

14.5.1 Methodology

To initiate sensitization, the stimulation site is outlined by tracing the thermode (22.8 cm^2) on the volar t of the dominant forearm or anterior thigh. Sensitization is initiated by heating the skin to 45°C for 5 minutes using the thermode. Immediately following heat application, 0.075% topical capsaicin cream is applied to the heated skin for 30 minutes. After this period, the capsaicin is removed, and the areas of secondary hyperalgesia are quantified.

Quantification of secondary hyperalgesia involves stimulating the skin using a 1 in foam brush and a 26-gauge von Frey filament along four linear paths around the sensitization site. Stimulation begins outside the hyperalgesic area and moves toward the treated area in 5 mm steps at 1-second intervals until the subject reports a significant change in sensation, such as burning, tenderness, or pricking. The boundaries of the hyperalgesic area are marked, and the rostral-caudal and lateral-medial dimensions are measured to calculate the surface area of hyperalgesia. Throughout the study day, reactivation is performed at 50-minute intervals, reheating the sensitized area to 40°C for 5 minutes using the same thermode. Reactivation is typically repeated four times during the day, with areas of secondary hyperalgesia to both brush and von Frey filament stimulation being reassessed after each reactivation period.

The ability of this model to produce reproducible areas of hyperalgesia, combined with its sensitivity to various analgesic agents, underscores its clinical significance for pain research. This model allows for a controlled and repeatable examination of pain mechanisms, particularly the effects of pharmacological agents on peripheral sensitization and central sensitization, without inducing excessive discomfort or injury in subjects.

14.6 INTRADERMAL CAPSAICIN PAIN MODEL: METHODOLOGY AND CLINICAL UTILITY

The intradermal capsaicin pain model is a widely utilized and safe method for inducing both primary and secondary hyperalgesia. In contrast to the heat/capsaicin sensitization model, which involves prolonged stimulation and rekindling, intradermal capsaicin results in a brief yet intense painful stimulus, followed by a long-lasting area of secondary hyperalgesia. The injection of capsaicin produces an immediate, intense stinging sensation at the injection site, which rapidly dissipates but is followed by a persistent tactile hypersensitivity in the surrounding area, commonly referred to as secondary tactile allodynia. This model is particularly significant in testing the analgesic efficacy of a broad range of pharmacological agents, delivered via oral, intravenous, or intraspinal routes. Its utility spans multiple drug classes, including opioids, NMDA antagonists, cannabis derivatives, sodium channel antagonists, and tricyclic antidepressants. Notably, opioids and NMDA antagonists have shown significant efficacy in reducing both pain and allodynia in this model, underscoring their role in pain modulation. Interestingly, cannabis has demonstrated a dose-dependent effect, with medium doses (4%) reducing pain, while higher doses (7%) paradoxically increased pain. In contrast, intravenous lidocaine and tricyclic antidepressants have shown minimal effect in this model, highlighting its specificity for certain analgesic mechanisms [54].

14.6.1 Methodology

Using a 27-gauge or 30-gauge hypodermic needle, 10–25 μl of capsaicin solution (10 mg/ml in 20% cyclodextrin or 10 mg/ml in 15% Tween-80) is injected intradermally on the forearm or anterior thigh. Following the injection, spontaneous pain intensity is measured using the visual analog scale (VAS), with assessments conducted immediately after injection (time 0) and at 5-minute intervals for the first 20 minutes, followed by 15-minute intervals up to 60 minutes. Additionally, elicited pain intensity can be assessed using von Frey filament stimulation, stroking with a 1 in foam brush and a 40°C thermal stimulus applied to the injection site, following the same time intervals as earlier. To quantify secondary hyperalgesia, a 1 in foam brush and 26-gauge (5.8) von Frey hair are used to stimulate the area surrounding the injection site. Stimulation is performed along 4 to 8 linear paths (vertical, horizontal, and diagonal) around the injection site in 5 mm steps at 1-second intervals. The stimulation begins well outside the hyperalgesic area (where no pain response is reported) and continues toward the treated area until the subject reports a definite change in sensation (e.g., burning, tenderness, or increased pricking). The boundaries of the hyperalgesic area are marked on the skin, and both rostral-caudal and lateral-medial dimensions are measured to calculate the total surface area of hyperalgesia. If the subject experiences intolerable pain following the injection, ice can be applied until the pain subsides. For consistency, and to improve reproducibility, it is recommended that subjects undergo a training session prior to formal testing. During this session, they are educated on the methodology and exposed to intradermal capsaicin to familiarize themselves with the procedure. Subjects who report a pain score of 4 or less following the injection should be excluded, as their responses may not reflect sufficient hyperalgesic sensitivity. The ability to discriminate between normal and hyperalgesic skin is critical for accurate assessment. Moreover, it has been suggested that maintaining consistent room and skin temperatures during testing may reduce variability across subjects. This can be achieved by controlling the room temperature or by using an infrared heat lamp with adjustable settings to standardize skin temperature for all participants.

14.7 DISCUSSION

The integration of HEPMs into the drug development process offers a transformative approach to evaluating analgesic compounds. By simulating specific pain mechanisms, these models allow for early-phase insights into the efficacy, safety, and pharmacodynamics of potential therapeutics. This is particularly relevant for pain therapies, where the high failure rate in phase II and III trials underscores the need for robust preclinical and early clinical tools to predict therapeutic success. The models discussed in this chapter, ranging from the UV-B hyperalgesia model to the intradermal capsaicin model, highlight the breadth and utility of HEPMs in targeting both peripheral and central sensitization pathways. From a clinical perspective, these models provide critical data on dose–response relationships, onset of action, and duration of efficacy, which are key determinants in the success of analgesic agents. For example, the UV-B model has shown clear differentiation between drugs targeting primary hyperalgesia, such as COX-2 inhibitors and opioids, while the intradermal capsaicin model has proven to be effective in assessing drugs targeting secondary hyperalgesia, particularly for agents like NMDA antagonists and cannabis derivatives. The ability to test compounds in controlled settings allows for precise modulation of pharmacological parameters, thereby improving the likelihood of clinical success.

Commercially, the value of HEPMs lies in their ability to de-risk the development of analgesic drugs. Given the significant financial investments required for the development of novel pain therapies, these models provide early go/no-go decision points, minimizing the risk of costly failures in later trial phases. For instance, the heat/capsaicin sensitization model and CPT have shown sensitivity to opioid analgesics, allowing researchers to evaluate tolerance development and synergistic effects when combined with other agents, such as gabapentin. Such insights can guide commercial decisions and inform regulatory submissions, particularly in the increasingly competitive market for pain therapeutics.

While these models offer substantial advantages, several challenges remain. For one, the reproducibility of results across different patient populations and settings requires careful attention to experimental design and methodological consistency. Variability in factors such as skin temperature and pain tolerance thresholds can influence outcomes, emphasizing the need for rigorous control of experimental conditions. In models like UV-B hyperalgesia and intradermal capsaicin, ensuring accurate subject selection and adequate recovery periods between tests is crucial for obtaining valid data.

Further, the CPT and thermal sensitization models demonstrate the complexity of pain mechanisms, particularly the involvement of central sensitization. The role of NMDA receptor activation and glutamate release in these models underscores the challenge of developing therapies that can address both acute and chronic pain mechanisms. These findings highlight the need for further refinement of these models to better predict long-term clinical outcomes, particularly in chronic pain conditions where central sensitization plays a dominant role.

14.8 CONCLUSION

HEPMs represent a critical innovation in the development of pain therapeutics, offering detailed insights into the mechanisms of pain modulation and enabling early evaluation of pharmacological interventions. By incorporating these models into the early stages of drug development, pharmaceutical companies can reduce the risks associated with late-stage trial failures and streamline the pathway from preclinical research to clinical implementation.

The models explored in this chapter, ranging from UV-B hyperalgesia to intradermal capsaicin and CPT, demonstrate their unique contributions to assessing the efficacy and safety of analgesic agents. By targeting peripheral sensitization and central pain pathways, these models provide a nuanced understanding of pain mechanisms and facilitate the development of therapies tailored to specific pain conditions, including osteoarthritis, post-surgical pain, and inflammatory pain disorders.

Despite the challenges of ensuring reproducibility and managing variability, the future of pain research will undoubtedly continue to rely on these models for their ability to simulate human pain experiences in a controlled, ethical, and scientifically valid manner. As the demand for effective and safer pain treatments grows, HEPMs will remain integral to the discovery and development of novel analgesics, ultimately improving patient outcomes and addressing the unmet needs in pain management.

REFERENCES

1. Sedgwick, P., *What are the four phases of clinical research trials*? BMJ, 2014. **348**: p. g3727.
2. Froney, M.M., et al., *Behind the screen: drug discovery using the big data of phenotypic analysis*. Front Educ (Lausanne), 2024. **9**.
3. Pibiri, I., *Recent advances: heterocycles in drugs and drug discovery*. Int J Mol Sci, 2024. **25**(17).
4. Dal-Re, R., et al., *Using the phases of clinical development of medicines to describe clinical trials assessing other interventions is widespread but not useful*. J Clin Epidemiol, 2023. **161**: p. 157–63.
5. Nguyen, V., B.V. Sweet, and T. Macek, *Defining the phases of clinical trials*. Am J Health Syst Pharm, 2006. **63**(8): p. 710–1.
6. Rodrigues, J., et al., *Strategies for pain management after extraction of primary teeth: a systematic review of randomized clinical trials*. Curr Pediatr Rev, 2024.
7. Pedersen, J.R., et al., *Clinical improvements due to specific effects and placebo effects in conservative interventions and changes observed with no treatment in randomized controlled trials of patients with chronic nonspecific low back pain: a systematic review and meta-analysis*. Pain, 2024. **165**(6): p. 1217–32.
8. Langford, D.J., et al., *Use of patient-reported global assessment measures in clinical trials of chronic pain treatments: ACTTION systematic review and considerations*. Pain, 2024.
9. Barakji, J., et al., *Tramadol for chronic pain in adults: protocol for a systematic review with meta-analysis and trial sequential analysis of randomised clinical trials*. Syst Rev, 2023. **12**(1): p. 145.
10. Petersen-Felix, S. and L. Arendt-Nielsen, *From pain research to pain treatment: the role of human experimental pain models*. Best Pract Res Clin Anaesthesiol, 2002. **16**(4): p. 667–80.
11. Staahl, C. and A.M. Drewes, *Experimental human pain models: a review of standardised methods for preclinical testing of analgesics*. Basic Clin Pharmacol Toxicol, 2004. **95**(3): p. 97–111.

12. Hayley, A.C., et al., *The acute and residual effects of escalating, analgesic-range doses of ketamine on driving performance: a simulator study*. Prog Neuropsychopharmacol Biol Psychiatry, 2018. **86**: p. 83–8.
13. Hayley, A.C., et al., *Neurocognitive performance under combined regimens of ketamine-dexmedetomidine and ketamine-fentanyl in healthy adults: a randomised trial*. Prog Neuropsychopharmacol Biol Psychiatry, 2019. **94**: p. 109647.
14. Hayley, A.C., et al., *Driving simulator performance after administration of analgesic doses of ketamine with dexmedetomidine or Fentanyl*. J Clin Psychopharmacol, 2019. **39**(5): p. 446–54.
15. Hayley, A., et al., *Neurocognitive and behavioural performance of healthy volunteers receiving an increasing analgesic-range infusion of ketamine*. Psychopharmacology (Berl), 2018. **235**(4): p. 1273–82.
16. Svensson, P., *What can human experimental pain models teach us about clinical TMD*? Arch Oral Biol, 2007. **52**(4): p. 391–4.
17. Enggaard, T.P., et al., *The effects of gabapentin in human experimental pain models*. Scand J Pain, 2010. **1**(3): p. 143–8.
18. Oertel, B.G. and J. Lotsch, *Clinical pharmacology of analgesics assessed with human experimental pain models: bridging basic and clinical research*. Br J Pharmacol, 2013. **168**(3): p. 534–53.
19. Magerl, W. and T. Klein, *Chapter 33 Experimental human models of neuropathic pain*. Handb Clin Neurol, 2006. **81**: p. 503–16.
20. Modir, J.G. and M.S. Wallace, *Human experimental pain models 2: the cold pressor model*. Methods Mol Biol, 2010. **617**: p. 165–8.
21. Skaper, S.D., *TRPV-ing up pain for a long life*. CNS Neurol Disord Drug Targets, 2014. **13**(6): p. 926.
22. Sato, J., et al., *Expression of capsaicin receptor TRPV-1 in synovial tissues of patients with symptomatic internal derangement of the temporomandibular joint and joint pain*. Oral Surg Oral Med Oral Pathol Oral Radiol Endod, 2005. **100**(6): p. 674–81.
23. Medeiros, P., et al., *CB(1)-cannabinoid-, TRPV(1)-vanilloid- and NMDA-glutamatergic-receptor-signalling systems interact in the prelimbic cerebral cortex to control neuropathic pain symptoms*. Brain Res Bull, 2020. **165**: p. 118–28.
24. Lakshmi, S. and P.G. Joshi, *Co-activation of P2Y2 receptor and TRPV channel by ATP: implications for ATP induced pain*. Cell Mol Neurobiol, 2005. **25**(5): p. 819–32.
25. Umeda, M. and A. Okifuji, *Prediction of pain responses to subsequent cold pressor test via baseline heart rate variability in healthy adults*. Eur J Pain, 2022. **26**(8): p. 1811–20.
26. Stephens, B.Y., et al., *Sympathetic transduction at rest and during cold pressor test in young healthy non-Hispanic Black and White women*. Am J Physiol Regul Integr Comp Physiol, 2023. **325**(6): p. R682–91.
27. Stavres, J., et al., *Hemodynamic responses to the cold pressor test in individuals with metabolic syndrome: a case-control study in a multiracial sample of adults*. J Hum Hypertens, 2024. **38**(9): p. 655–62.
28. Siegel, E.Y., G.P. Cassidy, and M.J. Telch, *Validity of the distress tolerance inventory in predicting response to the Cold-Pressor Test*. Cogn Behav Ther, 2024. **53**(5): p. 508–523.
29. Kogelman, L.J.A., et al., *Multi-omics to predict changes during cold pressor test*. BMC Genomics, 2022. **23**(1): p. 759.
30. Fanninger, S., et al., *Water temperature during the cold pressor test: a scoping review*. Physiol Behav, 2023. **271**: p. 114354.
31. Ege, F., et al., *Effects of the cold pressor test on popliteal vein diameter, flow velocity, and blood flow in the lower limb in 60 healthy individuals*. Med Sci Monit, 2024. **30**: p. e944560.
32. Wolfe, D., B. Rosenstein, and M. Fortin, *The effect of EMS, IFC, and TENS on patient-reported outcome measures for chronic low back pain: a systematic review and meta-analysis*. Front Pain Res (Lausanne), 2024. **5**: p. 1346694.

33. Vance, C.G.T., et al., *Using TENS for pain control: update on the state of the evidence.* Medicina (Kaunas), 2022. **58**(10).
34. Ogren, C., et al., *High-frequency, high-intensity TENS compared to standard treatment with opioids for postoperative pain relief after laparoscopic cholecystectomy: a multicentre randomized controlled trial.* Eur J Pain, 2024.
35. Patel, A., V. Palayeker, and P. Shekane, *Optimal perioperative pain management of the transgender patient for gender affirming surgery: a scoping review.* Curr Pain Headache Rep, 2024. **28**(7): p. 663–671.
36. Haque, R., et al., *Age and gender differences in the relationship between chronic pain and dementia among older australians.* Value Health, 2024.
37. Chang, J.H., et al., *Role of ERK in gender difference of fibromyalgia pain.* Mol Pain, 2024. **20**: p. 17448069241261940.
38. Hansen, M.S., et al., *Is heat pain detection threshold associated with the area of secondary hyperalgesia following brief thermal sensitization? A study of healthy volunteers—design and detailed plan of analysis.* BMC Anesthesiol, 2016. **16**(1): p. 28.
39. Hansen, M.S., et al., *Heat pain detection threshold is associated with the area of secondary hyperalgesia following brief thermal sensitization: a study of healthy male volunteers.* J Pain Res, 2017. **10**: p. 265–74.
40. Mukhomedzyanov, A.V., et al., *The Role of delta(2)-Opioid Receptors in the Regulation of Tolerance of Isolated Cardiomyocytes to Hypoxia and Reoxygenation.* Bull Exp Biol Med, 2024. **176**(4): p. 433–6.
41. Han, X., et al., *Opioid-induced hyperalgesia and tolerance are driven by HCN Ion channels.* J Neurosci, 2024. **44**(6).
42. Echeverria-Villalobos, M., et al., *The role of neuroinflammation in the transition of acute to chronic pain and the opioid-induced hyperalgesia and tolerance.* Front Pharmacol, 2023. **14**: p. 1297931.
43. Coffey, K.R. and J.F. Neumaier, *A unique role for cAMP signaling in microglia during opioid tolerance and withdrawal.* Neuropsychopharmacology, 2024. **49**(1): p. 331–2.
44. Stine, C., et al., *Heat shock protein 90 inhibitors block the antinociceptive effects of opioids in mouse chemotherapy-induced neuropathy and cancer bone pain models.* Pain, 2020. **161**(8): p. 1798–807.
45. Rukwied, R., et al., *Slow depolarizing stimuli differentially activate mechanosensitive and silent C nociceptors in human and pig skin.* Pain, 2020. **161**(9): p. 2119–28.
46. Prato, V., et al., *Functional and molecular characterization of mechanoinsensitive "Silent" nociceptors.* Cell Rep, 2017. **21**(11): p. 3102–15.
47. Lynn, B., *'Silent' nociceptors in the skin.* Trends Neurosci, 1991. **14**(3): p. 95.
48. Sycha, T., et al., *Rofecoxib attenuates both primary and secondary inflammatory hyperalgesia: a randomized, double blinded, placebo controlled crossover trial in the UV-B pain model.* Pain, 2005. **113**(3): p. 316–22.
49. Rossler, B., et al., *Central origin of pinprick hyperalgesia adjacent to an UV-B induced inflammatory skin pain model in healthy volunteers.* Scand J Pain, 2013. **4**(1): p. 40–5.
50. Modir, J.G. and M.S. Wallace, *Human experimental pain models 1: the ultraviolet light UV-B pain model.* Methods Mol Biol, 2010. **617**: p. 159–64.
51. von Ardenne, M. and P.G. Reitnauer, *[Erythema formation as a cause of cell damage chain reaction with poisoning of lysosomal enzymes in low skin pH-Erythema prevention by multiphased therapy by hyperthermy with a two chamber tub].* Z Naturforsch B, 1970. **25**(8): p. 872–84.
52. Valtonen, E.J., *Studies of the mechanism of ultra-violet erythema formation. V. Changes in the fine structure of mast cells of the skin during the process of ultra-violet erythema caused by waveband UV-C.* Acta Derm Venereol, 1968. **48**(3): p. 203–11.
53. Kockott, D., et al., *New approach to develop optimized sunscreens that enable cutaneous vitamin D formation with minimal erythema risk.* PLoS One, 2016. **11**(1): p. e0145509.
54. Modir, J.G. and M.S. Wallace, *Human experimental pain models 3: heat/capsaicin sensitization and intradermal capsaicin models.* Methods Mol Biol, 2010. **617**: p. 169–74.

15 Psychological Aspects of Pain
A Focus on Depression

Thomas Rutledge

15.1 INTRODUCTION

Depression is among the most frequent psychiatric comorbidities of chronic pain. Although depression is known to be common in the United States, associated with increased medical costs, and established as a predictor of disability and premature death, these patterns appear magnified among patients with chronic pain (1). For example, the 6–7% rate of depression in the general US population estimated by the National Institute of Mental Health is dwarfed by the 30–60% rate of depression among patients with chronic pain reported in the most widely cited reviews on the topic (2). Research using large populations of military veterans in the United States has further shown that depression is linked with a twofold or higher incidence of opioid prescriptions in the context of chronic pain compared to veterans with chronic pain but no depression (3). This same research also observed substantially higher rates of adverse outcomes, such as suicide, among patients with both chronic pain and depression. Given the broad and severe impact of depression on overall health, hospital systems now routinely require depression screenings in general medical settings, such as primary care (4). Despite higher depression rates among pain clinic patients compared to primary care, routine depression assessment has yet to be implemented in pain clinic settings.

This chapter will assimilate evidence from epidemiological, laboratory, and interventional research to suggest that anesthesiologists and other pain specialists can benefit from incorporating regular measurement of depression in the context of their clinical service delivery. Furthermore, this chapter will describe practical approaches to depression measurement and treatment that can be conducted by pain specialists even without the presence of mental health professionals, where these latter resources as not available. These goals will be pursued by identifying converging themes from different areas of pain research.

15.1.1 Theme 1: Epidemiology—Depression Is Distributed Unevenly across Pain Treatment Settings and May Not Present in Traditional Ways among Patients with Chronic Pain

Due to our emphasis on mean-based statistics (e.g., using averages and measures of central tendency as our metrics for evaluating efficacy), even well-trained scientists and health-care providers are prone to certain errors in applying published pain

DOI: 10.1201/9781003094302-15

research to patient care. For example, observational studies and reviews report statistics such as that 30–60% of patients with chronic pain endorse comorbid depression (5, 6). Because these papers provide limited information about variability, it is natural—and often misleading—to conclude that this average statistic applies globally to patients with chronic pain and across different medical contexts in which patients with chronic pain receive care. In contrast, papers that include data concerning patterns of variation in the depression–chronic pain relationship sometimes yield more focused conclusions. These latter insights enable data interpretations that are more accurate and actionable and are possible only when means and central tendency measures are combined with corresponding information about sources of variability.

One of the most widely cited reviews of depression in chronic pain, for example, examined how depression rates vary across levels of pain intensity and across different medical clinics (2). As seen in Figure 15.1, these results should be alarming for providers working in pain clinics. Although an already-high 27% of patients in primary care clinics met criteria for concurrent depression, the range (i.e., variability) spanned from 13% of patients in gynecology clinics receiving care for pelvic pain to 87% of patients in dental clinics receiving care for facial pain. More than 50% of patients receiving care in pain clinics and orthopedic clinics met criteria across multiple studies. Practically, this means that roughly 1 out of every 2 patients seeing a provider in the pain clinic is likely to be experiencing clinically significant depression. As in the world of real estate, when it comes to understanding the overlap between depression and chronic pain, location matters.

Why does the location of care influence rates of comorbid depression so strongly among patients with chronic pain? The simple answers are chronicity and intensity. Patients receiving their pain care from primary care providers alone tend to be patients with less complex etiologies, less intense and shorter duration of their pain symptoms, and enjoying better responses to first-line pain treatments. Since depression rates correlate with pain duration, intensity, and interference, they tend to be higher among patients receiving chronic pain treatments in more specialized clinics. Pain intensity

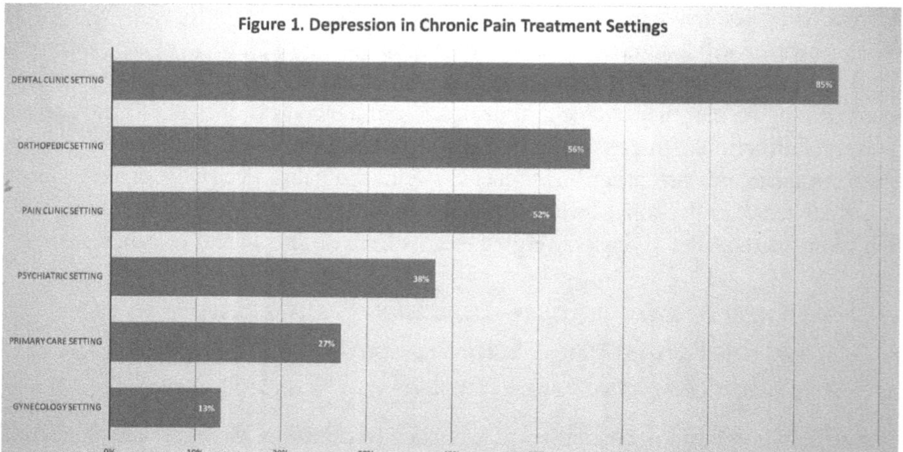

FIGURE 15.1 DEPRESSION IN CHRONIC PAIN TREATMENT SETTINGS.

Source: Thomas Rutledge. Adapted from results reported in Bair et al. (2003[2]).

alone is a reliable predictor of comorbid depression (7). Reviews indicate that depression may be prevalent at a 2–3 times greater rate among patients reporting higher intensity versus lower or moderate pain, for example, even among otherwise-similar populations of patients with chronic pain. In most cases, patients spend months or even years receiving conventional pain therapies before graduating to these specialized pain services, during which time their symptoms may progress and cause increasing levels of dysfunction. A result is higher rates of depression and more severe symptoms.

The more complex answer to the higher rates of comorbid depression seen in specialized pain clinics involves the "black hole of chronic pain." The "black hole" metaphor effectively describes the vicious cycle that frequently accompanies chronic pain. Recurrent medical visits, an ongoing focus on pain symptoms, loss of recreational activities, disruptions to lifestyle, deconditioning from reduced physical activity, weight gain, sleep impairment, and disruptions in relationships are just some of the routine consequences of chronic pain capable of independently worsening the effects of a pain condition (8). Add several of these factors together—often in negative feedback loops that sustain or progress in severity—and a significant impact on emotional health becomes increasingly likely.

Because depression is not routinely assessed in most pain clinic settings, many of the comorbid depression cases are missed (see **Table 15.1**). Research

TABLE 15.1
Depression Summary for Pain Specialists

1. What is depression?	*Depression* is a heterogeneous psychiatric condition characterized by severe, chronic, and dysfunctional changes in emotions, thinking, and behaviors. As a medical condition, depression is distinct from sadness or grief, with symptoms requiring a minimum two-week duration and adverse impact on the patient's ability to function.
2. What are the common symptoms of depression?	According to the DSM-V, depression symptoms include: • Feeling sad or having a depressed mood • Loss of interest or pleasure in activities once enjoyed • Changes in appetite—weight loss or gain unrelated to dieting • Trouble sleeping or sleeping too much • Loss of energy or increased fatigue • Increase in purposeless physical activity (e.g., inability to sit still, pacing, handwringing) or slowed movements or speech (these must be severe enough to be observable by others) • Feeling worthless or guilty • Difficulty thinking, concentrating, or making decisions • Thoughts of death or suicide Notably, a diagnosis of depression requires either sadness or loss of interest, while overall endorsing five or more of the aforementioned symptoms.
3. Did you know?	Depressive symptoms can be categorized into groups of somatic and cognitive symptoms. Somatic symptoms include loss of interest, low energy levels, and changes in weight, appetite, sleep, and sex drive. This distinction is important for patients with chronic pain and pain providers because somatic symptoms of depression are often higher among patients with medical conditions, such as chronic pain. Some research also indicates that somatic symptoms may better predict functional status and treatment outcomes for patients with chronic medical conditions.

demonstrates that medical providers frequently overlook signs of depression and other mental health conditions without a system in place for identifying them (e.g., clinical reminders, depression measures completed as part of the check-in process, etc.; 9). Although some pain providers are hesitant to systematically measure depression in their patients due to concerns about managing suicidal ideation and a lack of mental health treatment resources, it is also critical to recognize that failing to measure depression has consequences that are equally, if not more, severe. As shown in Figure 15.2, unrecognized depression undermines the efficacy of the pain provider's treatment efforts in multiple ways. Considering again that these effects may manifest in half or more of patients enrolled in pain clinic care, their cumulative toll may be enormous in the form of excess medical costs, missed appointments, impaired treatment responses, and adverse outcomes. A 2012 observational study on more than 100,000 veterans provided a demonstration of the relative effects of depression on chronic pain (3). In this sample, patients with chronic pain and comorbid depression were 1.8 (during the initial year of their pain diagnosis) to 2.7 (in their first year of VA care) times more likely to receive an opioid diagnosis compared to veterans with chronic pain and no mental health diagnosis.

Higher rates of opioid prescriptions among veterans with comorbid depression were, unfortunately, just one of many concerning implications for pain providers.

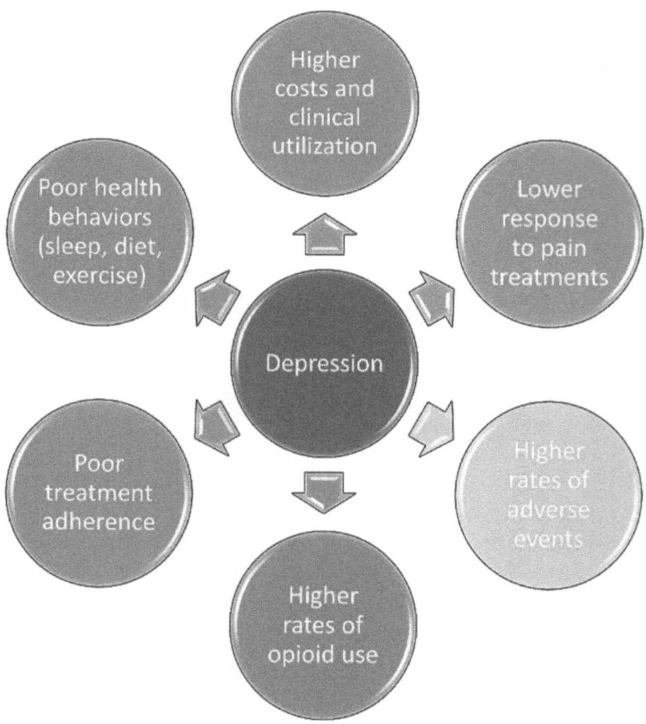

FIGURE 15.2 How unrecognized depression undermines the treatment of chronic pain.

Similar statistical patterns were evident, for example, in requests for early opioid refills and concurrent use of other sedating medications. Worse still were the markedly higher rates of adverse events, such as self-inflicted injuries, opioid and alcohol-related accidents and overdoses, and violence-related injuries. The collective picture drawn from these findings is grim. The presence of comorbid depression in patients with chronic pain is associated with a host of behavioral, psychiatric, and ethical-legal outcomes that may mitigate the effects of chronic pain treatments. These epidemiological results strongly reinforce the need to measure and monitor depression among patients participating in specialized pain clinics, where depression is more likely to be present and more likely to be severe (10).

Epidemiological research on depression and chronic pain offers one more important finding for pain providers. This is because depression often appears in disguise. Summarized at the bottom of Table 15.1 (Subsection 3), depressive symptoms among patients with chronic pain are frequently more somatic than among patients without pain or other chronic medical conditions. Instead of stereotypical sadness or tearfulness, for instance, patients with chronic pain endorse depressive symptoms, such as lack of energy, poor sleep, weight and appetite changes, and guilt. This common somatic symptom presentation is important because these symptoms are generally not captured in popular depression screening tools, such as the PHQ2, and even intentionally omitted in common depression measures, such as the HADS and GDS. For this reason, even the well-intended pain clinic provider can miss many cases of comorbid depression in their patients due to measurement systems that are designed to capture depression in its standard psychiatric form. Alternative depression measures such as the Beck Depression Inventory excel at capturing the kinds of somatic symptoms common among patients with chronic pain but are somewhat longer to administer (see Table 15.2 for expanded information about common depression measures and their relative advantages and disadvantages for pain clinic use).

This opening section scrutinized the large body of epidemiological research addressing the chronic pain and depression relationship to identify practical applications. Some of the epidemiological findings suggested applications directly counter to current practices. For example, although it is common knowledge that depression is a frequent, if unwanted, companion to chronic pain, an analysis of reviews and higher-quality observational studies indicated that specialists in pain clinics may be twice as likely to encounter depression as a comorbid condition than care providers in primary care. From this stable and replicated finding, logic would predict—erroneously—that depression would be routinely assessed in pain clinic settings. Primary care providers are more likely to measure depression in their patients with chronic pain than their pain clinic colleagues due to factors such as mandatory clinical reminders.

This section also offered findings from the epidemiological literature suggesting that the costs of overlooking depression in chronic pain settings outweigh the challenges of measuring depression by a considerable margin. Even suicidal ideation—arguably the single most common reason that pain providers may hesitate to ask about depression—is a symptom that can be managed and treated in most cases when identified. The use of a validated depression assessment tool such as those summarized in this chapter can make the measurement of depressive symptoms "painless" for patients

TABLE 15.2
Common Measures of Depression and Their Relative Advantages and Disadvantages in Pain Clinic Settings

Depression Assessment Tool	Primary Advantage/Primary Disadvantage
Patient Health Questionnaire (PHQ2 and PHQ9)	• Advantage: Among the briefest measures of depression and assesses the same symptoms used by the DSM-V for diagnosing depression • Disadvantage: High false-positive rate with PHQ2 and does not assess many somatic depressive symptoms that are common among patients with chronic pain
Beck Depression Inventory (I and II)	• Advantage: Contains a more comprehensive selection of depressive symptoms, including somatic symptoms • Disadvantage: 21 items in length, more than twice as long as the PHQ9
Hospital Anxiety and Depression Scale (HADS)	• Advantage: Brief measure designed for medical patient populations • Disadvantage: Intentionally excludes somatic symptoms based on the perspective that these may confound the accuracy of depression diagnosis in medical patients
Hamilton Depression Rating Scale (HAM-D)	• Advantage: Effective tool for diagnosing depression and assessing changes over treatment • Disadvantage: Must be administered by a health-care provider rather than completed by the patient
Geriatric Depression Scale (GDS)	• Advantage: Designed for older-age patients, making it potentially a good fit for many patients with chronic pain • Disadvantage: Minimizes somatic symptoms of depression, potentially underestimating depression in pain and other medical populations

and pain providers by building it into routine clinic care and reviewing the measures during visits. In contrast, ignorance of suicidality and other depressive symptoms can undermine pain treatment participation and outcomes through multiple pathways.

15.1.2 Theme 2: The Depression—Chronic Pain Relationship Functions Less Like a Bidirectional Association and More Like a Möbius Strip

The traditional scientific perspective on the depression–chronic pain relationship is to describe it as bidirectional. This is to say that depression may predispose or exacerbate chronic pain and that chronic pain may enable or worsen depression (11). As reviewed in this section, there is substantial data from epidemiological, laboratory, and interventional research to support this conventional relationship model. However, this section will also offer an alternative model that arguably more accurately represents the dynamic and often synergistic interplay between depression and chronic pain (Figure 15.3). This latter alternative model is the Möbius strip. A Möbius strip is a cylindrical, one-sided shape without boundaries that mathematicians frequently use to represent unbounded relationships or infinite loops. Following a summary of

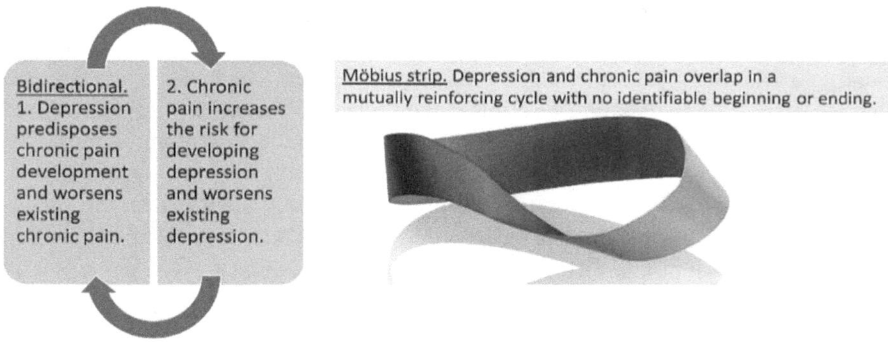

FIGURE 15.3 Pathways connecting depression and chronic pain.

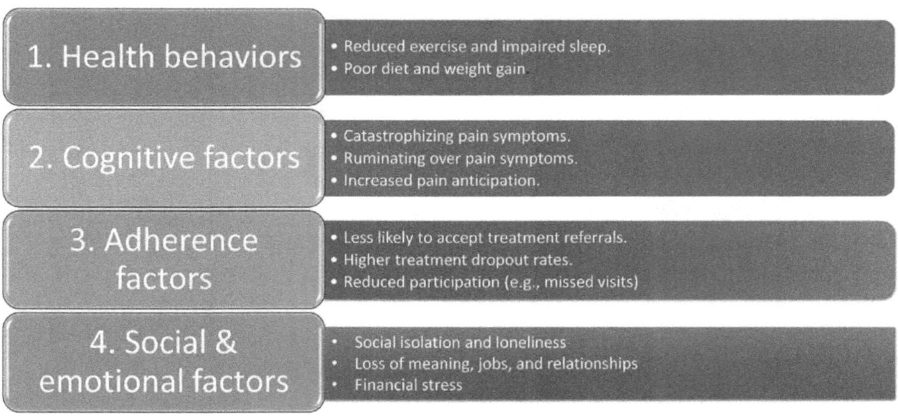

FIGURE 15.4 Pathways connecting depression to chronic pain.

depression–chronic pain research, the reader may determine for themselves whether the bidirectional or Möbius strip model offers a superior account.

Observations that psychological, behavioral, and social factors could influence the perception of pain predate Melzack and Hall's gate control theory by many decades (12). For instance, it had been frequently observed that pain intensity reports by US soldiers in wars during the 19th and early 20th centuries varied markedly based on situational and emotional factors. In some cases, psychosocial factors appeared to greatly reduce the perception of pain even in the face of grave injuries. In others, psychosocial factors seemed to turn up the intensity of pain experienced in a manner akin to a volume knob on a radio or television. These and related observations about pain that defied a simple biological account for pain contributed greatly to Melzack and Hall's eventual theory identifying a prominent role for psychosocial factors in the experience, effects, and treatment of pain (13).

In contrast, it required decades of research after the publication of the gate control theory for the multiple pathways for psychosocial factor–pain relationships to be elucidated. In a summary form (Figure 15.4), psychosocial factors such as depression may cause or contribute to pain across categories of impaired health behaviors, pain-enhancing cognitions, by undermining treatment adherence, and social and emotional processes that increase pain perceptions and worsen the dysfunction associated with pain. The clinical symptom overlap between depression and pain conditions is numerous. In addition to common somatic symptoms identified in the previous section—fatigue, weight gain, sleep impairment, etc.—patients with depression and chronic pain also frequently endorse guilt, social isolation, sedentary lifestyles, sexual dysfunction or loss of sexual interest, and suicidal ideation. This substantial symptom overlap offers a practical explanation for why patients with either depression or chronic pain may be more likely to meet diagnostic criteria for the other condition in the future.

Epidemiological researchers identified an initially curious finding. Among large numbers of people experiencing ostensibly similar injuries, only a fraction went on to develop chronic pain associated with significant dysfunction and disability. Medical and demographic factors proved to be unreliable predictors of chronic pain development. However, histories of psychiatric conditions—including trauma and depression, among others—were often associated with long-term outcomes of injuries and procedures such as back surgeries (14). This body of epidemiological evidence in the 1980s and 1990s helped shape insurance company policies and clinical practice standards to recommend pre-procedural psychological evaluations of patients for implantable pain device procedures (15, 16). Despite a substantial body of observable evidence linking depression to chronic pain development and poorer treatment outcomes, however, the mechanisms and nature of the relationship were unclear. Could depression cause chronic pain? And if so, how? Or were other factors—such as loss of employment, relationship distress, and decreased sleep and exercise that could cause both depression and chronic pain—instead responsible?

One of the defining features of clinical depression is alterations in patients' thinking. Depression is, for example, associated with distorted thinking patterns, such as black-and-white thinking, overgeneralizing, mind reading, minimization of good events and maximization of bad events, and the tendency to catastrophize or exaggerate the meanings of events, conversations, and even medical symptoms (17). Depression—surprising to many—is among the leading causes of disability in the United States, in part due to these profound changes in thinking. In this respect, depression is associated with more disability than most medical conditions. Rather than from injuries or progressive disease processes, however, the disability associated with depression results from changes in behavior and thinking. Thinking patterns characteristic of depression, for example, result in widespread dysfunction in relationships ("Nobody likes me"), health habits ("Why bother?"), and employment ("I'm dragging the company down, anyway"). The adverse consequences of depression for conditions such as chronic pain are not difficult to predict.

The clinical implications of depression as a comorbidity of chronic pain may initially seem counterintuitive. Although patients with depression are more likely to report struggles with pain symptoms, for instance, and to describe their pain symptoms as more distressing and interfering to their physicians, their ability to participate in treatment is relatively diminished. Patients with comorbid depression are more likely to decline treatment referrals, drop out of treatments, and participate less gainfully when enrolled.

In practice, depression and pain make natural dance partners. The thinking distortions commonly present among patients with depression, for instance, are mirrored by thinking patterns among patients with chronic pain. The latter patients also frequently endorse tendencies to ruminate over negative events, magnify the possibility of negative outcomes, struggle with feelings of guilt or being a burden to others, and feel less valuable than others, among multiple parallel thinking pattern similarities. As a result, depression and pain can each dispose or magnify dysfunctional thinking patterns that may have originated from the other condition or from an independent event (e.g., childhood trauma predisposing dysfunctional thinking patterns that later manifest in depression and chronic pain).

A combination of laboratory, interventional, and neuroimaging research from the past three decades has provided insight into perhaps the most powerful pathway explaining the relationship between depression and pain: shared biology (Figure 15.5). As summarized earlier, depression and pain share thinking patterns, behavioral symptoms, interpersonal effects, tendencies toward overreliance upon and abuse of medications, and even similarities in impairments in certain cognitive functions, such as memory and attention. Given their numerous overlapping symptoms,

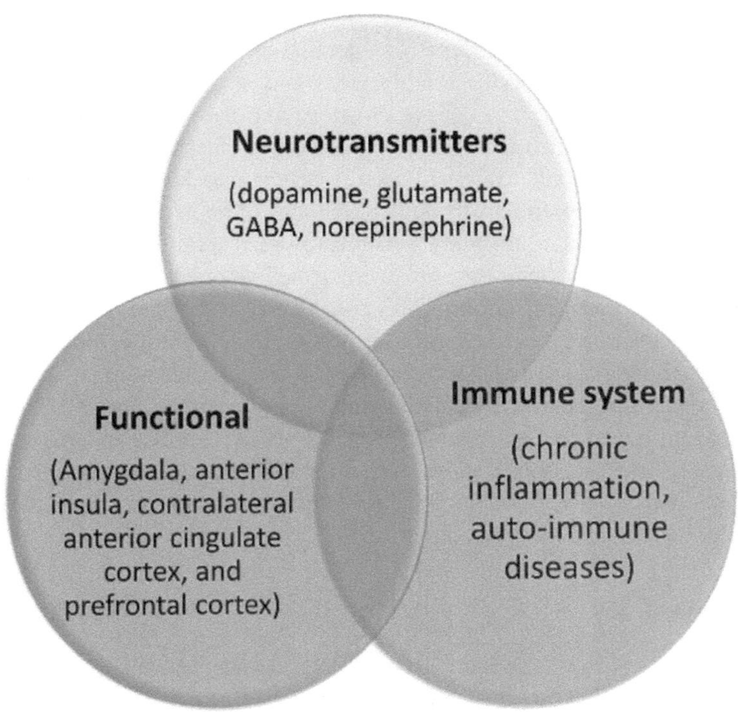

FIGURE 15.5 Biological pathways common to depression and chronic pain.

it would be puzzling if depression and chronic pain did not share similar neurotransmitters and demonstrate similar patterns of brain activation (18). Neurotransmitters such as dopamine, norepinephrine, GABA, and glutamate, for example, play roles in both depression and pain. Medications that affect these neurotransmitters (such as tricyclic antidepressants) are among the established treatments for both conditions. Serotonin, notably, is not on this list of overlapping neurotransmitters (playing an important role in depression, however). Serotonin reuptake inhibitors improve depressive symptoms but typically have little or no benefit for the treatment of chronic pain. Relative changes in these neurotransmitters in the central nervous systems of patients with depression are believed to explain symptoms such as decreased pleasure and motivation, poor self-esteem, and increased tendencies toward negative emotions. In chronic pain, they are associated with pain perception, pain interference, and pain disability.

Among prominent overlapping hormones, cortisol, thyroid, and sex hormones, such as testosterone, are affected in both depression and chronic pain. Chronic pain is associated with many types of hormone deficits and disorders, and hormonal dysfunction, such as thyroid, testosterone, and vitamin D deficiency, has been linked to the development of depression in multiple studies. Immune system dysfunction—such as chronic inflammation—is known to cause depressive symptoms as well as to contribute to some forms of chronic pain conditions. A still-growing body of research indicates from fMRI observations that areas such as the amygdala, anterior insula, contralateral anterior cingulate cortex, and prefrontal cortex play functional roles in the affective components of both depression and pain (19). In the cases of depression and chronic pain, these brain areas may become relatively more or less active, affecting sensitivity to negative emotions and pain symptoms. Neurological mechanisms also appear to account for the effects of sleep and exercise on depression and chronic pain. For example, sleep is believed to lower thresholds to emotional and physical pain, in part through alterations of neurochemical pathways and brain activation (e.g., the amygdala becomes more responsive to negative stimuli after shortened sleep, as demonstrated in controlled laboratory studies). Exercise, in contrast, appears to trigger opposing functional and neurochemical responses that increase stress tolerance, reduce muscle tension, and lower emotional reactivity. This accumulating biological research substantiates the importance of including sleep (the evidence concerning cognitive behavior therapy for insomnia—or CBT-I—is particularly strong among sleep treatments) and physical exercise treatments as core components of interventions for patients with either depression or chronic pain. For patients with both depression and chronic pain, the evidence suggests that their potential to benefit could be even larger.

15.2 SUMMARY

This section summarizes research from observational, laboratory, neuroimaging, and intervention studies to highlight the complex interrelationship between depression and chronic pain. Although depression is associated with many chronic medical conditions, there is perhaps no other single chronic disease with which depression shares such an extensive list of common symptoms, behaviors, psychosocial effects, and biological mechanisms (20). The practical benefit of this condition overlap is that pain specialists—who we now know may be unsuspectingly co-treating depression in half or more of their patients on average—can confidently prescribe treatments such as exercise, weight loss, and sleep that simultaneously improve depression and pain. Given the evidence that depression and chronic pain frequently interact in vicious cycles to worsen a patient's function and treatment outcomes, the promise from initial treatment research that co-treatment of these conditions could reverse this pattern to produce a mutually beneficial virtuous cycle is considerable.

The evidence in this section also provides support for both the conventional bidirectional relationship model between depression and chronic pain and for the novel Möbius strip model introduced in this section. The primary advantage of the bidirectional model is parsimony. Depression may, in some cases, predispose patients to develop chronic pain, and chronic pain may sometimes predispose depression. The multiple symptom, behavioral, and biological pathways connecting the conditions offer compelling support for this interpretation, as does the large epidemiological literature documenting the high rates with which depression and chronic pain co-occur over time. The advantage of a simpler relationship model, however, is arguably equaled or even surpassed by the value of the more complex analogy of the depression and pain relationship as a kind of medical Möbius strip. In a Möbius strip, there exist no clear boundaries between sides, directions, or conditions. Arbitrary boundaries instead become continuous. For this reason, a Möbius strip model permits a more fluid and wider range of relationships between two or more conditions and better captures the many depression–pain variations present in research and clinical practice. The Möbius strip model also fits well with the epidemiological literature suggesting that depression and pain can synergistically cause, result from, or interact with each other through individual or combinations of mechanisms and over time intervals ranging from weeks to decades. Finally, the Möbius strip model is also consistent with the growing research concerning parallel biological pathways and the dual benefits of medication (tricyclic antidepressants; 21) and behavioral (exercise, CBT-i) treatments by conceptualizing depression and chronic pain as manifestations of similar underlying neurological, biochemical, genetic, and epigenetic causes.

15.2.1 Theme 3: Depression and Chronic Pain Research Offer Practical Methods for Enhancing the Future of Pain Clinic Care

Previous sections have established several themes important for pain clinic providers: (1) The close relationship between chronic pain severity and duration with depression translates into very high rates of comorbid depression in specialized pain treatment settings, such as pain clinics. (2) Depression can be practically measured by non–mental health providers in the content of pain clinic care using any of several well-validated questionnaires. (3) The price of ignoring comorbid depression is high, with research indicating that depression has substantial adverse effects rippling across domains of medical costs, treatment responsiveness and participation, medication adherence and misuse, and even rates of lawsuits. And (4) there is now compelling and relatively comprehensive data from biological and neuroscience research authenticating the physical basis of the depression–chronic pain relationship. It is no longer scientifically tenable to explain depression among patients with chronic pain solely as a failure to cope with the condition. Although this relationship can take many forms, mechanisms from cognitive, behavioral, biochemical, neurological, and genetic levels create increasingly clear pathways through which depression and chronic pain interact over time.

Based on these themes, what practical steps can pain providers take to optimize the quality of their care and patient experiences?

Implement a standardized form of depression assessment into pain clinic service delivery. In 2008, the American Heart Association recommended that depression be routinely assessed among patients surviving myocardial infarction (22). Although controversial at that time, this recommendation was not made lightly. Instead, it was based on nearly two decades of observational, interventional, and laboratory science documentation of high rates of depression among post-MI patients, relatively worsened morbidity and morbidity among post-MI patients with depression, and mechanisms providing biological plausibility to the relationship. More than a decade later, a similar tipping point to depression in chronic pain has arguably been achieved. In this case, however, no government agency or major pain society has yet championed the cause of integrating routine depression measurements into pain clinic services. This leaves individual pain providers and clinics to deliberate on the relative advantages, disadvantages, and practical plans for assessing comorbid depression in their patients.

Neither mental health professionals nor clinical diagnostic interviews are necessary to reliably identify the presence of clinically significant depression in patients. Many depression questionnaires accomplish this objective. These measures generally take no more than five minutes to complete (some as brief as 2 items), they do not require the presence of a clinician (i.e., they can be self-administered and returned to a clerk or nurse before a visit begins), and the scores can be recorded in the electronic medical record with no need for paper storage. There are advantages to using somewhat-longer measures of depression, such as the Beck Depression Inventory, due to its greater coverage of physical and somatic symptoms common to patients with chronic pain. However, any validated measure of depression can be a valuable resource for the pain provider.

A frequent question posed by pain providers considering a depression measure is how to interpret and use the results. Questionnaires offer information about mental health similar to what blood tests or imaging results generate for physical health. Specifically, questionnaires provide clues about diagnoses and data to improve decision-making about treatment. Elevated depression scores should signal the pain provider to (1) discuss pain psychology or mental health treatment referrals as part of their visit, (2) be alert for how depression symptoms may be affecting the patient's treatment participation and treatment response, and (3) consider recommending treatments that may dually assist the patient's pain and depressive symptoms when depression is present. These are powerful advantages for the pain provider, gained from a modest 5-minute investment.

Form a referral or consulting relationship with a pain psychologist or pain psychiatrist. One of the commonly cited barriers to greater attention to depression and other psychiatric concerns among patients with chronic pain is a lack of embedded mental health resource. Many pain specialists, for example, direct or work in private practice clinics, with no internalized mental health resources. Although most hospital systems contain psychiatry and psychology services in various forms for electronic referrals, the professionals comprising these latter services rarely have specific training or expertise with chronic pain. When mental health professionals reside in separate hospital services, they are less likely to participate in pain clinic rounds for case presentations and may not be familiar with standards for evaluating patients with chronic pain for procedures such as implantable pain devices. It is important to clarify that these limitations only partially mitigate their value to pain providers. Mental health professionals are generally well-trained for depression and can assist most patients with the condition, including those with chronic pain. However, there are unique advantages to cultivating a relationship with a board-certified pain psychologist/psychiatrist or clinical health psychologist, who may be able to conduct a full range of pain-specific psychological assessments and provide evidence-based pain psychology treatments. There are a growing number of pain psychology specialists in the United States, and their services are generally covered by insurance for treatment and pain-specific assessment purposes. For pain providers (and patients), there is also an expanding list of online resources for locating pain psychologists in their area. These include Psychology Today (https://www.psychologytoday.com/us/therapists/chronic-pain), the American Board of Professional Psychology (https://abpp.org/Directory), and the American Psychological Association (https://locator.apa.org/).

Make it standard practice to recommend exercise as a treatment for physical and emotional well-being, and recommend CBT-I to facilitate improvements in sleep. Even for pain providers without internal or local access to pain psychology services for the management of depression, good treatment options are available. Given the high rates of depression and sleep impairment among patients seeking treatment in pain clinic settings, it should arguably be standard practice to recommend forms of pain-friendly exercise and options for participating in CBT-i for sleep. No single exercise modality is appropriate for all patients with chronic pain (23). Aquatherapy, walking, bicycling, recumbent bicycling, and other lower-intensity options are most broadly suitable. This list is easily broadened by patients' own interests and preferences. More critical than having a standard exercise recommendation is setting a standard for talking about the importance of exercise during pain clinic visits. As reviewed in this chapter, the benefits of exercise extend to mental health as well as to general physical conditioning, pain management, and muscle strengthening rationales. Recent systematic reviews and meta-analyses (e.g., 24) show that exercise interventions improve depressive symptoms on par with antidepressants and psychotherapies, for example, and may be particularly useful for those with more severe depression. Further, the mechanistic pathways through which aerobic and resistance training facilitates mood improvements have been illuminated greatly over the previous decade of research. CBT-i, meanwhile, is the single most effective intervention for insomnia and sleep impairment (25). In contrast to sleep medications with many known side effects and that show only limited improvements in sleep quantity or quality in polysomnography studies, CBT-i improves sleep quantity and quality with no significant side effects. CBT-i can also be tailored to patients with chronic pain, among whom sources of sleep disruption differ from those of typical patients, and reliably improves depressive symptoms as well as sleep. Finally, CBT-i is increasingly available through smartphone apps (e.g., https://apps.apple.com/us/app/cbt-i-coach/id655918660, https://play.google.com/store/apps/details?id=gov.va.mobilehealth.ncptsd.cbti&hl=en_US&gl=US), circumventing any lack of local CBT-i resources.

15.3 SUMMARY

This chapter was written for providers working in specialized pain treatment settings. By combining themes from observational, laboratory, and treatment research, this chapter intended to (1) raise awareness among pain clinic providers regarding the ubiquity of depression among patients in their care; (2) appreciate the risks of overlooking comorbid depression in their patients; (3) improve pain providers' understanding of brief depression measurement tools applicable to their clinics; (4) expand their knowledge of the evidence demonstrating the biopsychosocial relationship between depression and chronic pain; and (5) consider practical applications from depression–chronic pain treatment research that could enhance the effectiveness of pain clinic care. Although pain clinic care is diverse and evolving rapidly with new research, treatments, and technologies, there is no evidence that rates of comorbid depression are declining. Instead, the effects, resources, and potential benefits reviewed in this chapter are more likely to remain stable or even expand in the decade ahead.

REFERENCES

1. Ericsson M, Poston II W, Linder J, Taylor JE, Haddock CK, Foreyt JP. Depression predicts disability in long-term chronic pain patients. Disabil Rehabil. 2002;24(6):334–40.
2. Bair M, Robinson R, Katon W, Kroenke K. Depression and pain comorbidity: A literature review. Arch Intern Med. 2003;163(20):2433–45.
3. Seal KH, Shi Y, Cohen G, et al. Association of mental health disorders with prescription opioids and high-risk opioid use in US veterans of Iraq and Afghanistan. *JAMA*. 2012;307(9):940–947. doi:10.1001/jama.2012.234.
4. O'Connor EA, Whitlock EP, Gaynes B, Beil TL. Screening for depression in adults and older adults in primary care: An updated systematic review [Internet]. Rockville (MD): Agency for Healthcare Research and Quality (US); 2009 Dec. Report No: 10–05143-EF–1.
5. Hilderink P, Burger H, Deeg D, Beekman A, Oude Voshaar R. The temporal relation between pain and depression: Results from the longitudinal aging study Amsterdam. Psychosom Med. 2012;74(9):945–51.
6. Turk DC, Audette J, Levy RM, Mackey SC, Stanos S. (2010). Assessment and treatment of psychosocial comorbidities in patients with neuropathic pain. Mayo Clin Proc. 2010;85(suppl), S42–50.
7. Currie SR, Wang J. Chronic back pain and major depression in the general Canadian population. Pain. 2004 Jan;107(1–2):54–60. doi: 10.1016/j.pain.2003.09.015.
8. Turk DC. A cognitive-behavioral approach to the treatment of chronic pain patients. Reg Anesth Pain Med. 2003; 28:573–9.
9. Goldman LS, Nielsen NH, Champion HC. Awareness, diagnosis, and treatment of depression. J Gen Intern Med. 1999;14(9):569–580. doi: 10.1046/j.1525–1497.1999.03478.x.

10. de Heer EW, Gerrits MMJG, Beekman ATF, Dekker J, van Marwijk HWJ, de Waal MWM, et al. (2014) The association of depression and anxiety with pain: A study from NESDA. PLoS ONE 9(10): e106907. doi: 10.1371/journal.pone.0106907.
11. Ehde DM, Dillworth TM, Turner JA. Cognitive-behavioral therapy for individuals with chronic pain: efficacy, innovations and directions for research. Amer Psychol. 2014;69(2):153–66.
12. Melzack R, Wall P. Pain mechanisms: A new theory. Science (80-). 1965;150(3699): 971 9.
13. Hoffman BM, Papas RK, Chatkoff DK, Kerns RD. Meta-analysis of psychological interventions for chronic low back pain. Health Psychol. 2007;26(1):1–9.
14. Tunks ER, Crook J, Weir R. Epidemiology of chronic pain with psychological comorbidity: Prevalence, risk, course, and prognosis. Can J Psychiatry 2008;53:224–34. doi: 10.1177/070674370805300403.
15. Beltrutti D, Lamberto A, Barolat G. The psychological assessment of candidates for spinal cord stimulation for chronic pain management. Pain Pr. 2004;4(3):204–21.
16. Block A, Ohnmeiss D, Guyer R, Rashbaum R, Hochschuler S. The use of presurgical psychological screening to predict the outcome of spine surgery. Spine J. 2001;1(4):274–82.
17. Quartana PJ, Campbell CM, Edwards RR. Pain catastrophizing: a critical review. Expert Rev Neurother. 2009;9: 745–58.
18. Flor H. Psychological pain interventions and neurophysiology: Implications for a mechanism-based approach. Am Psychol. 2014 Feb-Mar;69(2):188–96. doi: 10.1037/a0035254.
19. Sheng J, Liu S, Wang Y, Cui R, Zhang X. The Link between Depression and Chronic Pain: Neural Mechanisms in the Brain. Neural Plast. 2017;2017:9724371. doi: 10.1155/2017/9724371.
20. Yang S, Chang MC. Chronic Pain: Structural and Functional Changes in Brain Structures and Associated Negative Affective States. Int J Molec Sci. 2019;20(13):3130.
21. Atkinson JH, Slater MA, Capparelli EV, Wallace MS, Zisook S, Abramson I, Matthews SC, Garfin SR. Efficacy of noradrenergic and serotonergic antidepressants in chronic back pain. J Clin Psychopharmacol 2007;27:135–42.
22. Lichtman JH, Bigger JT Jr, Blumenthal JA, Frasure-Smith N, Kaufmann PG, Lespérance F, Mark DB, Sheps DS, Taylor CB, Froelicher ES; American Heart Association Prevention Committee of the Council on Cardiovascular Nursing; American Heart Association Council on Clinical Cardiology; American Heart Association Council on Epidemiology and Prevention; American Heart Association Interdisciplinary Council on Quality of Care and Outcomes Research; American Psychiatric Association. Depression and coronary heart disease. Recommendations for screening, referral, and treatment. A science advisory from the American Heart Association Prevention Committee of the Council on Cardiovascular Nursing, Council on Clinical Cardiology, Council on Epidemiology and Prevention, and Interdisciplinary Council on Quality of Care and Outcomes Research. Circulation. 2008;118:1768–75.
23. Geneen LJ, Moore RA, Clarke C, Martin D, Colvin LA, Smith BH. Physical activity and exercise for chronic pain in adults: an overview of Cochrane Reviews. Cochrane Database Syst Rev. 2017 Jan 14;1(1): CD011279. doi: 10.1002/14651858.CD011279.pub2.
24. Schuch, FB, Stubbs, B. The Role of Exercise in Preventing and Treating Depression, Current Sports Medicine Reports. 2019;18(8):299–304 doi: 10.1249/JSR.0000000000000620.
25. Trauer JM, Qian MY, Doyle JS, Rajaratnam SM, Cunnington D. Cognitive Behavioral Therapy for Chronic Insomnia: A Systematic Review and Meta-analysis. Ann Intern Med. 2015 Aug 4;163(3):191–204. doi: 10.7326/M14–2841.

16 Neuromodulation

Brooke Towne, Jacob Caylor, Imanuel Lerman, Sopyda Yin, and Rajiv Reddy

16.1 INTRODUCTION

Spinal cord stimulation (SCS), a form of neuromodulation, is an FDA-approved, minimally invasive implantable therapy for patients with treatment-refractory chronic pain syndromes.[1] First clinically trialed in 1967, electrical stimulation in the epidural space was applied by Shealy et al. to alleviate pain from a patient's lung cancer.[1, 2] Throughout the last half-century, spinal cord dorsal column stimulation has evolved to include multiple electrical waveforms and anatomical targets to optimize patient analgesia. By adjusting stimulation parameters, including the pulse width, amplitude, and frequency, patients may experience either a tingling sensation (paresthesia) over their painful area or a paresthesia-free effect replacing pain perception. Initially, it was thought that applying paresthesia over the patient's painful area would block nociceptive input, aligning with Melzack and Wall's gate control theory of pain, which hypothesized that AB input would block pain signals from ascending nociceptive fibers.[3] However, it is now known that multiple different mechanisms play a role in providing pain relief, and each mechanism is unique, depending on the type of spinal cord stimulation used in a patient.[1] Though there is substantial clinical data claiming that these devices are effective, preclinical basic science has lagged, and further investigation is needed to determine the underlying mechanisms of pain relief. Before investigating how each mode of SCS exerts its clinical effect, an understanding is needed of the intended anatomic neural targets; for further review, see Caylor et al. (2019).[1]

16.2 ANATOMICAL TARGETS OF NEUROMODULATION

Understanding the spinothalamic tract's pain signal transmission is crucial to appreciating SCS mechanisms of analgesia. Action potentials arising from the stimulation of peripheral nociceptors are transmitted to the central nervous system by thinly myelinated Aδ and unmyelinated C nerve fibers.[4] Aδ fibers carry signals for acute pain, temperature, and pressure to synapse in Rexed lamina I and III–V within the dorsal horn of the spinal cord.[4, 5] On the other hand, slower-conducting C fibers are polymodal that convey sensory signals from thermoreceptors, mechanoreceptors, and chemoreceptors.[6] C fibers carry a delayed pain response classically characterized as a dull, achy, or burning sensation, and synapse on Rexed laminae I–II in the dorsal horn.[6] Both primary afferent Aδ and C neurons project to interneuron circuitry as well as synapse directly onto two different types of second-order neurons:

DOI: 10.1201/9781003094302-16

multimodal wide dynamic range neurons and nociceptive-specific neurons. Wide dynamic range neurons are located in Rexed laminae III–V and receive input from Aβ, Aδ, and C fibers carrying inputs from both noxious and non-noxious stimuli.[5, 6] In addition, they also receive stimulation from independent sympathetic neurons.[7] Given they receive inputs from both noxious and non-noxious stimuli, it seems appropriate they have a graded firing frequency with repetitive stimuli.[6] This is in contrast to the nociceptive-specific neurons, which receive only noxious stimuli and do not exhibit a graded response or stimulation via sympathetic neurons. Second-order neurons from both the wide dynamic range and the nociceptive-specific decussate at the anterior commissure and ascend via the anterolateral spinothalamic tract, carrying sensations of crude touch, pain, and temperature up to third-order neurons located in the posterior, medial, and later thalamus. From the thalamus, third-order neurons ascend to the corresponding area of the somatosensory cortex in the brain, where the stimulus is perceived. The spinothalamic tract, which carries noxious stimuli from the periphery to the brain, serves as a modulatory target for spinal cord stimulation via both segmental spinal and supraspinal mechanisms.

Spinal cord stimulation has long been thought to work via stimulation of the dorsal columns, as they are the most superficial structure in close proximity to the current delivered from SCS—however, these axons do not carry pain sensations. The dorsal column medial lemniscus pathway carries fine touch, vibration, and proprioceptive afferents from peripheral mechanoreceptors to the brain.[6] Thus, it seems intuitive that activation of these dorsal column axons elicits paresthesia. First-order pseudounipolar neurons enter via the dorsal root ganglion and ascend the dorsal columns via the dorsal column medial lemniscus pathway to synapse on second-order neurons located in the ipsilateral medulla. Fibers from the upper extremities enter the cervical spinal cord and ascend via the fasciculus cuneatus to synapse on the medullary nucleus cuneataus laterally, and fibers from the lower extremities ascend via the fasciculus gracilis to synapse on the medullary nucleus gracilis medially.[5] Axons from each nucleus join to form the internal arcuate fibers and decussate in the brain stem before proceeding to ascend to synapse on the ventral posterior lateral and ventral posterior medial nuclei in the thalamus. While these fibers ascend through the brain stem, they acquire inputs from the trigeminal nerve. From the ventral posterior lateral and ventral posterior medial nuclei, third-order neurons run through the posterior third of the internal capsule to the primary and secondary somatosensory cortex.[5] While SCS may activate these fibers and elicit perceived paresthesia, it is unclear if the analgesic effect works through antidromic or orthodromic activation.

The descending modulatory systems (DMS) are responsible for tuning, amplifying, and inhibiting ascending pain signals—these are largely comprised of descending projections from the periaqueductal gray and the locus coeruleus. Signals from the periaqueductal gray project to the rostral ventromedial medulla, which is comprised of the nucleus raphe magnus and the nuclei of the reticular formation. Both the periaqueductal gray and rostral ventromedial medulla have inputs arising from pain modulatory centers in cortical and subcortical structures which contribute to the emotional and stress response to pain.[8–11] These structures also receive ascending sensory inputs from projection neurons, creating a feedback loop for noxious stimuli.[8–11] Signals from the rostral ventromedial medulla travel to the dorsal lateral funiculus to ultimately project onto interneurons within the dorsal horn of the spinal cord, primarily utilizing the neurotransmitter serotonin.[6, 12] This system also utilizes GABAergic and opioidergic mechanisms at the supraspinal and segmental levels.[13] Neurons from the raphe nucleus magnus projecting to the dorsal horn can have several different classifications: ON, OFF, serotonin-like, or neutral. ON cells are typically found in an inactivated state and are activated by a nociceptive stimulus, which prompts an enhancement of dorsal horn nociceptive transmission.[14] On

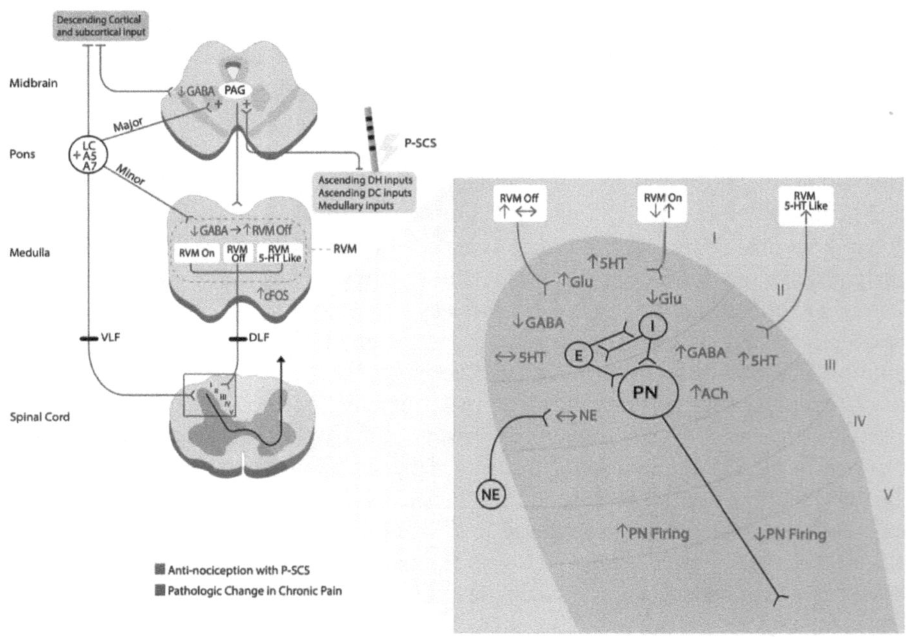

FIGURE 16.1 Changes in dorsal horn circuitry to chronic pain and SCS. In the development of chronic pain, neural circuitry undergoes rewiring, wherein abnormal enhancement of excitatory pathways and loss of inhibition facilitate nociceptive transmission to sub-threshold stimuli. Increased excitatory interneuron (E) input, decreased inhibitory interneuron (I) input, and local factors contribute to pathologic destabilization of normal input balance to the projection neuron. SCS changes the balance of nociceptive and antinociceptive inputs through the activation of local segmental and descending supraspinal mechanisms to restore balance to this network. "Up" arrows represent increased concentration or activity, whereas "down" arrows represent the opposite. "Sideways" arrows represent no change. Acronyms: PAG, periaqueductal gray; RVM, rostral ventromedial medulla; LC, locus coeruleus; A5, noradrenergic cell group A5; A7, noradrenergic cell group A7; DH, dorsal horn; DC, dorsal column; VLF, ventrolateral funiculus; DLF, dorsolateral funiculus; RVM ON, RVM ON cells projecting from the RVM to the DH; RVM OFF, RVM OFF cells projecting from the RVM to the DH; RVM 5-HT like, RVM 5-HT like cells projecting from RVM to DH; cFOS, a proto-oncogene; E, excitatory interneuron; I inhibitory interneuron; PN, projection neuron; Glu, glutamate; 5-HT, 5-hydroxytryptamine; Ach, acetylcholine; NE, norepinephrine; GABA, gamma-aminobutyric acid.

the other hand, OFF cells play a role in suppressing dorsal horn pain transmission, which is enhanced by opioids. Fibers from the rostral ventral medulla regulate the OFF cells. Pathological activation of ON cells or deactivation of OFF cells leads to increased pain transmission in the dorsal horn as well and is believed to play a role in central sensitization and opioid-induced hyperalgesia.[14] Exogenous opioids activate OFF cells and suppress ON cells at the rostral ventral medulla as well, via a GABAergic mechanism.[5] It has been demonstrated that SCS can lead to dorsal horn antinociception via activation of rostral ventral medulla OFF cells as well as serotonin-like cells, an analgesic pathway shared in part with opioids.[15] This SCS antinociceptive property was also shown to be diminished with GABA antagonism.[15] Another descending pain pathway relies on norepinephrine for descending pain modulation. The locus coeruleus receives inputs from ascending pain signals originating in the dorsal horn, as well as via pathways from the insular cortex, amygdala, and hypothalamus. Because of its notable inputs from these cortical and subcortical structures, the locus coeruleus creates a pain-signaling pathway that's responsive to emotion and stress.[16, 17] Axons from the locus coeruleus provide signals to interneurons found in laminae I–III in the dorsal horn via the neurotransmitter norepinephrine.[18] Together, these opioidergic, serotonergic, GABAergic, and noradrenergic circuits create a plastic, adaptive modulatory system that regulates those signals seen by the supraspinal pain centers. As these circuits and pathways remain incompletely elucidated with regard to SCS, we will overview the evidence for neuromodulation about each involved neurotransmitter. For the following, these basic sciences investigations utilize classic tonic SCS as opposed to the new paradigms and waveforms, which we will discuss later in the chapter.

16.3 NEUROTRANSMITTERS OF NEUROMODULATION

Gamma-aminobutyric acid (GABA) is a critical inhibitory CNS neurotransmitter that SCS is likely to utilize when providing analgesia to the patient. GABA binds to two known receptors: $GABA_A$ and $GABA_B$.[19] $GABA_A$ is a post-synaptic receptor complex created from a binding domain and a chloride ionophore. Activation of $GABA_A$ leads to an influx of Cl^-, which hyperpolarizes the post-synaptic nerve and increases the firing threshold.[19] On the other hand, $GABA_B$ is a post-synaptic G protein–coupled receptor that, when activated, leads to the opening of K^+ channels, also yielding hyperpolarized post-synaptic neurons with an increased firing threshold.[19] In addition to their role in post-synaptic hyperpolarization, $GABA_B$ receptors also play a role in pre-synaptic inhibition via a Ca^{2+}-dependent process.[6, 19] GABAergic interneurons found in laminae I–III receive projections from Aβ, Aδ, and C fibers.[6, 20] These interneurons play a role in inhibiting excitatory neurotransmitter release, and dysfunction in this pathway leads to WDR neuron hyperexcitability.[21, 22] It has been shown that SCS activates GABAergic interneurons of the spinal cord dorsal horn directly, likely through pre-synaptic suppression of excitatory glutamate release.[21] In addition, SCS also plays a central role in increasing GABA at the dorsal horn by decreasing GABAergic signaling in the periaqueductal gray—this leads to the activation of the serotonergic DMS.[23, 24] To support this theory, it has been shown that administration of intrathecal baclofen, a $GABA_B$ receptor agonist, not only enhances the analgesic effects of SCS but can also transform non-responding SCS-treated patients into responders.[21] In addition to its central role played at the periaqueductal gray, SCS also has been shown to activate thalamic GABAergic neurons, which could indicate modulation of cortical processing and thalamocortical dysrhythmia.[25, 26] Taken together, this shows that SCS neuromodulation likely works, at least partially, through GABAergic circuits, both at segmental and supraspinal locations.

Serotonin (5HT) is a monoamine neurotransmitter originating from the rostral ventral medulla and supraspinal nuclei—it is transported in an anterograde fashion, to be released in the dorsal horn, and is the namesake of the serotonergic DMS.[27–30] Several studies have been conducted that demonstrate SCS therapy activates the serotonergic DMS. As the serotonergic DMS innervates the interneuron circuitry of the dorsal horn, SCS activation of this pathway leads to segmental (local) spinal cord pain inhibition.[27–30] It has also been found that intrathecal serotonin potentiates the antinociceptive effects of SCS.[31] Serotonin-mediated analgesia in the spinal cord acts through a GABAergic intermediary. Studies have shown that SCS works through primarily $5HT_3$ receptors with a $GABA_B$ receptor link, reinforcing this pathway.[32] Although it is known that SCS activates the DMS in an orthodromic manner, the exact degree of serotonin contribution to pain relief derived from SCS is unknown. However, serotonergic DMS plays a greater role in pain relief when compared to its noradrenergic DMS counterpart, which we will discuss next.[33]

Norepinephrine is a catecholamine produced by the locus coeruleus, trafficked caudally, and released in the dorsal horn, where it exhibits its antinociceptive effects.[34] In the dorsal horn, norepinephrine acts to modulate pain sensations via several different mechanisms. Norepinephrine acts pre-synaptically to inhibit primary Aδ and C fibers, and post-synaptically to inhibit wide dynamic range and nociceptive-specific neurons.[35, 36] In addition, it also activates inhibitory neurons, which leads to an increase in GABAergic and glycinergic currents.[37, 38] Although norepinephrine itself plays a role at the spinal cord segmental level, SCS has been proposed to exhibit noradrenergic antinociceptive properties at a central level by orthodromic activation of the locus coeruleus.[33, 39] The locus coeruleus relays this signal through the periaqueductal gray and enhances the serotonergic descending antinociceptive pathway.

Although not completely understood, acetylcholine is also believed to play a role in modulating nociceptive signals in the dorsal horn. Cholinergic modification of nociceptive signals has been identified mainly by studies involving clonidine, a pre-synaptic alpha 2 adrenergic receptor agonist, which utilizes acetylcholine at the spinal level to exert its analgesic effects.[40] After this was discovered, several studies were performed, revealing that acetylcholine levels in the dorsal horn were decreased in nerve-lesioned animals, and acetylcholine levels were increased in P-SCS-responding animals.[41] Further, it was found that specifically muscarinic 1 and 4 receptors contributed to the analgesic properties, and administration of muscarinic 2 and 4 receptor agonists reversed P-SCS non-responders.[41] It's important to note that these effects are independent of the serotonergic descending antinociceptive pathway described previously. More work is needed to clarify the role of the cholinergic influence in SCS.

Endogenous β-endorphins, enkephalins, and dynorphins are peptides that activate μ-, κ-, δ-opioid receptors, and exert their analgesic properties through direct receptor activation at the segmental level, as well as centrally via the recruitment of both serotonergic and noradrenergic descending antinociceptive pathways.[42] G protein–coupled μ-, κ-, and δ-opioid receptors are largely present on both pre- and post-synaptic neurons within the dorsal horn.[42] Activation of these receptors leads to hyperpolarization and decreased signaling.[42] These receptors are also found in the periaqueductal gray and recruit both the serotonergic and noradrenergic DMS via communication with this pathway, the medulla, the dorsal raphe nucleus, and the locus coeruleus. Activation of the serotonergic DMS has been shown to increase endogenous opioids in the dorsal horn.[43] Given that SCS results in increased endogenous opioids in the dorsal horn as well, it has been suggested that SCS may activate κ opioid receptors within the dorsal horn to contribute to its analgesic effects.[44] Studies have shown that frequency-specific P-SCS activation of opioidergic analgesic effects is reversed with the administration of naloxone and naltrindole.[45] This recruitment of opioidergic pathways is likely temporally limited to the first few days of stimulation, as studies have revealed naloxone administration attenuated early but not late hyperalgesia.[46] The lack of sustained effect is thought to be due to opioid tolerance, and there appears to be a ceiling effect that SCS provides via the opioidergic pathway.[47] Thus, it does not seem that SCS achieves long-lasting pain relief through mechanisms of altering endogenous opioids, even though changes are seen early in SCS; however, these mechanism may contribute to analgesia experienced during the SCS trial. Further investigation is required to evaluate the role of opioidergic mechanisms in SCS and to specifically evaluate waveform- and paradigm-specific endogenous opioid release.

TABLE 16.1A
Measured Neurotransmitters in Response to Spinal Cord Stimulation (SCS)

	Tissue Sampled and Measured Change To:			
Neurotransmitter	**P-SCS**	**B-SCS**	**HF-SCS**	**DRG-S**
Glu	SC: ↓ [21] PAG: ↓ [48]			
5-HT	SC: ↑ [31, 32] PAG: ↔ [48]			
GABA	SC: ↑ [21, 22] PAG: ↓ [48] RVM: ↓? [49] Plasma: ↑ [50]	Plasma: ↔ [50]		
NE	SC: ↔ [39] CSF: ↑ [51, 52] Plasma: ↑ [51]			
ACh	SC: ↑ [41]			
SP	SC: ↑ [31] PAG: ↔ [48]			

TABLE 16.1B
Spinal Cord Stimulation Exerts Analgesia by Activating Specific Receptor Subtypes

		Analgesia Response To			
Neurotransmitter	**Receptor Subtype**	**P-SCS**	**B-SCS**	**HF-SCS**	**DRG-S**
5-HT	5-HT_1:	↔ [53]			
	5-HT_2:	↑ [54]			
	5-HT_3:	↑ [53,54]			
	5-HT_4:	↑↑ [53]			
	5-HT_6:	↑ [53]			
	5-HT_7:	↔ [53]			
		↔ [53]			
GABA	$GABA_A$:	↑ [23,53,54]			
	$GABA_B$:	↔ [55]			
		↑↑ [32,53–55]			
NE	α1 adrenergic:	↑ ? [54]			
	α2 adrenergic:	↑↑ [54,56]			
	β1 adrenergic:	↑ ? [54]			
	β2 adrenergic:	↑ ? [54]			
Dopamine	D2	↑? [54]			
	D3	↑? [54]			
ACh	M1 mAChR:	↑ [41]			
	M2 mAChR:	↑ [41,57]			
	M3 mAChR:	↔ [41]			
	M4 mAChR:	↑↑ [41,57]			
	nAChR:	↔ [32]			
		↔ [41]			

16.4 NEUROMODULATION AND NEUROINFLAMMATION

One emerging hypothesis of pain relief in SCS is that it modulates the inflammatory milieu in the CNS, leading to decreased pain. We know from basic science research that CNS inflammation is a critical point in the development of pain hypersensitivity. Glial cells are nonneuronal cells found in both the central and peripheral nervous system and provide protection and support to neurons. Glia in the central nervous system includes microglia, astrocytes, oligodendrocytes, and ependymal cells, while glia in the peripheral nervous system is comprised of satellite glial cells and Schwann cells.[58] These cells do not produce electrical impulses and, instead, maintain an environment that provides homeostasis to the neuronal cells. Their main functions include providing nutrients, insulation, protection, and oxygen to neurons, in addition to fighting foreign pathogens. Interestingly, these cells also play an important role in neurotransmission and aid with modulating signal transduction and synaptic pruning.[59] The release of cytokines and glial modulators at nerve terminals leads to changes in the signal transmissions within that synapse. These glial cells also respond to tissue injury and nerve inflammation through the process of "gliosis." This reactivity is characterized by alterations in morphology, cellular signaling, receptor regulation, and mediator release.[58] Neuronal injury resulting in reactive gliosis specifically has been shown to lead to an increase in excitatory post-synaptic potentials and a decrease of inhibitory post-synaptic potentials, ultimately resulting in an increased projection neuron firing and pathologic nociception.[58] Since it is known that glial activation contributes to the formation of neuropathic pain and inactivation leads to improvement in allodynia, it is reasonable to assume that glial modulation could play a role in SCS.[60, 61] Studies have shown that SCS effectively decreased microglia and astrocyte markers within the superficial and deep dorsal horn lamina after treatment.[62] These changes observed in glial cell activation can also be seen within the dorsal root ganglia. A subset of glial cells, satellite glial cells are involved in nociceptive modulation within the dorsal root ganglia (DRG).[6, 63] These cells have been shown to alter neuronal transmission via the P2X3 pathway, which leads to increased abnormal nociception.[64, 65] Given this information, it has been hypothesized that DRG stimulation may modulate satellite glial cell activation.[66] Studies have shown that DRG stimulation leads to decreases in markers of glial activation and neuronal injury, specifically, glial fibrillary acidic protein (GFAP) and activating transcription factor 3 (ATF-3).[66] Although it is known that glial inflammatory mechanisms play a role in the development and maintenance of chronic pain, work is now just emerging to evaluate the role of neuromodulation on inflammation in the CNS.

Cytokine and inflammatory mediatory dysregulation play a key component in the generation of chronic pain. While mounting a strong immune response after injury is initially advantageous, chronic and continued activation of the inflammation cascade transforms into a maladaptive process. When observing disease processes such as osteoarthritis, CRPS, fibromyalgia, and postherpetic neuralgia, studies have found increased inflammatory markers within the CSF of patients with these diseases.[67] This finding is also consistent with disease processes that have indications for SCS therapy, including lumbar radiculopathy, failed back surgery syndrome, and chronic lower back pain.[67] Of the pro-inflammatory cytokines known, interleukin-1β and TNF-α have been shown to act via a positive feedback mechanism to further the immune response and reinforce glial activation.[67] If SCS is effectively modulating the inflammation in the CNS, then one would expect there to be changes in biomarker profiles.

With regards to inflammatory mediator levels with SCS, data is inconclusive. Studies have shown increases of IL-1B and IL-10 within the dura matter of P-SCS patients.[68] Of note, the concentration of IL-6 has been shown to be inversely related to the delivered current of stimulation, creating a bell-shaped relationship.[68] When observing the immunomodulatory effects of SCS in patients with CRPS, it was shown to have reduced interferon-γ-inducible protein 10 and vascular endothelial growth factor (VEGF), but no significant differences in pro- or anti-inflammatory cytokines.[69] These results highlight the future work that needs to be done regarding inflammatory mediator modulation in chronic pain syndromes. Neurotrophic factors such as nerve growth factor, brain-derived neurotrophic factor, and glial cell line–derived neurotrophic factor are essential for homeostasis and regeneration after

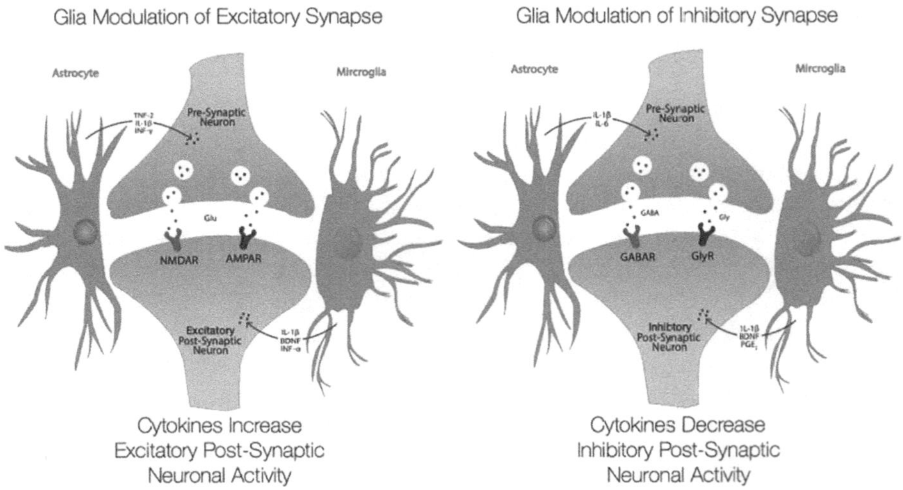

FIGURE 16.2 Local glia modulate synaptic transmission after nerve injury. Glia is intimately associated with spinal excitatory and inhibitory synapses. The release of cytokines and glial mediators on pre- and post-synaptic terminals modulates the activity of that synapse. Cytokines released at glutaminergic excitatory synapses augment transmission, while cytokines released at GABAergic and glycinergic synapses attenuate the signal. The net effect of gliosis, and the release of glial mediators, is an increase in spinal cord pain transmission. Novel modes of SCS may modulate glial activity, thereby enacting their antinociceptive mechanisms through this pathway. Acronyms: Glu, glutamate; GABA, gamma-aminobutyric acid; Gly, glycine; TNF-α, tumor necrosis factor alpha; IL-1β, interleukin 1β; IFN-γ, interferon gamma; NMDAR, NMDA receptor; AMPAR, AMPA receptor; BDNF, brain-derived neurotrophic factor; GABAR, GABA receptor; GlyR, glycine receptor; PGE_2, prostaglandin E_2.

neuron injury and are triggered by inflammation.[70] These neurotrophic factors are present at increased levels in patients with lumbar radiculopathy, failed back surgery syndrome, and chronic lower back pain.[70] Studies have revealed increased expression of these factors in inflammatory and neuropathic pain states, but no change in levels with the application of SCS.[71] Although the evidence is not completely established, there is data to support the theory that SCS acts to modulate neuroinflammation, and thus nociception. Additional preclinical work aimed to clarify the response of these neuroinflammatory signaling pathways to SCS is underway and greatly needed in this space.

16.5 MECHANISMS OF ACTION BY ELECTRICITY WAVEFORM

16.5.1 Paresthesia-Based Spinal Cord Stimulation (P-SCS)

Originally hypothesized to operate under the gate control theory of pain, the P-SCS mechanism of action was thought to be due to stimulation of Aβ fibers and inhibitory interneurons, leading to inhibition of nociceptive signaling from pathologic wide dynamic receptors to Aδ and C fibers.[72, 73] P-SCS is comprised of a baseline frequency that ranges between 40 and 60 Hz, with pulse widths ranging between 150 and 500 μs. The amplitude and positioning of the leads is adjusted so the patient receives a non-painful paresthesia over the target dermatome. P-SCS delivers pulsatile frequency that activates dorsal horn inhibitory interneurons, which ultimately release GABA and glycine within the dorsal horn.[33, 74] How P-SCS achieves this, though, is not entirely clear. Theories on inhibitory interneuron activation include direct modulation by a localized electric field, activation of descending inputs to the interneurons, and antidromic activation via Aβ afferents.[75] More than one of these methods may be at play, with studies arguing for multiple contributions to the dorsal horn inhibitory circuit from P-SCS.[14, 76, 77] In addition to activating inhibitory interneurons, P-SCS is thought to attenuate inflammatory mediator release and gliosis, which contribute to allodynia and hyperalgesia.[58] Although this theory has yet to be completely explored, current evidence suggests P-SCS decreases microglia and astrocyte activation, but the effect on local glial inflammatory mediators is unknown.[78, 79] P-SCS also may play a role in the activation of the dorsal columns and subsequent stimulation and activation of the serotonergic and noradrenergic DAS.[33, 80] Triggering of these descending supraspinal inhibitory loops leads to increases in GABA and glycine within the dorsal horn via

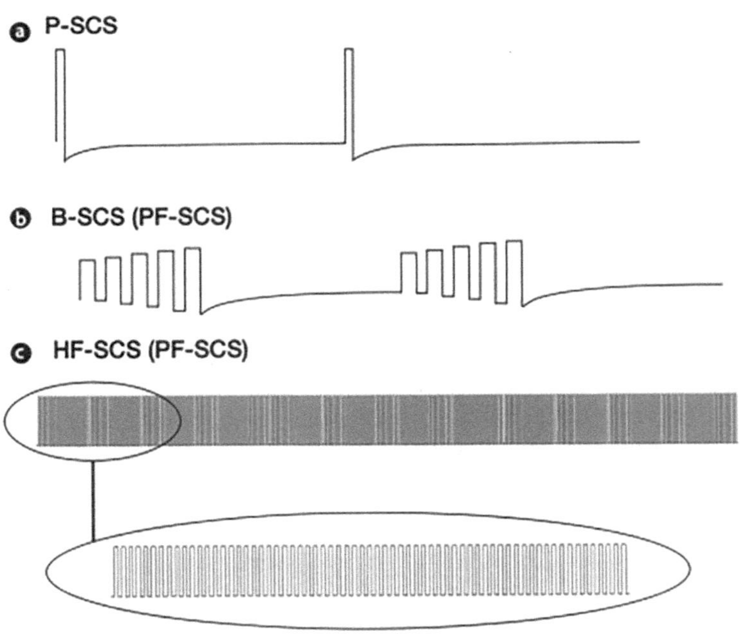

FIGURE 16.3 Stimulation patterns in paresthesia and paresthesia-free SCS paradigms. (a) Traditional SCS comprised of tonic or repetitive low-frequency SCS usually in the range of 40–60 Hz produces paresthesia of P-SCS. (b) Paresthesia-free burst spinal cord stimulation (B-SCS) employs an incremental increase in amplitude with each burst. Interburst frequency is 40 Hz, while intraburst frequency is 500 Hz. (c) Between each burst, there is a passive recharge phase. Paresthesia-free, high-frequency SCS employs an ultra-high frequency of 10 kHz in continuous mode.

serotonin and norepinephrine.[21, 22, 55] In addition to activation of the serotonergic and noradrenergic DAS, P-SCS also activates opioidergic mechanisms via a time-limited, frequency-dependent mechanism.[33] This opioidergic recruitment likely has a ceiling effect, and further studies need to be done to determine the mechanism of this recruitment.[47, 81] In summary, P-SCS likely exerts its analgesia through modulation of multiple endogenous pathways—the full extent of these contributions remains to be elucidated.

16.5.2 High-Frequency Spinal Cord Stimulation (HF-SCS)

High-frequency, paresthesia-free SCS delivers high-frequency and low-amplitude pulses via percutaneously placed epidural electrodes and is used for the management of failed back surgery syndrome and chronic axial back pain. Unlike P-SCS, HF-SCS maximizes total charge delivery without generating paresthesia, and pain relief with HF-SCS does not correspond to an area of paresthesia, revealing a likely novel mechanism of action.[82] Traditionally, HF-SCS utilizes 10 kHz stimulation; however, lower-frequency subthreshold models of 1, 1.15, and 5 kHz have all shown benefit.[83–85] Regardless of the frequency delivered, HF-SCS has shown superiority to P-SCS in several clinical trials.[82, 86] Several hypotheses have been developed to explain the beneficial effects of HF-SCS, including: (1) HF-SCS stimulation creates a reversible depolarization blockade, (2) HF-SCS causes desynchronization of neural signaling, and (3) HF-SCS stimulation results in membrane integration.[87] While these hypotheses are still being developed, both computer and animal models suggest that, in contrast to traditional SCS, paresthesia-free HF-SCS does not activate or modulate fibers within the dorsal column.[88, 89] In traditional SCS, the gracile nucleus is activated via inputs from the dorsal column fibers. However, Song et al. revealed no activation of gracile nucleus neurons from the dorsal column afferents in response to HF-SCS.[89] Studies have also demonstrated that the antinociceptive effects of HF-SCS exhibit a delayed onset when compared to P-SCS, which has become known as the "wash-in period."[90] It is not surprising that the peak pain inhibition of HF-SCS also occurred later than P-SCS in animal models.[89] While the mechanisms and effects of P-SCS have been studied, further work is needed to clarify these properties of HF-SCS.

16.5.3 Burst Spinal Cord Stimulation (B-SCS)

Providing a predominantly paresthesia-free delivery, B-SCS utilizes a stacked pulse model of energy delivery.[91–94] The burst model mimics endogenous physiologic neuronal burst firing within the central nervous system and results in either activation of membrane potential and subsequently, an action potential or supra-threshold conductance that initiates two or more action potentials. The action potentials occur during an "active phase," while the period between these potentials is known as the "silent phase." These action potentials exhibiting burst firing have been identified within the thalamus, dorsal horns, and C fibers, indicating they may play a role in nociceptive pathways.[95] Certain neurons undergo "multiplexing," and depending on the neuron, some will activate when receiving particular burst frequencies, while others will remain silent.[96] B-SCS emulates these physiologic burst patterns and is comprised of 40 Hz bursts with five spikes at 500. This is accompanied by a pulse width of 1,000 μs and an interburst interval of 1,000 μs. Studies have revealed that increased bulse widths increase B-SCS analgesia, and the number of pulses per burst increases the buildup of post-synaptic potential and improves signals comparative to noise.[97, 98] In addition, increasing the number of pulses per burst leads to enhanced neuroplasticity.[97] These effects, however, exhibit a ceiling effect of around 6–7 spikes per burst.[99] It has also been discovered that an intraburst frequency of 500 Hz was optimal, and this higher frequency can lead to maximal opioidergic effects.[100]

Although the mechanism of action isn't entirely understood, it has been postulated that B-SCS may operate by modulating antinociceptive C fibers in addition to modulating multiplexing and cortical attentional mechanisms.[96, 98, 101] It has been described that the reward system within the CNS is responsible for regulating the descending pain inhibitory system. It is no surprise that in chronic pain states, an imbalance between ascending pain pathways (medial and lateral pain pathways) and the descending pain inhibitory pathway exists, likely caused by a disruption in the reward system.[102–105] In a study done by De Ridder et al. using EEG analysis in human subjects with SCS, it was revealed that both burst and traditional SCS lead to alterations in the ascending lateral pathway in addition to the descending pain inhibitory pathway. However, burst stimulation also leads to alterations in the medial pain pathway, indicating a novel mechanism.[106] Despite both traditional SCS and B-SCS mitigating the increase in signaling in pain-related areas of the brain, B-SCS leads to the apparent normalization of this pathologic brain activity.[106] These results could explain the improved results from patients utilizing B-SCS as compared to traditional tonic SCS.

16.5.4 Dorsal Root Ganglion Stimulation (DRG-S)

The dorsal root ganglion contains the cell bodies of first-degree sensory neurons that carry pain signals to the spinal cord.[107, 108] In chronic pain states, inflammation leads to maladaptive increased firing rates. What makes DRG-S unique is that the dorsal root ganglion lies within the lateral epidural space, and DRG-S targets the sensory neurons themselves, as compared to other types of SCS which target the posterior spinal cord tracts. This allows DRG-S for a more specified target of therapy to precise dermatomes or pain regions. DRG-S is thought to reduce sensory neuron excitability and reduce action potential propagation from the periphery.[107] In addition, DRG-S is believed to decrease inflammatory markers and markers of glial cell activation and neuronal injury.[66] Despite trials showing superiority to traditional SCS in certain pain conditions, one obvious drawback would be the technically difficult placement required to target specific dorsal root ganglions.

16.6 CONCLUSION

Currently, the evolution of SCS waveforms and neuroanatomical targets is outpacing the preclinical basic science research for these therapies. With each platform adopting and developing new waveforms at a rapid pace, it is challenging to determine which mechanism of action underlies a given SCS's analgesia. This becomes even more challenging when different electrical waveforms are layered on one another (known as multiplexing). It is understood that SCS potentially modulates a patient's chronic pain through multiple mechanisms. These include locally, (1) by altering neurotransmitters at the level of the dorsal horn, (2) by activating ascending projections, (3) by activating the descending modulatory systems, and (4) by modulating cortical and subcortical pain processing centers. Though further work is needed to characterize how these therapies provide analgesia, their demonstrated clinical benefit ensures that the space will continue to rapidly evolve and warrants further preclinical study.

REFERENCES

1. Tilley D, Benyamin R, Vallejo R. Dose-Dependent Changes in Gene Expression Using Spinal Cord Stimulation (SCS). Paper presented at: North American Neuromodulation Society 2019; Las Vegas.
2. Caylor J, Reddy R, Yin S, et al. Spinal cord stimulation in chronic pain: evidence and theory for mechanisms of action. *Bioelectronic Medicine*. 2019;5(1):1–41.
3. Shealy CN, Taslitz N, Mortimer JT, Becker DP. Electrical inhibition of pain: experimental evaluation. *Anesthesia & Analgesia*. 1967;46(3):299–305.
4. Melzack R, Wall PD. Pain assessment, a new theory. *Science*. 1965;150(3699):971–975.
5. Benzon HT, Raja SN, Fishman SM, Liu SS, Cohen SP. *Essentials of Pain Medicine*. Elsevier Health Sciences; 2017.
6. Wall PD, Melzack R. Textbook of Pain. In. 6th Editio ed: Saunders; 2013.
7. Todd AJ. Neuronal circuitry for pain processing in the dorsal horn. *Nature Reviews Neuroscience*. 2010;11(12):823–836.
8. Roberts WJ, Foglesong ME. I. Spinal recordings suggest that wide-dynamic-range neurons mediate sympathetically maintained pain. *Pain*. 1988;34(3):289–304.
9. Dong YF, Tang JS, Yuan B, Jia H. Morphine applied to the thalamic nucleus submedius produces a naloxone reversible antinociceptive effect in the rat. *Neuroscience Letters*. 1999;271(1):17–20.
10. Hardy SG. Projections to the midbrain from the medial versus lateral prefrontal cortices of the rat. *Neuroscience Letters*. 1986;63(2):159–164.
11. Helmstetter FJ, Tershner SA, Poore LH, Bellgowan PS. Antinociception following opioid stimulation of the basolateral amygdala is expressed through the periaqueductal gray and rostral ventromedial medulla. *Brain Research*. 1998;779(1–2):104–118.
12. Sakata S, Shima F, Kato M, Fukui M. Dissociated mesencephalic responses to medial and ventral thalamic nuclei stimulation in rats. Relationship to analgesic mechanisms. *Journal of Neurosurgery*. 1989;70(3):446–453.
13. Basbaum AI, Clanton CH, Fields HL. Opiate and stimulus-produced analgesia: functional anatomy of a medullospinal pathway. *Proceedings of the National Academy of Sciences of the United States of America*. 1976;73(12):4685–4688.
14. Cui M, Feng Y, McAdoo DJ, Willis WD. Periaqueductal gray stimulation-induced inhibition of nociceptive dorsal horn neurons in rats is associated with the release of norepinephrine, serotonin, and amino acids. *The Journal of Pharmacology and Experimental Therapeutics*. 1999;289(2):868–876.
15. Mendell LM. Constructing and deconstructing the gate theory of pain. *Pain*. 2014; 155(2):210–216.
16. Song Z, Ansah O, Meyerson B, Pertovaara A, Linderoth B. The rostroventromedial medulla is engaged in the effects of spinal cord stimulation in a rodent model of neuropathic pain. *Neuroscience*. 2013;247:134–144.
17. Bernard JF, Bester H, Besson JM. Involvement of the spino-parabrachio -amygdaloid and -hypothalamic pathways in the autonomic and affective emotional aspects of pain. *Progress in Brain Research*. 1996;107:243–255.

18. Gauriau C, Bernard J-F. Pain pathways and parabrachial circuits in the rat. *Experimental Physiology*. 2002;87(2):251–258.
19. Kwiat GC, Basbaum AI. The origin of brainstem noradrenergic and serotonergic projections to the spinal cord dorsal horn in the rat. *Somatosensory & Motor Research*. 1992;9(2):157–173.
20. Olsen RW, DeLorey TM. GABA receptors have been identified electrophysiologically and pharmacologically in all regions of the brain. In: Siegel GJ, Agranoff BW, Albers RW, eds. 6 ed. Philadelphia: Lippincott-Raven; 1999.
21. Lekan HA, Carlton SM. Glutamatergic and GABAergic input to rat spinothalamic tract cells in the superficial dorsal horn. *The Journal of Comparative Neurology*. 1995;361(3):417–428.
22. Cui JG, O'Connor WT, Ungerstedt U, Linderoth B, Meyerson BA. Spinal cord stimulation attenuates augmented dorsal horn release of excitatory amino acids in mononeuropathy via a GABAergic mechanism. *Pain*. 1997;73(1):87–95.
23. Stiller CO, Cui JG, O'Connor WT, Brodin E, Meyerson BA, Linderoth B. Release of gamma-aminobutyric acid in the dorsal horn and suppression of tactile allodynia by spinal cord stimulation in mononeuropathic rats. *Neurosurgery*. 1996;39(2):365–367.
24. Duggan AW, Foong FW. Bicuculline and spinal inhibition produced by dorsal column stimulation in the cat. *Pain*. 1985;22(3):249–259.
25. Sivilotti L, Woolf CJ. The contribution of GABAA and glycine receptors to central sensitization: disinhibition and touch-evoked allodynia in the spinal cord. *Journal of Neurophysiology*. 1994;72(1):169–179.
26. Moens M, Mariën P, Brouns R, et al. Spinal cord stimulation modulates cerebral neurobiology: a proton magnetic resonance spectroscopy study. *Neuroradiology*. 2013;55(8):1039–1047.
27. Moens M, Sunaert S, Mariën P, et al. Spinal cord stimulation modulates cerebral function: an fMRI study. *Neuroradiology*. 2012;54(12):1399–1407.
28. Vera-Portocarrero L, Zhang E-T, Ossipov M, et al. Descending facilitation from the rostral ventromedial medulla maintains nerve injury-induced central sensitization. *Neuroscience*. 2006;140(4):1311–1320.
29. Suzuki R, Rahman W, Hunt SP, Dickenson AH. Descending facilitatory control of mechanically evoked responses is enhanced in deep dorsal horn neurons following peripheral nerve injury. *Brain Research*. 2004;1019(1–2):68–76.
30. Pertovaara A. Plasticity in descending pain modulatory systems. In: *Progress in Brain Research*. Vol 129. Elsevier; 2000:231–242.
31. Newton BW, Hamill RW. The morphology and distribution of rat serotoninergic intraspinal neurons: an immunohistochemical study. *Brain Research Bulletin*. 1988;20(3):349–360.
32. Linderoth B, Gazelius B, Franck J, Brodin E. Dorsal column stimulation induces the release of serotonin and substance P in the cat dorsal horn. *Neurosurgery*. 1992;31(2):287–289.
33. Song Z, Ultenius C, Meyerson BA, Linderoth B. Pain relief by spinal cord stimulation involves serotonergic mechanisms: an experimental study in a rat model of mononeuropathy. *Pain*. 2009;147(1–3):241–248.
34. Tazawa T, Kamiya Y, Kobayashi A, et al. Spinal cord stimulation modulates supraspinal centers of the descending antinociceptive system in rats with unilateral spinal nerve injury. *Molecular Pain*. 2015;11:36–36.
35. Hayashida K-I, Obata H, Nakajima K, Eisenach JC. Gabapentin acts within the locus coeruleus to alleviate neuropathic pain. *Anesthesiology*. 2008;109(6):1077–1084.
36. Hayashida K-I, DeGoes S, Curry R, Eisenach JC. Gabapentin activates spinal noradrenergic activity in rats and humans and reduces hypersensitivity after surgery. *Anesthesiology*. 2007;106(3):557–562.
37. Pertovaara A. Noradrenergic pain modulation. *Progress in Neurobiology*. 2006;80(2):53–83.

38. Baba H, Goldstein PA, Okamoto M, et al. Norepinephrine facilitates inhibitory transmission in substantia gelatinosa of adult rat spinal cord (part 2) effects on somatodendritic sites of gabaergic neurons. *Anesthesiology: The Journal of the American Society of Anesthesiologists*. 2000;92(2):485–485.
39. Baba H, Shimoji K, Yoshimura M. Norepinephrine facilitates inhibitory transmission in substantia gelatinosa of adult rat spinal cord (part 1): effects on axon terminals of GABAergic and glycinergic neurons. *Anesthesiology*. 2000;92(2):473–484.
40. Song Z, Ansah OB, Meyerson BA, Pertovaara A, Linderoth B. Exploration of supraspinal mechanisms in effects of spinal cord stimulation: role of the locus coeruleus. *Neuroscience*. 2013;253:426–434.
41. Foreman RD. *Neural Mechanisms of Spinal Cord Stimulation*. Vol 1072012.
42. Schechtmann G, Song Z, Ultenius C, Meyerson BA, Linderoth B. Cholinergic mechanisms involved in the pain-relieving effect of spinal cord stimulation in a model of neuropathy. *Pain*. 2008;139(1):136–145.
43. Benzon HT, Rathmel JP, Wu CL, Turk D, Argof CE, Hurley RW. *Practical Management of Pain*. 5 ed. Philadelphia: Mosby; 2014.
44. Wang YY, Wu SX, Liu XY, Wang W, Li YQ. Effects of c-fos antisense oligodeoxynucleotide on 5-HT-induced upregulation of preprodynorphin, preproenkephalin, and glutamic acid decarboxylase mRNA expression in cultured rat spinal dorsal horn neurons. *Biochemical and Biophysical Research Communications*. 2003;309(3):631–636.
45. Ding X, Hua F, Sutherly K, Ardell JL, Williams CA. C2 spinal cord stimulation induces dynorphin release from rat T4 spinal cord: potential modulation of myocardial ischemia-sensitive neurons. *American Journal of Physiology-Regulatory, Integrative and Comparative Physiology*. 2008;295(5):R1519–R1528.
46. Sato KL, King EW, Johanek LM, Sluka KA. Spinal cord stimulation reduces hypersensitivity through activation of opioid receptors in a frequency-dependent manner. *European Journal of Pain*. 2013;17(4):551–561.
47. Sun L, Tai L, Qiu Q, et al. Endocannabinoid activation of CB1 receptors contributes to long-lasting reversal of neuropathic pain by repetitive spinal cord stimulation. *European Journal of Pain*. 2017;21(5):804–814.
48. Inoue S, Johanek LM, Sluka KA. Lack of analgesic synergy of the cholecystokinin receptor antagonist proglumide and spinal cord stimulation for the treatment of neuropathic pain in rats. *Neuromodulation: Technology at the Neural Interface*. 2017;20(6):534–542.
49. Stiller CO, Linderoth B, O'Connor WT, et al. Repeated spinal cord stimulation decreases the extracellular level of gamma-aminobutyric acid in the periaqueductal gray matter of freely moving rats. *Brain Research*. 1995;699(2):231–241.
50. Song Z, Ansah OB, Meyerson BA, Pertovaara A, Linderoth B. The rostroventromedial medulla is engaged in the effects of spinal cord stimulation in a rodent model of neuropathic pain. *Neuroscience*. 2013;247:134–144.
51. Crosby ND, Weisshaar CL, Smith JR, Zeeman ME, Goodman-Keiser MD, Winkelstein BA. Burst and tonic spinal cord stimulation differentially activates GABAergic mechanisms to attenuate pain in a rat model of cervical radiculopathy. *IEEE Transactions on Bio-Medical Engineering*. 2015;62(6):1604–1613.
52. Levin BE, Hubschmann OR. Dorsal column stimulation: effect on human cerebrospinal fluid and plasma catecholamines. *Neurology*. 1980;30(1):65–65.
53. Liu JT, Tan WC, Liao W-J. Effects of electrical cervical spinal cord stimulation on cerebral blood perfusion, cerebrospinal fluid catecholamine levels, and oxidative stress in comatose patients. In: *Reconstructive Neurosurgery*. Springer; 2008:71–76.
54. Song Z, Meyerson BA, Linderoth B. Spinal 5-HT receptors that contribute to the pain-relieving effects of spinal cord stimulation in a rat model of neuropathy. *Pain*. 2011;152(7):1666–1673.

55. Barchini J, Tchachaghian S, Shamaa Fa, et al. Spinal segmental and supraspinal mechanisms underlying the pain-relieving effects of spinal cord stimulation: an experimental study in a rat model of neuropathy. *Neuroscience*. 2012;215:196–208.
56. Cui JG, Linderoth B, Meyerson BA. Effects of spinal cord stimulation on touch-evoked allodynia involve GABAergic mechanisms. An experimental study in the mononeuropathic rat. *Pain*. 1996;66(2–3):287–295.
57. Schechtmann G, Wallin J, Meyerson BA, Linderoth B. Intrathecal clonidine potentiates suppression of tactile hypersensitivity by spinal cord stimulation in a model of neuropathy. *Anesthesia & Analgesia*. 2004;99(1):135–139.
58. Song Z, Meyerson BA, Linderoth B. Muscarinic receptor activation potentiates the effect of spinal cord stimulation on pain-related behavior in rats with mononeuropathy. *Neuroscience Letters*. 2008;436(1):7–12.
59. Ji R-R, Berta T, Nedergaard M. Glia and pain: is chronic pain a gliopathy? *Pain*. 2013;154 Suppl:S10–28.
60. Tremblay M-E, Stevens B, Sierra A, Wake H, Bessis A, Nimmerjahn A. The role of microglia in the healthy brain. *The Journal of Neuroscience: The Official Journal of The Society for Neuroscience*. 2011;31(45):16064–16069.
61. Watkins LR, Milligan ED, Maier SF. Glial activation: a driving force for pathological pain. *Trends in Neurosciences*. 2001;24(8):450–455.
62. Watkins LR, Milligan ED, Maier SF. Spinal cord glia: new players in pain. *Pain*. 2001;93(3):201–205.
63. Mika J, Zychowska M, Popiolek-Barczyk K, Rojewska E, Przewlocka B. Importance of glial activation in neuropathic pain. *European Journal of Pharmacology*. 2013;716(1–3):106–119.
64. Rozanski GM, Li Q, Stanley EF. Transglial transmission at the dorsal root ganglion sandwich synapse: glial cell to postsynaptic neuron communication. 2013(1460–9568 (Electronic)).
65. Chen Y, Zhang X, Wang C, Li G, Gu Y, Huang L-YM. Activation of P2X7 receptors in glial satellite cells reduces pain through downregulation of P2X3 receptors in nociceptive neurons. *Proceedings of the National Academy of Sciences of the United States of America*. 2008;105(43):16773–16778.
66. Hanani M. Satellite glial cells in sensory ganglia: from form to function. *Brain Research Brain Research Reviews*. 2005;48(3):457–476.
67. Pan B, Yu H, Fischer GJ, Kramer JM, Hogan QH. Dorsal root ganglionic field stimulation relieves spontaneous and induced neuropathic pain in rats. *Journal of Pain*. 2016;17(12):1349–1358.
68. Bjurstrom MF, Giron SE, Griffis CA. Cerebrospinal fluid cytokines and neurotrophic factors in human chronic pain populations: a comprehensive review. *Pain Practice*. 2016;16(2):183–203.
69. Kriek N, Schreurs MW, Groeneweg JG, et al. Spinal cord stimulation in patients with complex regional pain syndrome: a possible target for immunomodulation? *Neuromodulation: Technology at the Neural Interface*. 2018;21(1):77–86.
70. Pezet S, McMahon SB. Neurotrophins: mediators and modulators of pain. *Annual Review of Neuroscience*. 2006;29:507–538.
71. Tilley DM, Cedeño DL, Kelley CA, DeMaegd M, Benyamin R, Vallejo R. Changes in dorsal root ganglion gene expression in response to spinal cord stimulation. *Regional Anesthesia and Pain Medicine*. 2017;42(2):246–251.
72. Melzack R, Wall P. Pain mechanisms: a new theory. *Science*. 1965;150(3699):971–979.
73. Sivanesan E, Maher DP, Raja SN, Linderoth B, Guan Y. Supraspinal mechanisms of spinal cord stimulation for modulation of pain. *Anesthesiology*. 2018(Xxx):1–1.
74. Yakhnitsa V, Linderoth B, Meyerson BA. Spinal cord stimulation attenuates dorsal horn neuronal hyperexcitability in a rat model of mononeuropathy. *Pain*. 1999;79(2–3):223–233.

75. Zhang TC, Janik JJ, Grill WM. Mechanisms and models of spinal cord stimulation for the treatment of neuropathic pain. *Brain Research*. 2014;1569:19–31.
76. Hochman S, Shreckengost J, Kimura H, Quevedo J. Presynaptic inhibition of primary afferents by depolarization: observations supporting nontraditional mechanisms. 201 (1749–6632 (Electronic)).
77. Szentagothai J. Neuronal and synaptic arrangement in the substantia gelatinosa rolandi. *The Journal of Comparative Neurology*. 1964;122:219–239.
78. McCarthy KF, McCrory C. Cerebrospinal fluid levels of glial cell-derived neurotrophic factor correlate with spinal cord stimulation frequency in patients with neuropathic pain: a preliminary report. *Spinal Cord*. 2014;52 Suppl 2:S8–10.
79. Sato KL, Johanek LM, Sanada LS, Sluka KA. Spinal cord stimulation reduces mechanical hyperalgesia and glial cell activation in animals with neuropathic pain. *Anesthesia and Analgesia*. 2014;118(2):464–472.
80. Saade NE, Tabet MS, Soueidan SA, Bitar M, Atweh SF, Jabbur SJ. Supraspinal modulation of nociception in awake rats by stimulation of the dorsal column nuclei. *Brain Research*. 1986;369(1–2):307–310.
81. Chandran P, Sluka KA. Development of opioid tolerance with repeated transcutaneous electrical nerve stimulation administration. *Pain*. 2003;102(1–2):195–201.
82. Kapural L, Yu C, Doust MW, et al. Novel 10-kHz High-frequency Therapy (HF10 Therapy) Is Superior to Traditional Low-frequency Spinal Cord Stimulation for the Treatment of Chronic Back and Leg Pain: The SENZA-RCT Randomized Controlled Trial. *Anesthesiology*. 2015;123(4):851–860.
83. North JM, Hong K-SJ, Cho PY. Clinical outcomes of 1 kHz subperception spinal cord stimulation in implanted patients with failed paresthesia-based stimulation: results of a prospective randomized controlled trial. *Neuromodulation: Journal of the International Neuromodulation Society*. 2016;19(7):731–737.
84. Perruchoud C, Eldabe S, Batterham AM, et al. Analgesic efficacy of high-frequency spinal cord stimulation: a randomized double-blind placebo-controlled study. *Neuromodulation: Journal of the International Neuromodulation Society*. 2013;16(4):363–369; discussion 369.
85. Youn Y, Smith H, Morris B, Argoff C, Pilitsis JG. The effect of high-frequency stimulation on sensory thresholds in chronic pain patients. *Stereotactic and Functional Neurosurgery*. 2015;93(5):355–359.
86. Kapural L, Yu C, Doust MW, et al. Comparison of 10-kHz high-frequency and traditional low-frequency spinal cord stimulation for the treatment of chronic back and leg pain: 24-month results from a multicenter, randomized, controlled pivotal trial. *Neurosurgery*. 2016;79(5):667–677.
87. Linderoth B, Foreman RD. Conventional and novel spinal stimulation algorithms: hypothetical mechanisms of action and comments on outcomes. *Neuromodulation*. 2017;20(6):525–533.
88. Lempka SF, McIntyre CC, Kilgore KL, Machado AG. Computational analysis of kilohertz frequency spinal cord stimulation for chronic pain management. *Anesthesiology*. 2015;122(6):1362–1376.
89. Song Z, Viisanen H, Meyerson BA, Pertovaara A, Linderoth B. Efficacy of kilohertz-frequency and conventional spinal cord stimulation in rat models of different pain conditions. *Neuromodulation: Technology at the Neural Interface*. 2014;17(3):226–235.
90. Shechter R, Yang F, Xu Q, et al. Conventional and kilohertz-frequency spinal cord stimulation produces intensity-and frequency-dependent inhibition of mechanical hypersensitivity in a rat model of neuropathic pain. *Anesthesiology*. 2013;119(2):422–432.
91. De Ridder D, Vanneste S, Plazier M, van der Loo E, Menovsky T. Burst spinal cord stimulation: toward paresthesia-free pain suppression. *Neurosurgery*. 2010;66(5):986–990.

92. Deer T, Slavin KV, Amirdelfan K, et al. Success using neuromodulation with BURST (SUNBURST) study: results from a prospective, randomized controlled trial using a novel burst waveform. *Neuromodulation: Journal of the International Neuromodulation Society*. 2018;21(1):56–66.
93. Schu S, Slotty PJ, Bara G, von Knop M, Edgar D, Vesper J. A prospective, randomized, double-blind, placebo-controlled study to examine the effectiveness of burst spinal cord stimulation patterns for the treatment of failed back surgery syndrome. *Neuromodulation: Journal of the International Neuromodulation Society*. 2014;17(5):443–450.
94. Tang R, Martinez M, Goodman-Keiser M, Farber JP, Qin C, Foreman RD. Comparison of burst and tonic spinal cord stimulation on spinal neural processing in an animal model. *Neuromodulation: Journal of the International Neuromodulation Society*. 2014;17(2):143–151.
95. Hodaie M, Cordella R, Lozano AM, Wennberg R, Dostrovsky JO. Bursting activity of neurons in the human anterior thalamic nucleus. *Brain Research*. 2006;1115(1):1–8.
96. Izhikevich EM, Desai NS, Walcott EC, Hoppensteadt FC. Bursts as a unit of neural information: selective communication via resonance. *Trends in Neurosciences*. 2003;26(3):161–167.
97. Crosby ND, Goodman Keiser MD, Smith JR, Zeeman ME, Winkelstein BA. Stimulation parameters define the effectiveness of burst spinal cord stimulation in a rat model of neuropathic pain. *Neuromodulation: Technology at the Neural Interface*. 2015;18(1):1–8.
98. De Ridder D, Vancamp T, Vanneste S. Fundamentals of burst stimulation of the spinal cord and brain. In: *Neuromodulation*. Elsevier; 2018:147–160.
99. Snider R, Kabara J, Roig B, Bonds A. Burst firing and modulation of functional connectivity in cat striate cortex. *Journal of Neurophysiology*. 1998;80(2):730–744.
100. Song B, Marvizón JCG. Dorsal horn neurons firing at high frequency, but not primary afferents, release opioid peptides that produce μ-opioid receptor internalization in the rat spinal cord. *Journal of Neuroscience*. 2003;23(27):9171–9184.
101. Liljencrantz J, Olausson H. Tactile C fibers and their contributions to pleasant sensations and tactile allodynia. *Frontiers in Behavioral Neuroscience*. 2014;8:37.
102. Baliki MN, Petre B, Torbey S, et al. Corticostriatal functional connectivity predicts transition to chronic back pain. *Nature Neuroscience*. 2012;15(8):1117.
103. De Ridder D, Vanneste S, Menovsky T, Langguth B. Surgical brain modulation for tinnitus: the past, present, and future. *Journal of Neurosurgical Sciences*. 2012;56(4):323–340.
104. Denk F, McMahon SB, Tracey I. Pain vulnerability: a neurobiological perspective. *Nature Neuroscience*. 2014;17(2):192.
105. Mansour AR, Baliki MN, Huang L, et al. Brain white matter structural properties predict transition to chronic pain. *PAIN®*. 2013;154(10):2160–2168.
106. De Ridder D, Vanneste S. Burst and tonic spinal cord stimulation: different and common brain mechanisms. *Neuromodulation: Technology at the Neural Interface*. 2016;19(1):47–59.
107. Koopmeiners AS, Mueller S, Kramer J, Hogan QH. Effect of electrical field stimulation on dorsal root ganglion neuronal function. *Neuromodulation*. 2013;16(4):304–311.
108. Van Buyten JP. Dorsal Root Ganglion Stimulation. *Essentials of Pain Medicine*. 2018: 683–692.

17 Mechanisms of Action of Clinically Relevant Analgesics (Opioids)

Jennifer Tram, Jacob Ezell, and Timothy Furnish

All figures were created by the authors and allowed for use for this publication.

17.1 INTRODUCTION

Opioid analgesics have been the gold standard for the treatment of pain for centuries. The most commonly prescribed opioids in the United States are morphine, oxycodone, hydrocodone, and codeine. Opioids have unique pharmacokinetics, depending on the specific opioid as well as other factors, including route of administration (oral, sublingual, intravenous, transdermal, etc.), dosage, opioid–receptor interactions, and duration of usage.

In this chapter, we will discuss the history of opioids, opioid–receptor subclasses, mechanism of action, adverse effects of opioids, endogenous opioid ligands, opioid subtypes, and future directions of opioid drug development.

17.2 HISTORY OF OPIOID ANALGESICS

Although opioids are primarily used as analgesics today, throughout history, they served various purposes in different civilizations and societies. The opium poppy was first cultivated in lower Mesopotamia around 3400 BC.[1] Hundreds of years later, Arabic physicians prescribed opium and opioid derivatives for the treatment of dysentery.[2] Later, in the 1600s, Thomas Sydenham, an English pharmacist who created an opium tincture called *laudanum*, commented on the enduring history of opioid usage:[3,4]

> Among the remedies which it has pleased Almighty God to give to man to relieve his sufferings, none is so universal and so efficacious as opium.

The German pharmacist Friedrick Sertürner first isolated opioid crystals from a resin derived from poppy seed juice. He studied the properties of this new substance in animals and published his findings in 1805.[5] He named the drug *morphium*, after the Greek god of dreams.[4,5] Further studies in humans identified the analgesic properties of this drug as well as other effects, such as dose-dependent euphoria, drowsiness,

DOI: 10.1201/9781003094302-17

and somnolence. In modern medicine, this same derivative is known as morphine. Commercial development of morphine began in 1827 by the German manufacturer Merck & Company.

The use of morphine continued to grow after the development of hypodermic needles in the mid-1800s.[4, 6] Shortly after this development, the production of codeine started. Due to morphine's increased availability in the late 1800s, its addictive properties became apparent. In 1895, the Bayer Company developed diacetylmorphine, sold under the trade name heroin, and marketed as a more efficacious and less-addictive form of morphine.[7] Obviously, history has shown this to be false.

The availability of opioids over the past 150 years has varied between easily obtained and highly restricted. In the late 19th century, *laudanum* and morphine were widely available and resulted in significant opioid addiction among the United States Civil War veterans, but also marketed and prescribed for insomnia, dysentery, headaches, menstrual cramps, and other maladies.[4] As the problems of opioid addiction became more apparent, the first laws restricting the use of opioids and other controlled substances were passed in the early 20th century. This resulted in restrictions on the availability and use of opioids through the early and middle 20th century. Starting in the 1970s, the expansion of hospice and palliative care services led to more widespread use of opioids for cancer and end-of-life pain management. As a possible consequence, less-restrictive prescribing of opioids spread to the treatment of non-cancer pain in the 1990s.[8] As opioid use for non-cancer pain expanded, so did opioid addiction, and the resulting opioid epidemic led to a resurgence of restrictive prescribing laws and practices in the early 21st century.

17.3 OPIOID RECEPTORS

The first three opioid receptors, mu (μ), delta (∂), and kappa (κ), were identified in the 1970s.[9, 10] In 1994, a fourth receptor, the nociception opioid peptide (NOP) receptor, was identified. The NOP receptor is related to other opioid receptors in function but does not bind to any class of exogenous opioid ligands such as morphine.[10] The NOP receptor is believed to play a role in the homeostasis of the endogenous opioid system and is inhibitory.[11] Investigations of the NOP receptor show promise in the study of alcohol abuse disorder and depression.[11] The sigma (σ) receptor was previously believed to be an opioid receptor but has no opioid agonism. It only has two transmembrane proteins compared to seven other opioid receptors.[10, 12, 13] The major agonists for the σ-receptor are the drugs of abuse phencyclidine (PCP), methamphetamine, and cocaine.[13]

The vast majority of clinically useful opioid agonists are μ-agonists.[14] There are no selective δ or NOP receptor agonists in clinical use. Two exogenous opioid agonists, butorphanol and pentazocine, have κ-opioid receptor preference.[15] Similarly, specific antagonists have been developed for each receptor, but only naloxone and naltrexone, which have strong μ-, κ-, and δ-receptor antagonism, are used clinically.[10, 11]

Activity at each receptor is represented in Table 17.1. There is an overlap in the activity of each receptor, with important differences in the adverse effects attributable

TABLE 17.1
Opioid Receptors with Their Associated Endogenous Peptides, Peptide Agonists, Clinical Agonists, and Clinical Antagonists

Opioid Receptor	Endogenous Peptide	Peptide Agonist	Clinical Agonists	Clinical Antagonists
Mu (μ)	Endomorphin-1, Endomorphin-2, B-endorphin	DAMGO, PL 017	Morphine, fentanyl, oxycodone, methadone	Naloxone, naltrexone
Delta (δ)	Leu-enkephalin, met-enkephalin, deltorphin I and II	DADLE, DPDPE, DSLET	None	Naloxone, naltrexone
Kappa (κ)	Dynorphine A, dynorphine B	Dynorphin 1a	Butorphanol	Naloxone, naltrexone
NOP	Nociceptin, orphanin FQ	ZP120	None	None

Source: [12], [13].

to each receptor. Activation of the receptors μ, κ, and δ results in supraspinal and spinal analgesia.[10, 15, 16] Additionally, the μ- and δ-receptors modulate hormone and neurotransmitter release.

Side effects of μ-receptor agonism include sedation, respiratory depression, slowed gastrointestinal transit times, physical dependence, and euphoria.[10] Activation of the δ-receptor results in anxiolysis but generally has fewer adverse effects, especially in comparison to μ-opioid receptor agonism. κ-receptor adverse effects include dysphoria, hallucinations, and slowed gastrointestinal transit times.[10, 15]

17.4 OPIOID RECEPTOR FUNCTION AND SIGNALING

All the opioid receptors are G protein–coupled receptors. There are several characteristics that all opioid receptors share, including an external amino terminus with glycosylation sites, a long intracellular carboxy-tail for phosphorylation, and interactions with arrestin proteins. All opioid receptors are also encoded by a single separate gene, composed of 370–400 amino acids, and have seven transmembrane-spanning segments.[16, 17] When activated, the G protein receptors have an inhibitory effect on the adenylyl cyclase (AC) pathway.[17, 18]

The G protein signaling pathway is activated by an opioid agonist binding to the extracellular G inhibitory (G_i) receptor. The intracellular G protein alpha (G_i-α) and beta/gamma (G_i-βγ) subunits dissociate after receptor activation and propagate an intracellular chain reaction. The G_i-α subunit inactivates AC and stops the conversion of adenosine triphosphate (ATP) to cyclic adenosine monophosphate (cAMP). Decreased cAMP levels result in decreased calcium influx into the cell.[10, 18] The G_i-α subunit also interacts with G protein–gated, inward-directed potassium channels to increase the efflux of potassium. The net transcellular electrical current changes are the hyperpolarization of the cell membrane resulting in less cellular signal transmission (net negative).

Activation of the G_i-α pathway also initiates the mitogen-activated protein kinase (MAPK) cascade.[18] The MAPK cascade activates extracellular signal–related kinase (ERK), which may lead to some of the adverse effects of opioid agonism, such as tolerance, dependence, and addiction, as well as constipation.[19] MAPK/ERK activation also contributes to analgesia and sedation.[11] Changes to the signaling components of the MAPK/ERK contribute to long-term changes in opioid receptor activation.

At the same time as the G_i-α cascade, the G_i-βγ subunit binds to and inhibits the opening of voltage-gated calcium channels to decrease calcium ion influx. Decreased intracellular calcium levels inhibit neurotransmitter release by blocking the fusion of neurotransmitter-filled synaptic vesicles in the synaptic cleft.[18] This occurs on the pre-synaptic terminal.

Overall, this shift in ion movement across the cell membrane decreases the excitability of the membrane, inhibits the adenyl cyclase pathway, and stimulates the mitogen-associated protein kinase (MAPK) pathway.[11] Inhibition of the AC pathway causes decreased cAMP levels in the cell, reduced protein kinase A (PKA), and altered transcription of RNA. The cAMP/PKA signaling pathway is important in pain modulation and plays a role in the induction and maintenance of long-term

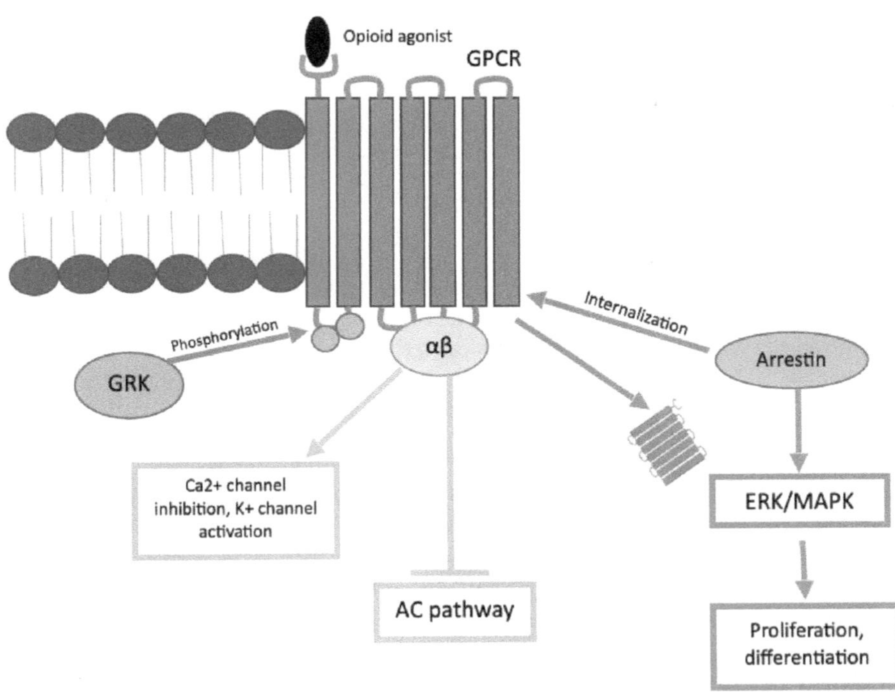

FIGURE 17.1 Opioid agonist binding to a GPCR causes Ca^{2+} channel inhibition, K+ channel activation, and adenylate cyclase pathway activation. It also activates arrestin, which causes internalization of the GPCR and leads to tolerance.[18]

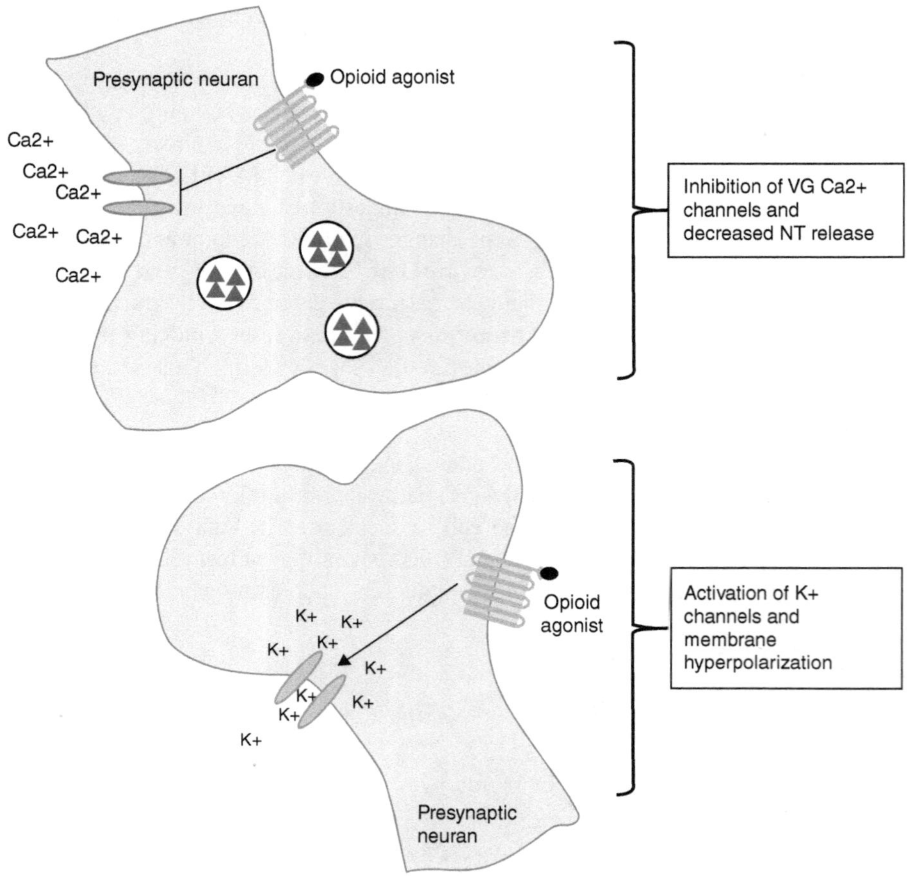

FIGURE 17.2 Pre-synaptic activation of opioid receptors causes inhibition of voltage-gated (VG) calcium (Ca^{2+}) channels and decreased neurotransmitter release, while post-synaptic activation of opioid receptors causes activation of potassium (K^{+}) channels and membrane hyperpolarization. The net effect is decreased synaptic activity and, thus, decreased pain transmission.[18]

potentiation and synaptic plasticity.[14, 18] Alterations in the PKA subunit with chronic painful stimuli can lead to elevated inflammatory responses and N-methyl-D-aspartate (NMDA)–dependent synaptic plasticity.[20]

Finally, within the brain, opioids can activate μ-receptors in hippocampal interneurons and decrease γ-aminobutyric acid (GABA) release.[21] The hippocampal neurons with μ-receptors are involved with the enhancement of noxious stimuli signaling. The reduced GABA levels lead to decreased inhibition of hippocampal pyramidal neurons, effectively resulting in neuronal excitation.[21, 22] This mechanism influences synaptic plasticity and contributes to addiction memory formation.

17.5 OPIOID ANALGESIC MECHANISM OF ACTION

Opioid receptors are located in multiple sites within and outside of the central nervous system. The three main divisions where opioid receptor activation is known to play a role in the modulation of nociception are the supraspinal central nervous system (CNS), the spinal dorsal horn of the CNS, and peripheral nociceptor nerve terminals.

17.5.1 Supraspinal Mechanisms of Action

Positron emission tomography has been used to identify opioid receptors or binding sites in the striatum, locus coeruleus (LC), amygdala, habenula, and periventricular gray.[23–25] However, the presence of an opioid receptor does not definitively correlate to relevance in pain processing. To determine the relevance of these CNS structures to pain processing, animal models were used. Thermal escape modeling is a laboratory pain model that applies heat to the hind paw of rodents until they lift their paw off a hot plate.[11, 26] By injecting opioids into various CNS sites, applying the thermal escape model, and using advanced imaging techniques, the opioid-modulated pain processing centers were mapped. Relevant central nervous system sites involved in opioid receptor–related pain transmission include the amygdala, substantia nigra, reticular formation, rostral ventral medulla, and nucleus raphe magnus (NRM).[25, 27] At the spinomedullary level, the substantia gelatinosa and medullary dorsal horn are involved.[10]

Recent studies suggest that most of these locations contain μ-, δ-, and κ-receptor types, but some receptors are expressed in relatively higher concentrations in certain structures of the brain than in others. For example, there are more μ-receptors in the amygdala, κ-receptors in the basal anterior forebrain, and δ-receptors in the olfactory tract.[28, 29] There are several structures in the brain that only express one receptor type as well; the lateral posterior nucleus of the thalamus only contains μ-receptors, while the arcuate nucleus and supraoptic nucleus only contain κ-receptors.[29] Besides analgesia, opioid receptors are involved in a variety of physiological pathways, including respiratory control, hormone secretion, reward behavior, and feeding patterns.[30, 31]

In the supraspinal CNS, the most common means to modulate pain transmission is via the bulbospinal descending pathway.[32] This occurs in the periaqueductal gray of the brain stem, where activation of opioid receptors results in decreased release of the inhibitory neurotransmitter GABA.[27] The decreased concentration of GABA in the neural synapses at this level decreases the tonic inhibition of inhibitory pain pathways (increases the inhibition) in the LC and NRM.[27, 33]

The net effect of decreased inhibition in the inhibitory LC and NRM is an increase in descending inhibition of pain transmission. This increase in inhibitory descending modulation from the LC and NRM in the medulla travels via bulbospinal projections to the dorsal horn inhibitory interneurons in the spinal cord, which then release serotonin (5HT) and noradrenaline (NOR).[27, 33] Activation of 5HT (by 5HT) and alpha-2 (by NOR) receptors in the dorsal horn nociceptors results in the inhibition of ascending spinal projections to the forebrain processing of pain.[27]

There is also evidence of limbic system activity on pain processing. Patients with chronic pain conditions have decreased gray matter in the amygdala and the hippocampus, which regulate emotional response to pain.[34] This reorganization of the corticolimbic system may explain the emotional responses to persistent pain and chronic pain states. Patients treated with morphine for severe pain report feeling pain but have an emotional indifference to the painful experience, possibly attributable to the loss of tissue in these centers. The presence of abundant opioid receptors in the limbic system, particularly in the amygdala, possibly explains the emotional response (pleasure and euphoria) caused by opiates.[34]

Opioid receptors modulate bulbo-cephalad regulation of pain. All forebrain NOR originates in the noradrenergic neurons of the LC, and all forebrain 5HT originates in the dorsal raphe of the brain stem. Outflow from the periaqueductal gray decreases the excitability of the dorsal raphe and LC.[10, 27] This alters the serotonergic and noradrenergic projections to the limbic and forebrain regions to decrease pain transmission.

17.5.2 Spinal Mechanisms of Action

In the spinal cord, μ-, δ-, and to some degree, κ-opioid receptor density is high in the dorsal horn, especially in the regions containing terminal small unmyelinated afferent C fibers.[35] Following the G_i pathway described earlier, voltage-gated calcium channel opening is inhibited. The reduced calcium influx at the pre-synaptic terminal reduces the release of excitatory neurotransmitters, such as substance P, glutamate, and calcitonin gene–related peptide (CGRP) into the synaptic cleft.[35]

At the post-synaptic neuron (second-order), opioid receptor activation results in increased efflux of potassium from the cell, which hyperpolarizes the neuron.[10] The hyperpolarized second-order neuron becomes less excitable to the propagation of nociceptive transmission. This joint ability of spinal opiates to reduce the release of excitatory neurotransmitters from C fibers as well as decrease the excitability of second-order dorsal horn neurons accounts for the powerful effect of opioids on spinal nociceptive processing.[10, 35]

The effect of opioids in the spinal cord selectively depresses the discharge of spinal dorsal horn neurons normally activated by afferent C fibers, which have a high threshold, but not large A delta afferents, which have a low threshold.[35] This effect yields antinociception without affecting proprioception or touch. The spinal effects of opioids may be reversed by the administration of naloxone.

17.5.3 Peripheral Mechanisms of Action

Opioids are largely thought of as centrally acting medications, but they do have some peripheral effects. At high concentrations, direct application of opioids to peripheral nerves can produce a local anesthetic-like effect that is not reversed by the administration of naloxone.[27, 36] This is believed to reflect a "nonspecific" action unrelated to opioid receptor activation. This local anesthetic-like action of opioids is attributed, in part, to a direct effect on axonal conduction.[36] High concentrations of peripheral opioids slow conduction in a concentration-dependent manner. The potency of this peripheral local anesthetic-like effect does not correlate with the analgesic potency of the opioid but, rather, is related to the opioid's lipid solubility. For example, the lipophilic opioids sufentanil, fentanyl, and meperidine have equal potency on axonal conduction peripherally and are more potent than the hydrophilic opioid morphine.[36] However, the central analgesic effects of sufentanil are 5–7 times more potent than fentanyl, and meperidine is 7.5 times weaker than morphine.[37]

Unlike their nonspecific action on axonal conduction, opioids demonstrate a normalizing effect on exaggerated pain thresholds when they are injected into inflamed peripheral tissues that display hyperalgesia.[38] Peripheral opioids have a direct effect on terminal excitability in inflamed tissue through an opioid receptor–mediated pathway. In post–tissue injury states where spontaneous activity is present, the spontaneous activity in hyperexcitable neurons is attenuated by the local administration of morphine.[39] This effect on pain thresholds is not seen when opioids are injected into non-inflamed tissues.[40] This opioid-related decrease in the spontaneous activity of peripheral nociceptors in inflamed tissues is reversible by naloxone, indicating the effect is, in part, attributable to opioid receptor agonism.[40] A clinical example of the peripheral action of opioids is the use of intra-articular morphine after arthroscopic surgery to decrease post-operative pain.

Our understanding of the activity of opioid receptors largely comes from evidence generated in animal models. Similar opioid agonism experiments in humans are impossible due to unacceptable risks, such as neurological damage from placing a needle in the brain stem to administer opioids directly.[41] However, there are some studies where intracerebroventricular opioids have been used in cancer-related pain.[41] The spinal administration of opioids is a mainstay of many surgical cases, including obstetrics.[42] Correlations between human and animal models have been substantiated from these studies.

17.6 ADVERSE EFFECTS AND TOLERANCE OF OPIOIDS

Opioids have a variety of adverse effects on the human body. Perhaps the most well-known are the effects on the gastrointestinal system. Opioids decrease propulsive peristaltic contractions while increasing circular muscle tone and intraluminal pressure.[43] Opioids cause dose-dependent constipation that persists regardless of the duration of opioid treatment (there is no tolerance).[43] Nausea is another adverse effect that occurs in approximately 40% of patients but is usually transient with the initiation of opioid therapy.[44]

Sedation may occur in 20–60% of patients and is often limited to the initiation of therapy and dose escalation.[45] A less common side effect is pruritus, which is generally not caused by histamine release but, rather, by a central μ-receptor mechanism.[10] Itching due to opioids can be reversed by nalbuphine (mixed opioid receptor agonist/antagonist) or low-dose naloxone.[46] Pruritus is more common and more intense with neuraxial administration.

Other side effects of opioids include delirium, hyperalgesia, respiratory depression, hypogonadism, and impairment of immunity.[47–49] Studies of patients with pain on chronic intrathecal opioids compared to similar patients with pain not treated with intrathecal opioids demonstrated that most men and all women develop hypogonadotropic hypogonadism with chronic intrathecal opioids.[49] About 15% developed central hypocortisolism, and another 15% growth hormone deficiency.[49] Opioid receptors also participate in the function of immune cells, with evidence suggesting that opioids modulate both the innate and acquired immune response, which ultimately results in decreased function of the immune response.[50, 51]

Perhaps the most important non-analgesic effect of opioids is tolerance. Several systems contribute to modulating opioid tolerance. The most widely described mechanism of tolerance is the ability of opioids to inhibit the AC enzyme through the prior mentioned G_i mechanism.[10] Following chronic suppression, AC is upregulated to return cAMP levels to more physiologic concentrations. Thus, to achieve the same suppression of AC, escalating opioid concentration is required. Other mechanisms include receptor desensitization, phosphorylation, and internalization.[14, 52]

Several mechanisms also exist which may prevent or delay tolerance to opioids. N-methyl-D-aspartate (NMDA) receptor antagonists like ketamine can reverse tolerance, but clinical use of these agents is limited due to undesirable psychomimetic side effects.[53] Similarly, the absence of morphine tolerance in both δ-1 (DOR-1) and enkephalin knockout mice suggests the DOR-1 receptor/enkephalin system prevents tolerance to morphine.[54]

A final proposed mechanism was shown in β-arrestin-2 knock-out mice that have increased sensitivity to morphine and, consequently, delayed tolerance.[15] In humans, β-arrestin activation leads to subsequent receptor internalization and desensitization.[16] The clinical impacts of β-arrestin receptor internalization and the development of opioid tolerance are unclear. Cross-tolerance occurs amongst all opioids; switching to another opioid agonist does not eliminate tolerance.

17.7 ENDOGENOUS OPIOID LIGANDS

The human body has a complex system of endogenous opioid ligands that are widely distributed throughout the central and peripheral nervous system. Physiologically, these ligands act to regulate pain, emotion, reward, stress response, motivation, addiction, and autonomic control. The term *endorphin* is an umbrella term referring to all the endogenous opioid agonist peptides. The endogenous ligands [Met]-enkephalin and [Leu]-enkephalin, for the δ-receptor, are derived from the precursor pro-enkephalin.[10] The endogenous ligands dynorphin-A and dynorphin-B, for the κ-receptor, are derived from the precursor pro-dynorphin.[10] Endogenous ligands for the μ-receptors are β-endorphin, endomorphin-1, and endomorphin-2.[10] The precursor ligand for β-endorphin is pro-opiomelanocortin (POMC), while the precursor ligand for the endomorphins is currently unknown. The endogenous ligands for the NOP receptor are nociceptin and orphanin FQ, which are derived from the precursor protein pre-pro-nociceptin.[10] A complete list of these precursors and peptides is found in Table 17.2.

The endogenous opioid ligands have multiple functions. For example, endogenous endorphins are involved in maternal instincts and natural reward circuits. Additional studies suggest that nociception is implicated in stress and anxiety responses.[55] Physiologic concentrations of endogenous opioid agonists likely modulate survival responses. Additionally, endogenous opioids play a role in descending inhibition of

TABLE 17.2
Opioid Receptors with Their Peptides and Precursor Peptides

Opioid Receptor	Precursor	Peptide
DOP	Pro-enkephalin	[Met]-enkephalin [Leu]-enkephalin
KOP	Pro-dynorphin	Dynorphin-A Dynorphin-B
MOP	POMC Unknown	Β-endorphin Endomorphin-1 Endomorphin-2
NOP	Pre-pro-nociceptin	Nociceptin Orphanin FQ

Source: [10].

pain transmission in the periaqueductal gray and ventral medulla, as well as direct inhibition of the substantia gelatinosa in the dorsal horn of the spinal cord.[10, 55]

Prolonged exogenous opioid therapy can inhibit the production of endogenous opioids and may even blunt receptor responsiveness to natural opioids, which increases the risk of dependence on exogenous opioids.[55] Current research in this field includes understanding the mechanism by which these endogenous opioids can contribute to tolerance, their role in the transition from acute to chronic pain, and their role in social bonding and sleep.[16]

17.8 OPIOID ANALGESIC SUBTYPES

Opioid analgesics can be categorized based on their action on the opioid receptors, composition (natural, semi-synthetic, or synthetic), and chemical structure.

In general, *opioids* are defined as any compound that binds an opioid receptor, while *opiates* are compounds that are derived from opium poppies. *Narcotics* is a legal term that is often taken to mean opioids but may also refer to any substance with addiction or abuse potential, like cocaine. *Endorphins* refer to any endogenous opioid, including enkephalins or dynorphins.

Opioids can be categorized based on their action on opioid receptors. Full opioid agonists bind to the receptor and induce its maximum response.[56] Examples include morphine, hydromorphone, codeine, hydrocodone, oxycodone, oxymorphone, fentanyl, meperidine, and methadone.[10] Opioid antagonists like naloxone and naltrexone inhibit opioid receptor activation.[56] Opioid agonist-antagonists are also known as partial agonists because they bind to the opioid receptor but induce a submaximal response; these include butorphanol, buprenorphine, nalbuphine, and pentazocine.[10, 56, 57]

Opioids may be natural alkaloids, semi-synthetic, or synthetics. Natural alkaloid derivatives of the opium poppy include morphine, codeine, papaverine, and thebaine.[10] Codeine and morphine are widely used in clinical practice, while thebaine is a precursor to several semi-synthetics.[11]

Semi-synthetic opioids are synthesized from natural alkaloids and possess similar chemical structures as their precursors. These include diacetylmorphine, hydromorphone, hydrocodone, oxycodone, oxymorphone, buprenorphine, butorphanol, and levorphanol.[10, 58]

Synthetic opioids, on the other hand, are entirely lab-synthesized, and many are very potent. Some examples of synthetic opioids are methadone, meperidine, fentanyl, sufentanil, alfentanil, remifentanil, tapentadol, and tramadol.[10, 58]

Opioid analgesics can also be separated into four categories based on chemical structure. The first category, the phenanthrenes, is comprised of three fused benzene rings. They can be further subdivided into morphine analogs (morphine, codeine, diacetylmorphine, hydromorphone, hydrocodone, dihydromorphine, oxycodone, oxymorphone, naloxone, naltrexone, and nalbuphine), morphinans (levorphanol and butorphanol), and oripavines, which are derived from thebaine (buprenorphine and etorphine).[6, 10]

Morphinins lack the 4,5-epoxy bridge seen in morphine and both the C7–C8 double bond and the 6-hydroxyl group. The second category is the benzomorphans, which have only one benzene ring. Two drugs in this class are ketocyclazocine, which was used to identify the κ-receptor, and pentazocine, which has mixed κ-agonist and μ-antagonist activity. Pentazocine is associated with a high incidence of dysphoria.[6] The third category of chemical structures is the diphenyl heptanes, which consist of the drugs methadone and propoxyphene.[10]

Finally, the phenylpiperidines can be broken down into the 4-phenylpiperidines, like meperidine, and the 4-aniliodopiperidines, such as fentanyl, loperamide, sufentanil, remifentanil, and alfentanil.[6, 10] Atypical synthetic opioid analgesics include

TABLE 17.3
Different Classifications of Opioids

Opioids	Action on Opioid Receptors	Full Agonists	Morphine, Codeine, Oxycodone, Hydromorphone, Fentanyl
		Antagonists	naloxone, naltrexone
		Agonist-antagonists	Butorphanol, buprenorphine, nalbuphine
	Composition	Natural alkaloids	Opium, morphine
		Semi-synthetics	Hydromorphone, hydrocodone, oxycodone, buprenorphine
		Synthetics	Methadone, fentanyl, tramadol
	Chemical Structure	Phenanthrenes	Morphine, codeine, naloxone
		Benzomorphans	Pentazocine
		Phenylethylamines	Methadone
		Phenylpiperidines	Meperidine, fentanyl, 1 r\ rv cv ro m i rJ cv
		Atypical synthetics	Tramadol, tapendadol

Source: [6, 10].

tramadol, which is a prodrug with weak μ-agonist and serotonin/norepinephrine reuptake inhibition activity, and tapentadol, which has μ-agonist and norepinephrine reuptake inhibition activity.[10]

Table 17.3 shows the aforementioned breakdown of classification types.

17.9 FUTURE DIRECTIONS

Future directions in opioid analgesic development involve research into biased agonists and receptor dimers, which include mixed opioid receptor agonists or agonists/antagonists.

Most opioid agonists interact with the G_i protein and activate β-arrestin, which leads to internalization of the opioid receptor and, subsequently, tolerance.[16] Biased opioid ligands, however, preferentially activate G_i over β-arrestin and thus may exhibit different tolerance developments and dependence.[15]

Some examples of biased agonists include oliceridine, PZM21, and SHR9352.[15] In vitro experiments of oliceridine showed G protein stimulation with reduction of β-arrestin recruitment and reduced internalization of μ-receptors.[15] Oliceridine was studied for acute pain in clinical trials and approved by the Food and Drug Administration (FDA) in 2020.[59] The FDA labeling of oliceridine includes the same adverse effects and risk of respiratory depression and dependence as other opioids. The FDA insisted on a maximum dose due to concerns that higher doses may cause QT interval prolongation and respiratory depression.[15, 60] PZM21 is another biased μ-receptor agonist that causes respiratory depression and has a similar tolerance profile to morphine.[61]

Another area of opioid analgesic research involves the development of receptor dimers. In the cellular membrane, opioid receptors form both homo- and heterodimers, thereby altering the pharmacological properties of the receptors.[16] The diversity of responses to opioid agonists is increased beyond those of the basic μ-, δ-, or κ-receptor monomers. Some examples of heteromers include δ-μ receptors that produce increased analgesia with decreased tolerance, δ-κ receptors that produce

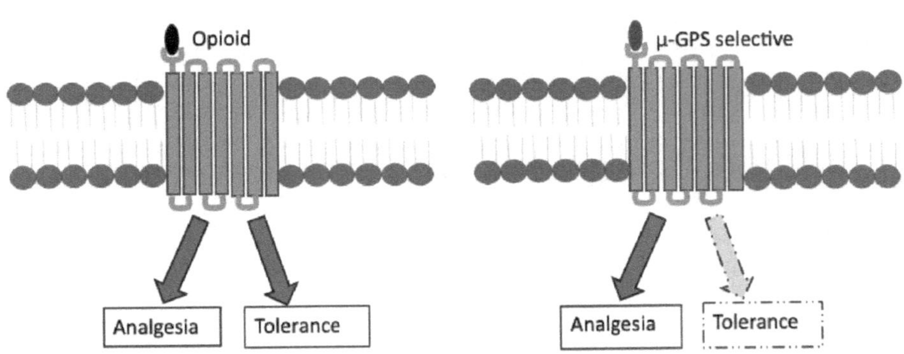

FIGURE 17.3 Opioid receptor activation leads to analgesia, but it can also cause tolerance via activation of the b-arrestin protein and subsequent receptor internalization.[16] One current research direction involves u-GPS selective agonists, which lead to analgesia by preferentially activating G_i instead of b-arrestin. Thus, the development of tolerance is delayed.

increased analgesia, especially in the spinal cord, and μ-NK1 receptors that cause increased analgesia with decreased tolerance.[16, 62]

Mixed μ/δ receptor agonists and mixed μ/NOP are another potential area of research. δ-receptor knockout mice demonstrate a lack of morphine tolerance.[11] Therefore, the administration of mixed μ-receptor agonists and δ-receptor antagonists in animal models can lead to antinociception with reduced tolerance development.[11] Mitragynine pseudoindoxy is a mixed μ-receptor agonist/δ receptor antagonist with a G protein pathway–signaling bias.[63] It forms the active compound of kratom, which is an herbal extract from the tropical tree *Mitragyna speciosa* found in Southeast Asia. Kratom has been used as a sedative and analgesic.[63, 64]

Similarly, mixed μ-receptor/NOP agonists demonstrate improved tolerance. NOP receptor activation provides the additional benefit of decreased respiratory depression.[11] In animal models, administration of mixed μ/NOP agonists like cebranopadol causes minimal respiratory depression, and tolerance only develops after long treatment periods.[11]

17.10 CONCLUSION

Opioids have been used to treat pain for centuries but became much more widely used with the development of morphine and heroin in the 1800s.[4, 7] It was not until the late 20th century, with the identification of the μ-, κ-, δ-receptors and nociceptin receptors that the mechanism of action of opioids came to be understood.[10] Side effects of opioids are generally caused by the μ-receptor and include sedation, nausea, respiratory depression, pruritus, hypogonadism, impaired immunity, decreased gastrointestinal motility, physical dependence, and tolerance.[10, 44, 49]

All opioids interact with G protein–coupled receptors and ultimately cause decreased calcium influx on the pre-synaptic membrane, as well as increased potassium influx on the post-synaptic membrane.[18] The net effect is decreased synaptic activity and decreased pain transmission. The different opioid receptors can be found in varying concentrations in the amygdala, substantia nigra, ventral medulla, substantia gelatinosa, and medullary dorsal horn.[10, 25, 27] Opioids also interact with the bulbospinal descending pathway in supraspinal sites and the limbic system to regulate the emotional response to pain.[32, 34] Peripherally, opioids can have a local anesthetic-like effect and normalize the exaggerated pain thresholds in inflamed tissue.[27, 36, 38]

Future directions in opioid development include biased agonists and receptor dimers to maximize the analgesic properties and limit the adverse effects and tolerance. In general, biased agonists preferentially inhibit G protein rather than β-arrestin and can delay the development of tolerance, and receptor dimers cause increased analgesia with decreased tolerance.[11, 15]

REFERENCES

1. Rosenblum A, Marsch LA, Joseph H, Portenoy RK. Opioids and the treatment of chronic pain: controversies, current status, and future directions. *Exp Clin Psychopharmacol*. Oct 2008;16(5):405–16. doi:10.1037/a0013628
2. Norn S, Kruse PR, Kruse E. [History of opium poppy and morphine]. *Dan Medicinhist Arbog*. 2005;33:171–84.

3. Reed MD. The balance between effective opioid-based pain management and patient safety: can it be achieved? *J Pediatr Pharmacol Ther*. Oct 2013;18(4):264–8. doi:10.5863/1551-6776-18.4.264
4. Stefano GB, Pilonis N, Ptacek R, Kream RM. Reciprocal evolution of opiate science from medical and cultural perspectives. *Med Sci Monit*. Jun 2017;23:2890–2896. doi:10.12659/msm.905167
5. Krishnamurti C, Rao SC. The isolation of morphine by Serturner. *Indian J Anaesth*. Nov 2016;60(11):861–862. doi:10.4103/0019–5049.193696
6. Williams J. Basic opioid pharmacology. *Rev Pain*. Mar 2008;1(2):2–5. doi:10.1177/204946370800100202
7. Hosztafi S. [The history of heroin]. *Acta Pharm Hung*. Aug 2001;71(2):233–42.
8. Manchikanti L, Helm S, Fellows B, et al. Opioid epidemic in the United States. *Pain Physician*. Jul 2012;15(3 Suppl):ES9–38.
9. Snyder SH, Pasternak GW. Historical review: opioid receptors. *Trends Pharmacol Sci*. Apr 2003;24(4):198–205. doi:10.1016/S0165–6147(03)00066-X
10. Pathan H, Williams J. Basic opioid pharmacology: an update. *Br J Pain*. Feb 2012;6(1):11–6. doi:10.1177/2049463712438493
11. Azzam AAH, McDonald J, Lambert DG. Hot topics in opioid pharmacology: mixed and biased opioids. *Br J Anaesth*. Jun 2019;122(6):e136-e145. doi:10.1016/j.bja.2019.03.006
12. Pasternak GW, Pan YX. Mu opioids and their receptors: evolution of a concept. *Pharmacol Rev*. 2013;65(4):1257–317. doi:10.1124/pr.112.007138
13. Matsumoto RR. Targeting sigma receptors: novel medication development for drug abuse and addiction. *Expert Rev Clin Pharmacol*. Jul 2009;2(4):351–8. doi:10.1586/ecp.09.18
14. Williams JT, Ingram SL, Henderson G, et al. Regulation of μ-opioid receptors: desensitization, phosphorylation, internalization, and tolerance. *Pharmacol Rev*. Jan 2013;65(1):223–54. doi:10.1124/pr.112.005942
15. Mores KL, Cummins BR, Cassell RJ, van Rijn RM. A review of the therapeutic potential of recently developed G protein-biased kappa agonists. *Front Pharmacol*. 2019;10:407. doi:10.3389/fphar.2019.00407
16. Valentino RJ, Volkow ND. Untangling the complexity of opioid receptor function. *Neuropsychopharmacology*. 12 2018;43(13):2514–2520. doi:10.1038/s41386-018-0225-3
17. Waldhoer M, Bartlett SE, Whistler JL. Opioid receptors. *Annu Rev Biochem*. 2004;73:953–90. doi:10.1146/annurev.biochem.73.011303.073940
18. Al-Hasani R, Bruchas MR. Molecular mechanisms of opioid receptor-dependent signaling and behavior. *Anesthesiology*. Dec 2011;115(6):1363–81. doi:10.1097/ALN.0b013e318238bba6
19. Duraffourd C, Kumala E, Anselmi L, Brecha NC, Sternini C. Opioid-induced mitogen-activated protein kinase signaling in rat enteric neurons following chronic morphine treatment. *PLoS One*. 2014;9(10):e110230. doi:10.1371/journal.pone.0110230
20. Li ZH, Cui D, Qiu CJ, Song XJ. Cyclic nucleotide signaling in sensory neuron hyperexcitability and chronic pain after nerve injury. *Neurobiol Pain*. 2019 Aug-Dec 2019;6:100028. doi:10.1016/j.ynpai.2019.100028
21. Borjkhani M, Bahrami F, Janahmadi M. Computational modeling of opioid-induced synaptic plasticity in the hippocampus. *PLoS One*. 2018;13(3):e0193410. doi:10.1371/journal.pone.0193410
22. Han H, Dong Z, Jia Y, et al. Opioid addiction and withdrawal differentially drive long-term depression of inhibitory synaptic transmission in the hippocampus. *Sci Rep*. May 2015;5:9666. doi:10.1038/srep09666
23. Koob GF, Volkow ND. Neurobiology of addiction: a neurocircuitry analysis. *Lancet Psychiatry*. Aug 2016;3(8):760–773. doi:10.1016/S2215–0366(16)00104–8
24. Cahill CM, Taylor AM, Cook C, Ong E, Morón JA, Evans CJ. Does the kappa opioid receptor system contribute to pain aversion? *Front Pharmacol*. 2014;5:253. doi:10.3389/fphar.2014.00253

25. Henriksen G, Willoch F. Imaging of opioid receptors in the central nervous system. *Brain.* May 2008;131(Pt 5):1171–96. doi:10.1093/brain/awm255
26. Morgan D, Carter CS, DuPree JP, Yezierski RP, Vierck CJ. Evaluation of prescription opioids using operant-based pain measures in rats. *Exp Clin Psychopharmacol.* Oct 2008;16(5):367–75. doi:10.1037/a0013520
27. Ossipov MH, Dussor GO, Porreca F. Central modulation of pain. *J Clin Invest.* Nov 2010;120(11):3779–87. doi:10.1172/JCI43766
28. Zhang J, Muller JF, McDonald AJ. Mu opioid receptor localization in the basolateral amygdala: an ultrastructural analysis. *Neuroscience.* Sep 2015;303:352–63. doi:10.1016/j.neuroscience.2015.07.002
29. Mansour A, Khachaturian H, Lewis ME, Akil H, Watson SJ. Autoradiographic differentiation of mu, delta, and kappa opioid receptors in the rat forebrain and midbrain. *J Neurosci.* Aug 1987;7(8):2445–64.
30. Nogueiras R, Romero-Picó A, Vazquez MJ, Novelle MG, López M, Diéguez C. The opioid system and food intake: homeostatic and hedonic mechanisms. *Obes Facts.* 2012;5(2):196–207. doi:10.1159/000338163
31. Nummenmaa L, Saanijoki T, Tuominen L, et al. μ-opioid receptor system mediates reward processing in humans. *Nat Commun.* 04 2018;9(1):1500. doi:10.1038/s41467-018-03848-y
32. Jensen TS. Opioids in the brain: supraspinal mechanisms in pain control. *Acta Anaesthesiol Scand.* Jan 1997;41(1 Pt 2):123–32. doi:10.1111/j.1399–6576.1997.tb04626.x
33. Bodnar RJ, Williams CL, Lee SJ, Pasternak GW. Role of mu 1-opiate receptors in supraspinal opiate analgesia: a microinjection study. *Brain Res.* Apr 1988;447(1):25–34. doi:10.1016/0006–8993(88)90962–6
34. Yang S, Chang MC. Chronic pain: structural and functional changes in brain structures and associated negative affective states. *Int J Mol Sci.* Jun 2019;20(13). doi:10.3390/ijms20133130
35. Heinke B, Gingl E, Sandkühler J. Multiple targets of μ-opioid receptor-mediated presynaptic inhibition at primary afferent Aδ- and C-fibers. *J Neurosci.* Jan 2011;31(4):1313–22. doi:10.1523/JNEUROSCI.4060–10.2011
36. Jaffe RA, Rowe MA. A comparison of the local anesthetic effects of meperidine, fentanyl, and sufentanil on dorsal root axons. *Anesth Analg.* Oct 1996;83(4):776–81. doi:10.1097/00000539-199610000-00021
37. Vardanyan RS, Hruby VJ. Fentanyl-related compounds and derivatives: current status and future prospects for pharmaceutical applications. *Future Med Chem.* Mar 2014;6(4):385–412. doi:10.4155/fmc.13.215
38. Godai K, Hasegawa-Moriyama M, Kurimoto T, et al. Peripheral administration of morphine attenuates postincisional pain by regulating macrophage polarization through a COX-2-dependent pathway. *Mol Pain.* Jun 2014;10:36. doi:10.1186/1744-8069-10-36
39. Hogan D, Baker AL, Morón JA, Carlton SM. Systemic morphine treatment induces changes in firing patterns and responses of nociceptive afferent fibers in mouse glabrous skin. *Pain.* Nov 2013;154(11):2297–309. doi:10.1016/j.pain.2013.05.033
40. Schreiter A, Gore C, Labuz D, et al. Pain inhibition by blocking leukocytic and neuronal opioid peptidases in peripheral inflamed tissue. *FASEB J.* Dec 2012;26(12):5161–71. doi:10.1096/fj.12–208678
41. Raffa RB, Pergolizzi JV. Intracerebroventricular opioids for intractable pain. *Br J Clin Pharmacol.* Jul 2012;74(1):34–41. doi:10.1111/j.1365–2125.2012.04201.x
42. DeBalli P, Breen TW. Intrathecal opioids for combined spinal-epidural analgesia during labor. *CNS Drugs.* 2003;17(12):889–904. doi:10.2165/00023210-200317120-00003
43. Akbarali HI, Inkisar A, Dewey WL. Site and mechanism of morphine tolerance in the gastrointestinal tract. *Neurogastroenterol Motil.* Oct 2014;26(10):1361–7. doi:10.1111/nmo.12443
44. Mallick-Searle T, Fillman M. The pathophysiology, incidence, impact, and treatment of opioid-induced nausea and vomiting. *J Am Assoc Nurse Pract.* Nov 2017;29(11):704–10. doi:10.1002/2327–6924.12532

45. Bourdeanu L, Loseth DB, Funk M. Management of opioid-induced sedation in patients with cancer. *Clin J Oncol Nurs*. Dec 2005;9(6):705–11. doi:10.1188/05.CJON.705–711
46. Jannuzzi RG. Nalbuphine for treatment of opioid-induced pruritus: a systematic review of literature. *Clin J Pain*. Jan 2016;32(1):87–93. doi:10.1097/AJP.0000000000000211
47. Khanna IK, Pillarisetti S. Buprenorphine—an attractive opioid with underutilized potential in the treatment of chronic pain. *J Pain Res*. 2015;8:859–70. doi:10.2147/JPR.S85951
48. Brennan MJ. The effect of opioid therapy on endocrine function. *Am J Med*. Mar 2013;126(3 Suppl 1):S12–8. doi:10.1016/j.amjmed.2012.12.001
49. Katz N, Mazer NA. The impact of opioids on the endocrine system. *Clin J Pain*. Feb 2009;25(2):170–5. doi:10.1097/AJP.0b013e3181850df6
50. McCarthy L, Wetzel M, Sliker JK, Eisenstein TK, Rogers TJ. Opioids, opioid receptors, and the immune response. *Drug Alcohol Depend*. Apr 2001;62(2):111–23. doi:10.1016/s0376–8716(00)00181–2
51. Liang X, Liu R, Chen C, Ji F, Li T. Opioid system modulates the immune function: a review. *Transl Perioper Pain Med*. 2016 2016;1(1):5–13.
52. Allouche S, Noble F, Marie N. Opioid receptor desensitization: mechanisms and its link to tolerance. *Front Pharmacol*. 2014;5:280. doi:10.3389/fphar.2014.00280
53. Cai YC, Ma L, Fan GH, Zhao J, Jiang LZ, Pei G. Activation of N-methyl-D-aspartate receptor attenuates acute responsiveness of delta-opioid receptors. *Mol Pharmacol*. Apr 1997;51(4):583–7. doi:10.1124/mol.51.4.583
54. Pradhan AA, Befort K, Nozaki C, Gavériaux-Ruff C, Kieffer BL. The delta opioid receptor: an evolving target for the treatment of brain disorders. *Trends Pharmacol Sci*. Oct 2011;32(10):581–90. doi:10.1016/j.tips.2011.06.008
55. Toubia T, Khalife T. The endogenous opioid system: role and dysfunction caused by opioid therapy. *Clin Obstet Gynecol*. 03 2019;62(1):3–10. doi:10.1097/GRF.0000000000000409
56. Helm S, Trescot AM, Colson J, Sehgal N, Silverman S. Opioid antagonists, partial agonists, and agonists/antagonists: the role of office-based detoxification. *Pain Physician*. 2008 Mar-Apr 2008;11(2):225–35.
57. Zola EM, McLeod DC. Comparative effects and analgesic efficacy of the agonist-antagonist opioids. *Drug Intell Clin Pharm*. Jun 1983;17(6):411–7. doi:10.1177/106002808301700601
58. LiverTox: Clinical and research information on drug-induced liver injury. 2012.
59. Viscusi ER, Webster L, Kuss M, et al. A randomized, phase 2 study investigating TRV130, a biased ligand of the μ-opioid receptor, for the intravenous treatment of acute pain. *Pain*. Jan 2016;157(1):264–272. doi:10.1097/j.pain.0000000000000363
60. Bergese SD, Brzezinski M, Hammer GB, et al. ATHENA: A Phase 3, open-label study of the safety and effectiveness of oliceridine (TRV130), A G-protein selective agonist at the μ-Opioid receptor, in patients with moderate to severe acute pain requiring parenteral opioid therapy. *J Pain Res*. 2019;12:3113–3126. doi:10.2147/JPR.S217563
61. Kudla L, Bugno R, Skupio U, et al. Functional characterization of a novel opioid, PZM21, and its effects on the behavioral responses to morphine. *Br J Pharmacol*. 12 2019;176(23):4434–4445. doi:10.1111/bph.14805
62. Ugur M, Derouiche L, Massotte D. Heteromerization modulates mu opioid receptor functional properties. *Front Pharmacol*. 2018;9:1240. doi:10.3389/fphar.2018.01240
63. Kruegel AC, Gassaway MM, Kapoor A, et al. Synthetic and receptor signaling explorations of the mitragyna alkaloids: mitragynine as an atypical molecular framework for opioid receptor modulators. *J Am Chem Soc*. 06 2016;138(21):6754–64. doi:10.1021/jacs.6b00360
64. Behnood-Rod A, Chellian R, Wilson R, et al. Evaluation of the rewarding effects of mitragynine and 7-hydroxymitragynine in an intracranial self-stimulation procedure in male and female rats. *Drug Alcohol Depend*. 10 2020;215:108235. doi:10.1016/j.drugalcdep.2020.108235

18 Mechanisms of Action of Clinically Relevant Analgesics (Non-Opiates)

Jacob Ezell, Jennifer Tram, and Timothy Furnish

All figures were created by the authors and are allowed for use in this chapter.

18.1 INTRODUCTION

Non-opioid analgesics are a broad class of medications that encompass many drug types and mechanisms of action. Historically, many of these medications were developed for the treatment of conditions other than pain and were later discovered to modulate pain transmission.

Drugs that increase the threshold required to induce pain after an acute painful stimulus are termed "analgesics." However, in post-injury pain states, many drugs do not affect acute pain but, instead, decrease hyperalgesia (increased sensitivity) or allodynia (pain in response to non-painful stimuli) that follows. These drugs are considered "anti-hyperalgesics.[1]"

In this chapter, we will discuss the analgesic and anti-hyperalgesic activity of nonsteroidal anti-inflammatory drugs (NSAIDs), acetaminophen, antidepressants, sodium channel blockers, ziconotide, gabapentinoids, N-methyl-D-aspartic acid (NMDA) antagonists, and capsaicin.

18.2 NONSTEROIDAL ANTI-INFLAMMATORY DRUGS

Nonsteroidal anti-inflammatory drugs (NSAIDs) are widely used due to their lack of addiction potential, efficacy, and favorable side effect profile.[2] This class of medications is anti-hyperalgesic, meaning, they work to decrease hyperalgesia and allodynia instead of decreasing the pain threshold. NSAIDs act via inhibition of cyclooxygenase-1 and -2 (COX) enzymes to decrease the synthesis of prostaglandins (PGs).[3]

After acute tissue damage, phospholipases, a class of enzymes that hydrolyze phospholipids, are activated in the injured area to increase the concentration of arachidonic acid (AA). Following the release of AA, COX enzymes catalyze the conversion of AA to PGs.[4] PGs increase the responsiveness of peripheral nerve terminals to stimuli by lowering the threshold for nociceptive nerve ending

DOI: 10.1201/9781003094302-18

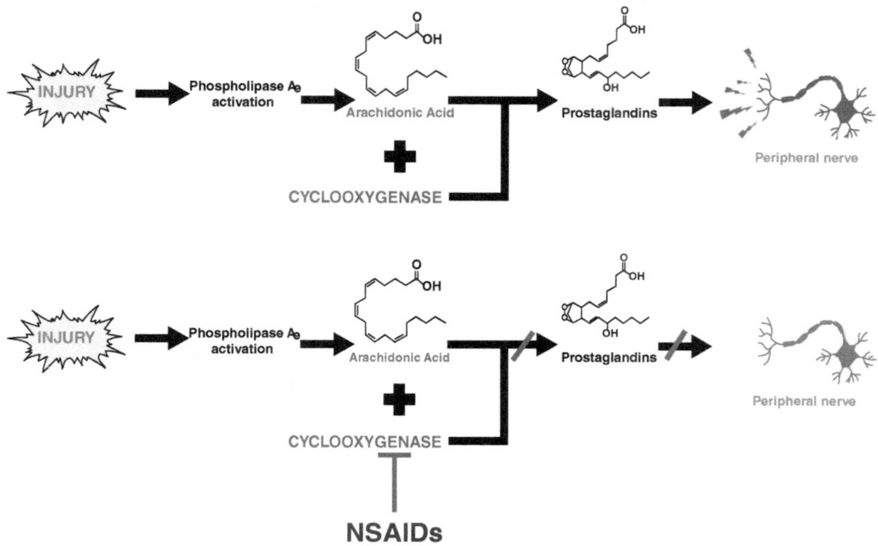

FIGURE 18.1 *Top*, following nerve injury, phospholipase A2 activation creates arachidonic acid that is converted to prostaglandins in the presence of cyclooxygenase. Prostaglandins lead to peripheral nerve sensitization. *Bottom*, NSAIDs block the conversion of arachidonic acid to prostaglandins to decrease nerve sensitization.

activation (Figure 18.1). This is termed a "leftward shift" in the stimulus–response curve, because a lower-intensity stimulus evokes a more intense, painful response.

Importantly, PGs and their analogs do not directly activate nociceptors but instead sensitize nerves to mechanical and chemical mediators of nociception, such as bradykinin.[5] By inhibiting the function of COX enzymes, the concentration of PGs at nerve terminals is decreased. This increases the threshold for nerve terminal activation, which decreases the responsiveness of peripheral nerve terminals to stimuli. NSAIDs cause a "rightward shift" in the stimulus–response curve for C fibers in the presence of PGs, meaning, a higher stimulus intensity is required to evoke a painful response.

COX enzymes have a variety of physiologic functions in the body. Classically, the COX enzymes exist as COX-1 and COX-2 subtypes.[3] COX-1 enzymes exist in the stomach, kidney, intestine, platelets, and most endothelial surfaces.[6] The COX-1 enzyme is "constitutively expressed" for the conversion of AA to prostaglandin E_2, prostaglandin I_2, and thromboxane A_2 (TXA_2). This means COX-1 is expressed at a constant rate regardless of demand in order to continuously maintain the protection of mucosal surfaces, renal homeostasis, and hemostasis.[4]

COX-2 enzymes are "inducibly expressed" in inflammatory sites, such as synovial tissues and macrophages. This means COX-2 is expressed only in response to inflammation.[6] In normal conditions, the gene expression of COX-2 is low; however, the addition of inflammatory stimuli (cytokines, chemokines, etc.) increases the expression of COX-2. The result is the creation of inflammatory PGs and proteases that mediate pain, inflammation, and fever.[7]

NSAIDs exhibit selectivity for the inhibition of COX-1 or COX-2 enzymes based on the physical properties of the NSAID. The COX-1/COX-2 inhibition for each NSAID is calculated using whole blood assays for concentration-dependent inhibition of COX-1 and COX-2 enzymes.[8, 9] NSAIDs that antagonize COX-1 and COX-2 with equal efficacy are termed "non-selective" NSAIDs. Examples of non-selective NSAIDs include naproxen, ibuprofen, sulindac, nabumetone, and diclofenac. The NSAIDs piroxicam, ketoprofen, apazone, flurbiprofen, and indomethacin exhibit COX-1 selectivity, while the NSAIDs rofecoxib, celecoxib, etoricoxib, valdecoxib, and meloxicam exhibit COX-2 selectivity (Table 18.1).[4]

Apart from peripheral COX inhibition, NSAIDs also have an anti-hyperalgesic effect on the central nervous system (CNS).[10] For instance, in the spinal cord, repeated C fiber activation results in increased prostaglandin E_2 (PGE_2) release. PGE_2 blocks glycine release and increases glutamate and substance P synaptic concentrations. Glycine inhibits nociceptive transmission. Glutamate and substance P increase nociceptive transmission. The cumulative effect of PGE_2 (decreased glycine, increased glutamate and substance P) in the spinal cord is a decrease in pain inhibition and an increase in pain transmission.[11, 12]

The effect of NSAIDs within the CNS is the inhibition of the conversion of AA to PGs. As a result, less substance P and glutamate are released at primary sensory neuron central terminals, and more glycine is released to activate inhibitory interneurons. This effectively decreases nociceptive signaling[11] (Figure 18.2).

Adverse effects of NSAIDs are typically caused by the inhibition of COX-1, which protects fragile mucosal surfaces through the creation of PGI_1 and PGE_2.[8]

Many of the adverse effects of NSAIDs occur in the gastrointestinal (GI) system and include dyspepsia and gastric mucosal ulceration. Ulceration due to NSAIDs has an annual prevalence of 5–10% and is correlated with specific NSAID, dosing, and patient comorbidities. Specific NSAIDs with a higher risk for gastric mucosal ulceration include ketorolac (RR 11.5), piroxicam (RR 7.43), indomethacin (RR 4.14), and naproxen (RR 4.10).[13] The risk of GI side effects is increased in NSAIDs

TABLE 18.1
NSAIDs Grouped by Selectivity for COX-2 Inhibition

Non-Selective	High COX-1 Selectivity	High COX-2 Selectivity
Naproxen	Piroxicam	Rofecoxib
Ibuprofen	Ketoprofen	Celecoxib
Sulindac	Apazone	Etoricoxib
Nabumetone	Flurbiprofen	Valdecoxib
Diclofenac	Indomethacin	Meloxicam

Note: Non-selective NSAIDs have equal affinity for COX-1 and COX-2. High COX-1-selective NSAIDs prefer COX-1 inhibition to COX-2. High COX-2-selective NSAIDs largely prefer COX-2 inhibition to COX-1.

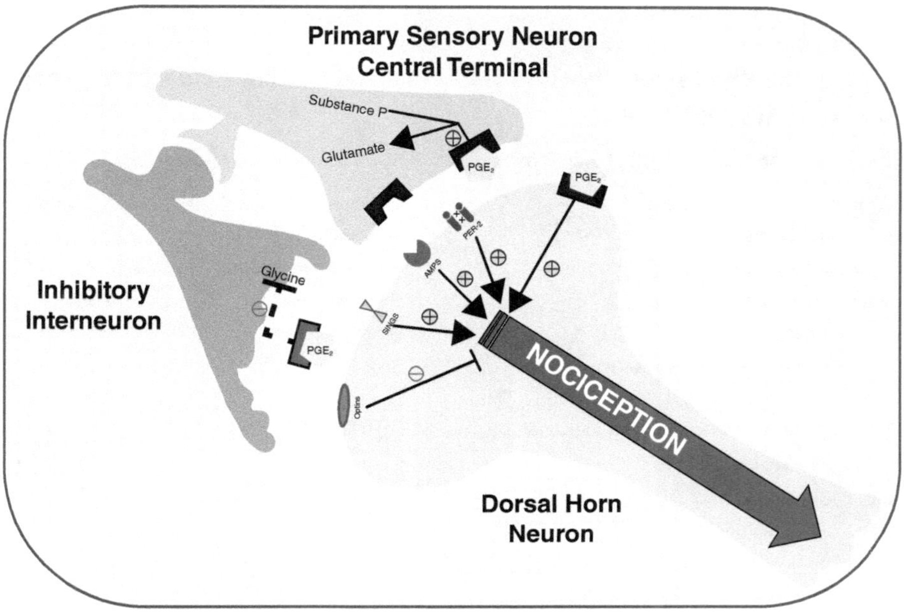

FIGURE 18.2 A peripheral sensory neuron synapse at the dorsal horn of the spinal cord. The primary sensory neuron central terminal (green) responds to PGE_2 to release substance P and glutamate that act on the dorsal horn neuron (orange) to promote nociception. The inhibitory interneuron (red) secretes glycine to stop nociceptive transmission; however, when PGE_2 occupies its binding site on the inhibitory interneuron, glycine secretion is prevented and the neuron is unable to prevent nociceptive transmission. *Note:* PGE_2 = prostaglandin E_2.

with a longer half-life (naproxen) and in NSAIDs taken at high doses.[14] High-risk comorbidities associated with gastric mucosal ulceration with NSAID use include concurrent *Helicobacter pylori* infection, co-existing corticosteroid use, and alcohol consumption.[4]

NSAIDs with a lower risk for gastric mucosal ulceration include celecoxib (relative risk (RR) 1.45), topical diclofenac, and ibuprofen (RR 1.84). The risk of gastric mucosal ulceration can also be mitigated with the concurrent use of a proton pump inhibitor or misoprostol.[13]

In the hematologic system, NSAIDs may interfere with platelet aggregation by disrupting the balance between TXA_2 and PGI_2.[15] TXA_2 is prothrombotic and promotes platelet adhesion and aggregation. PGI_2 is antithrombotic and disrupts platelet aggregation and adhesion. Depending on the specific NSAID, disruption of the balance between these two mediators may result in bleeding complications or a prothrombotic state.[13, 15] Most NSAIDs are associated with an increased risk of cardiovascular adverse events, such as hypertension, myocardial infarction, stroke, and hemostasis. In general, co-administration of NSAIDs, especially naproxen, with vitamin K antagonists, such as coumarins, should be avoided because NSAIDs can displace coumarin from plasma proteins, increasing the concentration of coumarin

TABLE 18.2
A List of the Risk Factors for Gastrointestinal and Cardiovascular Side Effects Due to NSAID Use

Risk Factors for Gastrointestinal Side Effects	Risk Factors for Cardiovascular Side Effects
>65 years old	Unstable angina
Peptic ulcer disease	Myocardial infarction
History of upper gastrointestinal bleeding	Recent coronary artery bypass surgery
Helicobacter pylori infection	Hypertension
Use of corticosteroids	Heart failure
Use of selective serotonin reuptake inhibitors (SSRIs)	Recent placement of a coronary artery stent
Use of antiplatelet therapy or other anticoagulants	High-dose NSAIDs
High-dose NSAIDs	
Tobacco smoking	
Alcohol consumption	

in plasma and the anticoagulant activity. This leads to an increased risk of bleeding complications. Risk factors for cardiovascular and gastrointestinal side effects due to NSAID use are summarized in Table 18.2.[4]

Aspirin (highly COX-1-selective) is cardioprotective due to its irreversible inhibition of COX-1 and modest COX-2 effects. This results in fewer thrombotic events and the creation of anti-inflammatory mediators through the modification of COX-2. However, NSAIDs with a high COX-1 selectivity may interfere with the antiplatelet activity of aspirin and increase the incidence of thrombosis. In contrast, NSAIDs with intermediate or high COX-2 selectivity do not exhibit the same effect. Celecoxib and naproxen are two other NSAIDs with lower risks for adverse cardiovascular reactions.[15, 16]

Finally, NSAIDs can have adverse effects on the renal system, including acute renal failure, acute interstitial nephritis, and renal papillary necrosis. These adverse effects are potentially reversible but can lead to chronic renal failure. Risk factors for renal injury due to NSAID use include age >65, duration of use, chronic renal failure, diabetes mellitus, hypertension, use of diuretics, and use of angiotensin-converting enzyme inhibitor.[17] Indomethacin is the NSAID most commonly associated with acute renal failure, but no NSAID is considered renally safe.[16] Therefore, routine monitoring of renal function is recommended in patients using NSAIDs for longer than 6 months.

Additional adverse reactions from NSAID use include hypersensitivity reactions, such as asthma exacerbation in patients with nasal polyposis and angioedema/urticaria. There is some evidence that NSAIDs may affect bone healing by COX inhibition.[18]

18.3 ACETAMINOPHEN

Acetaminophen was discovered in 1887 and is the most commonly used medication for pain and fever in the United States.[19] It is considered the first-line medication for the treatment of mild to moderate chronic pain.[4, 19] Acetaminophen lacks systemic anti-inflammatory effects and minimal COX-1/2 interactions.[19, 20] The mechanism of action is unclear, but hypothesized mechanisms include central anti-inflammatory effects, descending serotonergic pathway antagonism, and endocannabinoid system modulation.

In the CNS, acetaminophen inhibits prostaglandin synthesis ten times more effectively than in the periphery. Additionally, there is evidence of COX-3 inhibition in canine models; however, this enzyme is believed to be non-functional in humans.[21] Other studies offer conflicting support for the involvement of COX enzyme inhibition to explain this central effect.[22]

Acetaminophen has no activity at serotonin (5-HT) receptors, but there is evidence of an indirect effect that increases 5-HT levels in areas of the brain involved in the descending modulation of pain.[23] This is supported by human studies which demonstrate that serotonin receptor antagonists abolished the analgesic effect of acetaminophen. This data suggests the role of descending serotonergic pathways in acetaminophen's effectiveness.[24, 25] However, the combined effects of COX inhibition with descending serotonergic pathways have not been studied, nor do descending serotonergic pathways alone explain the complete analgesic effects of acetaminophen.

As a final mechanistic consideration, a metabolite of acetaminophen, N-arachidonoylphenolamine (AM404), has been shown to indirectly increase activity in the endocannabinoid system.[26, 27] AM404 is an activating ligand for cannabinoid receptors (CB_1) and vanilloid receptor subtype 1 (TRPV1), possibly explaining its analgesic effects. AM404 has also been shown to block the cellular reuptake of anandamide, an endogenous cannabinoid, thus increasing the concentration of ligand available for antinociceptive signaling in the spine and brain.[28]

While the mechanisms of acetaminophen as an analgesic remain unclear, it likely acts at multiple locations along multiple pain pathways. Further studies are required to understand the analgesic mechanisms and nociceptive pathway interactions of the drug.

When acetaminophen is used at doses lower than 4 g/24 hours, minimal side effects are reported.[19] Hepatotoxicity occurs above this dose because approximately 5% of acetaminophen undergoes N-hydroxylation by cytochrome p450 enzymes (CYP2E1) to create the toxic metabolite N-acetyl-p-benzoquinone imine (NAPQI). This metabolite is quickly neutralized with glutathione sulfhydryl groups and excreted in the urine. However, the depletion of glutathione stores due to high concentrations of acetaminophen results in a buildup of NAPQI. The NAPQI metabolite binds to hepatocytes, leading to potentially lethal hepatic necrosis.[29]

Caution is advised in patients with hepatic insufficiency due to malnutrition, hepatitis C infection, human immunodeficiency virus (HIV) infection, alcohol abuse, or concomitant use of cytochrome P450-inducing medications, such as rifampin, barbiturates, and some anti-epileptic medications.[19]

18.4 ANTIDEPRESSANTS

While not originally designed for analgesia, antidepressants have demonstrated a clinically useful ability to reduce hyperalgesia.[30] The anti-hyperalgesic effect of antidepressants is independent of their effects on mood. While antidepressants have little effect on acute thermal or mechanical nociception, they are considered first-line therapy for some neuropathic pain conditions.[30] Tricyclic antidepressants (TCAs), including amitriptyline and nortriptyline, and serotonin-norepinephrine reuptake inhibitors (SNRIs), such as duloxetine and venlafaxine, are effective for the treatment of chronic neuropathic pain syndromes.[31]

Generally, selective serotonin reuptake inhibitors (i.e., fluoxetine) have not been found useful for the treatment of chronic pain conditions.[32] Additionally, selective norepinephrine reuptake inhibitors are not used clinically in humans due to an unfavorable side effect profile. However, the use of norepinephrine reuptake inhibitors in preclinical animal models demonstrates the importance of norepinephrine in pain transmission.[33, 34] Other clinical studies support that norepinephrine plays a larger role in anti-hyperalgesic actions of antidepressants than serotonin.[30]

The mechanism of action of antidepressants in reducing hyperalgesia involves serotonergic and noradrenergic descending inhibitory pathways. Antidepressants inhibit reuptake of serotonin and norepinephrine in the neuronal synaptic cleft to increase the serotonin and norepinephrine available for receptor activation.[35] Serotonin primarily acts in the periaqueductal gray, resulting in the activation of the rostral ventral medulla and descending inhibition of nociception.[36] The serotonergic pathways are mediated by enkephalin and dynorphin release from inhibitory interneurons in the spinal cord.[37] Norepinephrine primarily acts in the locus coeruleus and nucleus reticularis to activate descending inhibitory pathways.[30] These pathways stimulate spinal cord inhibitory interneurons to release the inhibitory neurotransmitter γ-aminobutyric acid (GABA), which blocks nociceptive transmission.[38]

Additional effects include norepinephrine agonism of the α_2-adrenergic receptors that are coupled to inhibitory G proteins. Activation of the inhibitory G proteins prevents the opening of pre-synaptic, voltage-gated calcium channels in the dorsal horn.[39] This mechanism blocks the release of excitatory neurotransmitters. The cell membrane potassium channels on dorsal horn neurons are also opened, resulting in membrane hyperpolarization (net negative charge) and an increased activation threshold required for action potentials.[40] These combined mechanisms of norepinephrine make it more important than serotonin in producing the anti-hyperalgesic effects attributed to antidepressants.

Additional proposed analgesic mechanisms of antidepressants include opioid-mediated effects and neuro-immune modulation. It has been shown that antidepressants are active at δ-opioid receptors in supraspinal areas of the brain stem and μ-opioid receptors in the spinal cord.[30] This is supported by animal models where the administration of naloxone can block the analgesic effects of antidepressants.[40] Chronic antidepressant therapy has been associated with significantly reduced inflammatory cytokine levels.

Unfortunately, one of the most common reasons for the discontinuation of antidepressants is their poorly tolerated side effects. Adverse reactions to tricyclic

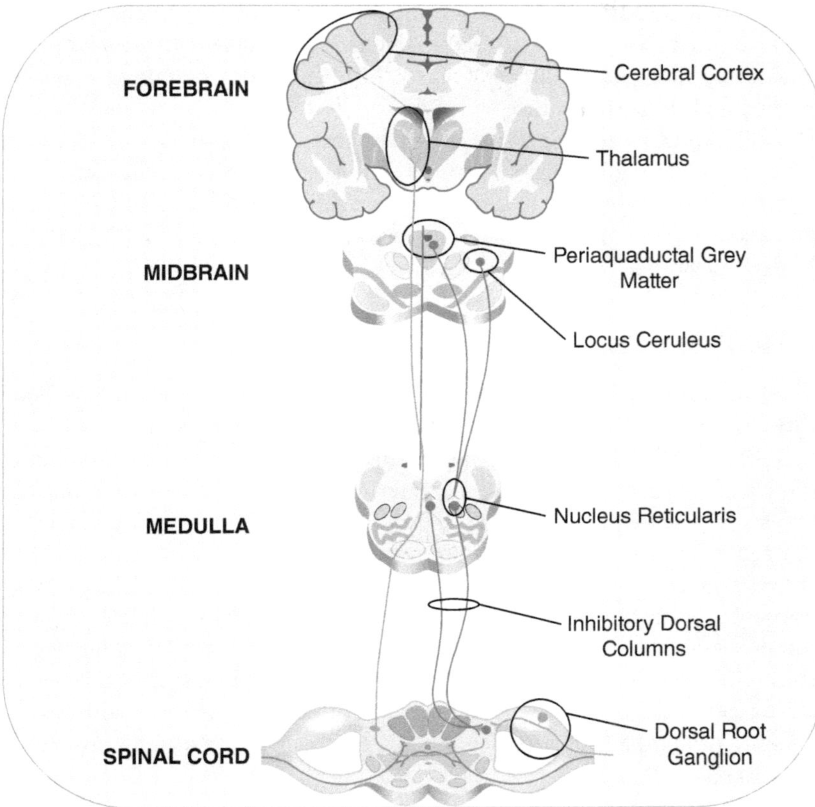

FIGURE 18.3 Descending inhibitory pathways involved in antidepressant mechanism of action for antinociception. Descending inhibitory pathways (blue) from the locus ceruleus, periaqueductal gray, and nucleus reticularis synapse in the spinal cord to inhibit the central transmission of pain sensation (green).

antidepressants include drowsiness, dizziness, dry mouth, constipation, nausea, urinary retention, sweating, headache, blurred vision, palpitations, irritability, and ataxia. Similarly, adverse reactions to SNRIs include nausea, dry mouth, headache, decreased libido, dizziness, somnolence or insomnia, reduced appetite, and hypertension.[41, 42]

Overactivation of both the peripheral and central post-synaptic serotonin receptors can lead to serotonin syndrome, which can be a life-threatening condition. Although variable, the classic presentation usually occurs within 24 hours of an increased dose of a serotonergic agent, the addition of another serotonergic agent such as tramadol or cyclobenzaprine, or overdose. The classic triad of symptoms includes altered mental status, neuromuscular abnormalities, and autonomic hyperactivity. However, serotonin syndrome can manifest in a wide variety of symptoms, such as agitation, disorientation, tremors, muscle rigidity, hypertension, tachypnea, shivering, vomiting, and arrhythmias. Prompt diagnosis is critical for survival. Treatment involves supplemental oxygen, continuous cardiac monitoring, sedation with benzodiazepines, and in extreme cases, serotonin antagonists. Mild cases may be managed with close observation and supportive care.[43]

Although typically minor and not life-threatening, discontinuation of antidepressants may result in withdrawal symptoms. Whenever possible, these agents should be tapered over several weeks to avoid discontinuation syndrome symptoms, such as nausea, headache, dizziness, chills, body aches, paresthesia, insomnia, and electric shock–like sensations.[44]

18.5 SODIUM CHANNEL BLOCKERS

There are many sodium channel blockers used in clinical practice today. The vast majority are local anesthetics, used for localized anesthesia by tissue infiltration, peripheral nerve blocks, and neuraxial anesthetic blockade.[45] These traditional local anesthetics act intracellularly along the axons of neurons to prolong the inactivated state of sodium channels and create a block of action potential conduction. The non-ionized form of the drug passes through the cell's lipid membrane and attaches to intracellular receptors on sodium channels, thus disrupting the influx of sodium ions through this channel.[46] The cumulative effect prevents the cell from depolarizing and effectively stops the propagation of an action potential along the axon, preventing the transmission of a painful stimulus to the spinal cord and central pain processing centers. Local anesthetic blockade of action potentials will also block transmission of non-painful stimuli, such as light touch and cold sensation, resulting in anesthesia as well as analgesia.

While sodium channel blockers used for peripheral or neuraxial blockade have high utility for acute pain, these drugs are not typically administered systemically or used long-term for chronic pain management. Lidocaine is the one exception, as it can be used short-term as a continuous intravenous infusion or topically as an anti-hyperalgesic in chronic neuropathic pain and post-operative somatic pain.[45]

The mechanisms of analgesia for systemic infusions of lidocaine are different than for peripheral nerve blockade. At low concentrations (1–3μg/ml serum), intravenous lidocaine can suppress glutamate-evoked excitation, DRG activity, and neuroma firing. It is not until systemic concentrations reach higher concentrations that spontaneous activity in injured nerves (5 μg/ml) and axonal conduction (5–10 μg/ml) is suppressed.[47–49] At typical analgesic infusions of IV lidocaine (1–2 mg/kg/hr), abnormal neuronal activity in peripheral neuromas, the dorsal root ganglion, and the dorsal horn of the spinal cord is suppressed. Axonal conduction and sensory blockade are not achieved at serum concentrations that are compatible with life.

There is some evidence for the efficacy of intravenous lidocaine in the treatment of neuropathic pain states, such as complex regional pain syndrome (CRPS) and neuropathic cancer-related pain.[50] These low-concentration infusions of lidocaine are able to effectively stop the transmission of aberrant nerve conduction. Additionally, a number of studies support the use of IV lidocaine to decrease pain and post-operative opioid consumption following abdominal surgery and complex spine surgery.[51, 52]

In addition to suppression of abnormal neuronal activity, systemic lidocaine infusions have several anti-inflammatory effects due to the inhibition of cytokine release, specifically the pro-inflammatory cytokines IL-4, IL-6, and TNF-α.[53] IV lidocaine also inhibits the production of pro-inflammatory cytokines in microglia of the CNS. It remains unclear to what extent the analgesic effects of lidocaine infusions could be related to the inhibition of these cytokines.[45]

Lidocaine is also administered topically in the form of sprays, gels, ointments, and patches. When applied topically, lidocaine permeates through the dermis for sodium conduction blockade, thus reducing peripheral nerve transmission and sensitization. There is no cutaneous anesthesia associated with most topical preparations of pure lidocaine, implying A delta fibers are unaffected. Typically, the maximum penetration level is 8–10 mm, which limits this application to superficial injury only, such as in post-herpetic neuralgia and other localized neuropathic conditions. There is some evidence for the use of topical lidocaine for non-neuropathic conditions, as well including post-operative incisional pain. Systemic absorption of lidocaine with topical applications is very low.[54]

Systemic side effects of sodium channel blockers are similar to those of the local anesthetics and are dependent on the total dose of the drug administered and the vascular uptake and distribution of the drug. When used within proper guidelines, adverse reactions are uncommon. However, when plasma concentrations rise, such as during inadvertent vascular injection, sodium channel blockers will affect peripheral nerves, the central nervous system, and cardiac conduction. Signs of local anesthetic systemic toxicity (LAST) include tinnitus, numbness around the mouth or metallic taste, and CNS excitatory or depressant effects that can lead to altered mental status and seizures; ultimately, cardiac conduction blockade can result in cardiac arrhythmias and cardiovascular collapse.[55] Therefore, it is recommended that patients receiving intravenous lidocaine infusions be monitored for signs of arrhythmia, cardiovascular instability, and local anesthetic toxicity with appropriately trained personnel and equipment. In extremely rare cases, such as those involving intentional ingestion, topical lidocaine can cause a similar presentation of systemic lidocaine toxicity. There is an exceedingly low chance of topical preparations leading to systemic toxicity.

18.6 ZICONOTIDE

Ziconotide is a non-opioid analgesic that is derived from the venom of a fish-eating marine cone snail, *Conus magus*.[56] The synthetic version of this conotoxin is a peptide drug which is FDA-approved for the treatment of chronic pain and is only available for administration via an intrathecal drug delivery device.[57]

Mechanistically, ziconotide has a high affinity for N-type, voltage-sensitive calcium channels on pre-synaptic neurons, where it creates a reversible inhibition and decrease in neurotransmitter release. These calcium channel receptors are located in the superficial, outermost laminae of the dorsal horn of the spinal column, where they mediate the mobilization of synaptic vesicles for the release of neurotransmitters. By preventing the release of neurotransmitters, ziconotide decreases nociceptive transmission.[58]

Spinal ziconotide is typically delivered via a continuous infusion for cancer pain and chronic neuropathic pain conditions such as CRPS, HIV neuropathy, and spinal cord injury.[59] Current data supports that ziconotide is anti-hyperalgesic and anti-allodynic. The drug has a narrow therapeutic range and is associated with several adverse reactions, including anxiety, ataxia, confusion, delusions/hallucinations, tremor, and difficulty with speech. At higher doses, it can cause psychosis and cataplexy. All these reactions are reversed with discontinuation of the drug. Unlike opioids, ziconotide does not cause respiratory depression or constipation. There are no dependence issues or tolerance to the analgesic effects.[50]

18.7 GABAPENTINOIDS

The gabapentinoids gabapentin and pregabalin were originally thought to be systemically active GABA analogs.[60] However, despite their name, neither possesses GABA receptor–binding properties or interactions. Instead, the gabapentinoids interact with the $\alpha_2\delta1$ subunit of voltage-gated calcium channels on pre-synaptic nerves to decrease the influx of calcium during depolarization.[61]

This mechanism was substantiated in animal models, where a non-functional point mutation in the $\alpha_2\delta$ subunit of voltage-gated calcium channels effectively eliminated the analgesic effects of gabapentinoids.[62] The net effect of this ligand–receptor relationship is reduced sensitization of spinal neurons, central neurons, and dorsal root ganglions, as well as a decrease in the release of excitatory neurotransmitters, such as glutamate, norepinephrine, and substance P. The receptors for glutamate, norepinephrine, and substance P are densely populated in the superficial dorsal horn of the substantia gelatinosa of the spinal cord.[63]

Other proposed mechanisms for the analgesic effects of gabapentinoids include decreased microglial activation, decreased creation of pro-inflammatory cytokines, nucleus accumbens descending modulation at high doses with an effect on the locus ceruleus, and supraspinal effects at centrally expressed voltage-gated calcium channels.[64]

Gabapentinoids have been shown to be efficacious for the treatment of fibromyalgia, neuropathic pain states like diabetic peripheral neuropathy, CRPS, post-herpetic neuralgia, and neuropathic cancer-related pain. There is some evidence for the use of gabapentinoids as an anti-hyperalgesic, but not as a primary analgesic, in the treatment of post-operative acute pain states.[63]

Gabapentinoids are typically well tolerated, but side effects can include dizziness, fatigue, drowsiness, ataxia, edema, nystagmus, and tremor. The class should be used cautiously in patients with chronic kidney disease, as it can lead to accumulation and toxicity.[63]

18.8 KETAMINE

Ketamine is a dissociative anesthetic that was derived from phencyclidine (PCP) and developed as an intravenous anesthetic agent that does not suppress respiration. At sub-anesthetic doses, ketamine is an analgesic medication. The mechanism of ketamine's analgesic properties is the non-competitive antagonism of the

N-methyl-D-aspartate (NMDA) receptors within the dorsal horn of the spinal cord, resulting in inhibition of central sensitization and anti-hyperalgesia.[65]

The NMDA receptor is involved in central sensitization, which makes the dorsal horn neurons more sensitive to incoming nociceptive signals. The process of NMDA receptor activation begins at the pre-synaptic nerve terminal through the opening of voltage-gated sodium and calcium channels by nociceptor activation. The increase in pre-synaptic calcium concentration results in the synaptic release of glutamate, which diffuses across to the post–synaptic nerve terminal and activates the α-amino-3-hydroxy-5-isoxazolepropionic acid (AMPA) receptors.[66] This results in sodium influx and depolarization of the post-synaptic neuron. In the resting state, magnesium ions "plug" the ionophore of the NMDA receptor to prevent the influx of calcium through the receptor.

In states of prolonged C fiber activation, multiple events occur that result in NMDA receptor activation and "windup," or sensitization of the post-synaptic dorsal horn neurons. Post-synaptic depolarization causes the release of the magnesium ion "plug" of the receptor. Glutamate and glycine bind and activate the NMDA receptor, allowing calcium influx via the NMDA receptor. This influx of calcium results in the activation of protein kinase C and the induction of nitric oxide synthase, which creates nitric oxide. Nitric oxide diffuses back across the synaptic cleft to the pre-synaptic nerve terminal and results in opioid resistance and the release of substance P. The released substance P diffuses back across to the post-synaptic terminal to increase activation of NK-1 receptors, thus resulting in increased sensitivity at the dorsal horn neuron. This renders the spinal cord neurons more responsive and efficient at transmitting nociceptive inputs, resulting in central sensitization to pain, a phenomenon described as "windup."[67]

Ketamine acts by preventing the removal of magnesium from the NMDA receptor, which prevents calcium influx. Ketamine shows efficacy in the treatment of neuropathic pain states such as CRPS and neuropathic cancer-related pain. Additionally, its use in the treatment of post-operative acute pain is growing.[66]

When administered in the appropriate setting, ketamine is safe and efficacious. However, it has significant adverse reactions that limit its utility, including tachycardia, hallucinations, psychosis, hypersalivation, diplopia, and increased bronchial secretions. In low-dose infusions for pain, the most common adverse reactions are blurry vision and hallucinations.

18.9 CAPSAICIN

Capsaicin is an active ingredient in chili peppers that causes the sensation of heat or burning. It has analgesic properties when applied topically. At low concentrations, these analgesic benefits require repeated applications. Typical over-the-counter concentrations range from 0.025% to 0.075%. A high-dose patch containing 8% capsaicin has FDA approval for the treatment of post-herpetic neuralgia and peripheral neuropathy.

Mechanistically, capsaicin causes initial activation of C fibers through TRPV1 receptors, influx of calcium into nerve cells, and release of substance P from nerve terminals. This process leads to a refractory period of reduced sensitization of nerve fibers. Persistent desensitization occurs with repeated low-dose application or with high-dose application. Desensitization is attributed to either substance P depletion or nerve fiber loss of function caused by cytoskeletal polymerization and mitochondrial dysfunction. These processes ultimately cause distal nerve terminal retraction from the dermis. This effect of topical capsaicin is reversible.[68]

Adverse reactions to topical formulations include mucosal membrane irritation, skin irritation, and capsaicin-induced erythema.

18.10 CONCLUSION

Non-opioid analgesics have varied mechanisms of action and side effect profiles. One of the most common classes of analgesics is NSAIDs, which inhibit cyclooxygenase enzymes and decrease the synthesis of prostaglandins. Another common analgesic, acetaminophen, has very minimal cyclooxygenase interaction and may act upon multiple pain pathways, although the specific mechanism remains unelucidated as of yet.

Several non-opioid analgesics were developed to treat another condition and are now used to treat chronic pain. This is especially true of drugs used to treat neuropathic pain. Antidepressants, such as TCAs and SNRIs, inhibit the reuptake of serotonin and norepinephrine. Both of these neurotransmitters enhance the descending inhibition of nociception. Similarly, gabapentinoids were originally approved as anticonvulsants and are now used as analgesics for neuropathic pain. They inhibit Ca^{2+} channels, resulting in a decrease in neurotransmitter release. Ketamine, a dissociative anesthetic, also prevents Ca^{2+} influx but, unlike the gabapentinoids, interacts with the NMDA receptor by preventing Mg^{2+} dissociation from the receptor.

Overall, non-opioid analgesics can be a powerful tool to treat pain as well as reduce or avoid opioid use. Most of the non-opioid analgesics work by decreasing hyperalgesia either peripherally or centrally. Side effect profiles and drug–drug interactions are specific to each analgesic or class of analgesics, and so care must be taken to select the appropriate medication and ensure optimal pain relief.

REFERENCES

1. Bickel A, Dorfs S, Schmelz M, Forster C, Uhl W, Handwerker OH. Effects of antihyperalgesic drugs on experimentally induced hyperalgesia in man. *Pain*. 1998 Jun;76(3):317–325. doi: 10.1016/S0304–3959(98)00062–1.
2. Conaghan PG. A turbulent decade for NSAIDs: Update on current concepts of classification, epidemiology, comparative efficacy, and toxicity. *Rheumatol Int*. 2012;32(6):1491–1502. doi:10.1007/s00296-011-2263-6.
3. Ricciotti E, Fitzgerald GA. Prostaglandins and inflammation. *Arterioscler Thromb Vasc Biol*. 2011;31(5):986–1000. doi:10.1161/ATVBAHA.110.207449.
4. Brune K, Patrignani P. New insights into the use of currently available non-steroidal anti-inflammatory drugs. *J Pain Res*. 2015;8:105–118. doi:10.2147/JPR.S75160.
5. Smyth EM, Grosser T, Wang M, Yu Y, FitzGerald GA. Prostanoids in health and disease. *J Lipid Res*. 2009;50(SUPPL.). doi:10.1194/jlr.R800094-JLR200.
6. Praveen Rao PN, Knaus EE. Evolution of nonsteroidal anti-inflammatory drugs (NSAIDs): Cyclooxygenase (COX) inhibition and beyond. *J Pharm Pharm Sci*. 2008;11(2). doi:10.18433/j3t886.

7. Simmons DL, Botting RM, Hla T. Cyclooxygenase isozymes: The biology of prostaglandin synthesis and inhibition. *Pharmacol Rev*. 2004;56(3):387–437. doi:10.1124/pr.56.3.3.
8. Atchison JW, Herndon CM, Rusie E. NSAIDs for musculoskeletal pain management: Current perspectives and novel strategies to improve safety. *J Manag Care Pharm*. 2013;19(9 Suppl A). doi:10.18553/jmcp.2013.19.s9.1.
9. Tacconelli S, Capone M, Patrignani P. Clinical pharmacology of novel selective COX-2 inhibitors. *Curr Pharm Des*. 2005;10(6):589–601. doi:10.2174/1381612043453108.
10. Vardeh D, Wang D, Costigan M, Lazarus M, Saper CB, Woolf CJ, et al. COX2 in CNS neural cells mediates mechanical inflammatory pain hypersensitivity in mice. *J Clin Invest*. 2009;119(2):287–294. doi:10.1172/JCI37098.
11. Yaksh TL, Dirig DM, Conway CM, Svensson C, Luo ZD, Isakson PC. The acute antihyperalgesic action of nonsteroidal, anti-inflammatory drugs and release of spinal prostaglandin E2 is mediated by the inhibition of constitutive spinal cyclooxygenase-2 (COX-2) but not COX–1. *J Neurosci*. 2001;21(16):5847–5853. doi:10.1523/jneurosci.21-16-05847.2001.
12. Abramson SB. Mechanisms of action of nonsteroidal anti-inflammatory drugs and therapeutic considerations. *Bull Hosp Jt Dis Orthop Inst*. 1990;50(2):107–115.
13. Castellsague J, Riera-Guardia N, Calingaert B, Varas-Lorenzo C, Fourrier-Reglat A, Nicotra F, et al. Individual NSAIDs and upper gastrointestinal complications: A systematic review and meta-analysis of observational studies (the SOS Project). *Drug Saf*. 2012;35(12):1127–1146. doi:10.2165/11633470-000000000-00000.
14. Baigent C, Bhala N, Emberson J, Merhi A, Abramson S, Arber N, et al. Vascular and upper gastrointestinal effects of non-steroidal anti-inflammatory drugs: Meta-analyses of individual participant data from randomised trials. *Lancet*. 2013;382(9894):769–779. doi:10.1016/S0140–6736(13)60900–9.
15. McGettigan P, Henry D. Cardiovascular risk and inhibition of cyclooxygenase: A systematic review of the observational studies of selective and nonselective inhibitors of cyclooxygenase 2. *J Am Med Assoc*. 2006;296(13):1633–1644. doi:10.1001/jama.296.13.jrv60011.
16. Brune K. Diclofenac: increase of myocardial infarctions at low doses? *Pharmacoepidemiol Drug Saf*. 2014;23(3):326–328. doi:10.1002/pds.3564.
17. Baker M, Perazella MA. NSAIDs in CKD: Are They Safe? *Am J Kidney Dis*. 2020; 76(4):546–557. doi:10.1053/j.ajkd.2020.03.023.
18. Sánchez-Borges M, Caballero-Fonseca F, Capriles-Hulett A. Cofactors and comorbidities in patients with aspirin/NSAID hypersensitivity. *Allergol Immunopathol (Madr)*. 2017;45(6):573–578. doi:10.1016/j.aller.2016.08.010.
19. Jozwiak-Bebenista M, Nowak JZ. Paracetamol: Mechanism of action, applications and safety concern. *Acta Pol Pharm—Drug Res*. 2014;71(1):11–23.
20. Hinz B, Brune K. Cyclooxygenase-2—10 Years later. *J Pharmacol Exp Ther*. 2002;300(2):367–375. doi:10.1124/jpet.300.2.367.
21. Dinchuk JE, Liu RQ, Trzaskos JM. COX-3: In the wrong frame in mind. *Immunol Lett*. 2003;86(1):121. doi:10.1016/S0165–2478(02)00268–7.
22. Kis B, Snipes JA, Busija DW. Acetaminophen and the cyclooxygenase-3 puzzle: Sorting out facts, fictions, and uncertainties. *J Pharmacol Exp Ther*. 2005;315(1):1–7. doi:10.1124/jpet.105.085431.
23. Alloui A, Chassaing C, Schmidt J, Ardid D, Dubray C, Cloarec A, et al. Paracetamol exerts a spinal, tropisetron-reversible, antinociceptive effect in an inflammatory pain model in rats. *Eur J Pharmacol*. 2002;443(1–3):71–77. doi:10.1016/S0014–2999(02)01578–9.
24. Pickering G, Loriot MA, Libert F, Eschalier A, Beaune P, Dubray C. Analgesic effect of acetaminophen in humans: First evidence of a central serotonergic mechanism. *Clin Pharmacol Ther*. 2006;79(4):371–378. doi:10.1016/j.clpt.2005.12.307.
25. Pickering G, Estève V, Loriot MA, Eschalier A, Dubray C. Acetaminophen reinforces descending inhibitory pain pathways. *Clin Pharmacol Ther*. 2008;84(1):47–51. doi:10.1038/sj.clpt.6100403.

26. Kelley BG, Thayer SA. Anandamide transport inhibitor AM404 and structurally related compounds inhibit synaptic transmission between rat hippocampal neurons in culture independent of cannabinoid CB1 receptors. *Eur J Pharmacol.* 2004;496(1):33–39. doi:10.1016/j.ejphar.2004.06.011.
27. Zygmunt PM, Chuang HH, Movahed P, Julius D, Högestätt ED. The anandamide transport inhibitor AM404 activates vanilloid receptors. *Eur J Pharmacol.* 2000;396(1):39–42. doi:10.1016/S0014–2999(00)00207–7.
28. Bertolini A, Ferrari A, Ottani A, Guerzoni S, Tacchi R, Leone S. Paracetamol: New vistas of an old drug. *CNS Drug Rev.* 2006;12(3–4):250–275. doi:10.1111/j.1527–3458.2006.00250.x.
29. Chowdhury A, Nabila J, Adelusi Temitope I, Wang S. Current etiological comprehension and therapeutic targets of acetaminophen-induced hepatotoxicity. *Pharmacol Res.* 2020;161. doi:10.1016/j.phrs.2020.105102.
30. Obata H. Analgesic mechanisms of antidepressants for neuropathic pain. *Int J Mol Sci.* 2017;18(11). doi:10.3390/ijms18112483.
31. Kremer M, Salvat E, Muller A, Yalcin I, Barrot M. Antidepressants and gabapentinoids in neuropathic pain: Mechanistic insights. *Neuroscience.* 2016;338:183–206. doi:10.1016/j.neuroscience.2016.06.057.
32. Finnerup NB, Attal N, Haroutounian S, McNicol E, Baron R, Dworkin RH, et al. Pharmacotherapy for neuropathic pain in adults: A systematic review and meta-analysis. *Lancet Neurol.* 2015;14(2):162–173. doi:10.1016/S1474–4422(14)70251–0.
33. Paqueron X, Conklin D, Eisenach JC. Plasticity in action of intrathecal clonidine to mechanical but not thermal nociception after peripheral nerve injury. *Anesthesiology.* 2003;99(1):199–204. doi:10.1097/00000542-200307000-00030.
34. Ito S, Suto T, Saito S, Obata H. Repeated administration of duloxetine suppresses neuropathic pain by accumulating effects of noradrenaline in the spinal cord. *Anesth Analg.* 2018;126(1):298–307. doi:10.1213/ANE.0000000000002380.
35. Micó JA, Ardid D, Berrocoso E, Eschalier A. Antidepressants and pain. *Trends Pharmacol Sci.* 2006;27(7):348–354. doi:10.1016/j.tips.2006.05.004.
36. Millan MJ. Descending control of pain. *Prog Neurobiol.* 2002;66(6):355–474. doi:10.1016/S0301–0082(02)00009–6.
37. Böhm C, Newrzella D, Herberger S, Schramm N, Eisenhardt G, Schenk V, et al. Effects of antidepressant treatment on gene expression profile in mouse brain: Cell type-specific transcription profiling using laser microdissection and microarray analysis. *J Neurochem.* 2006;97 Suppl 1:44–49. doi:10.1111/j.1471–4159.2006.03750.x.
38. Baba H, Kohno T, Okamoto M, Goldstein PA, Shimoji K, Yoshimura M. Muscarinic facilitation of GABA release in substantia gelatinosa of the rat spinal dorsal horn. *J Physiol.* 1998;508(1):83–93. doi:10.1111/j.1469–7793.1998.083br.x.
39. Pan HL, Wu ZZ, Zhou HY, Chen SR, Zhang HM, Li DP. Modulation of pain transmission by G-protein-coupled receptors. *Pharmacol Ther.* 2008;117(1):141–161. doi:10.1016/j.pharmthera.2007.09.003.
40. Isenberg KE, Cicero TJ. Possible involvement of opiate receptors in the pharmacological profiles of antidepressant compounds. *Eur J Pharmacol.* 1984;103(1–2):57–63. doi:10.1016/0014–2999(84)90189–4.
41. Ferguson JM. SSRI antidepressant medications: Adverse effects and tolerability. *Prim Care Companion J Clin Psychiatry.* 2001;3(1):22–27. doi:10.4088/pcc.v03n0105.
42. Santarsieri D, Schwartz TL. Antidepressant efficacy and side-effect burden: A quick guide for clinicians. *Drugs Context.* 2015;4. doi:10.7573/dic.212290.
43. Scotton WJ, Hill LJ, Williams AC, Barnes NM. Serotonin syndrome: Pathophysiology, clinical features, management, and potential future directions. *Int J Tryptophan Res.* 2019;12. doi:10.1177/1178646919873925.
44. Henssler J, Heinz A, Brandt L, Bschor T. Antidepressant withdrawal and rebound phenomena. *Dtsch Arztebl Int.* 2019;116(20):355–361. doi:10.3238/arztebl.2019.0355.

45. Hermanns H, Hollmann MW, Stevens MF, Lirk P, Brandenburger T, Piegeler T, et al. Molecular mechanisms of action of systemic lidocaine in acute and chronic pain: A narrative review. *Br J Anaesth.* 2019;123(3):335–349. doi:10.1016/j.bja.2019.06.014.
46. Lirk P, Hollmann MW, Strichartz G. The science of local anesthesia. *Anesth Analg.* 2018;126(4):1381–1392. doi:10.1213/ANE.0000000000002665.
47. Chabal C, Russell LC, Burchiel KJ. The effect of intravenous lidocaine, tocainide, and mexiletine on spontaneously active fibers originating in rat sciatic neuromas. *Pain.* 1989;38(3):333–338. doi:10.1016/0304–3959(89)90220–0.
48. Devor M, Wall PD, Catalan N. Systemic lidocaine silences ectopic neuroma and DRG discharge without blocking nerve conduction. *Pain.* 1992;48(2):261–268. doi:10.1016/0304–3959(92)90067-L.
49. Tanelian DL, MacIver MB. Analgesic concentrations of lidocaine suppress tonic A-delta and C fiber discharges produced by acute injury. *Anesthesiology.* 1991;74(5):934–936. doi:10.1097/00000542-199105000-00020.
50. Wallace MS, Ridgeway BM, Leung AY, Gerayli A, Yaksh TL. Concentration-effect relationship of intravenous lidocaine on the allodynia of complex regional pain syndrome types I and II. *Anesthesiology.* 2000;92(1):75–83. doi:10.1097/00000542-200001000-00017.
51. Farag E, Ghobrial M, Sessler DI, Dalton JE, Liu J, Lee JH, et al. Effect of perioperative intravenous lidocaine administration on pain, opioid consumption, and quality of life after complex spine surgery. *Anesthesiology.* 2013;119(4):932–940. doi:10.1097/ALN.0b013e318297d4a5.
52. Dunn LK, Durieux ME. Perioperative use of intravenous lidocaine. *Anesthesiology.* 2017;126(4):729–737. doi:10.1097/ALN.0000000000001527.
53. Taniguchi T, Shibata K, Yamamoto K, Mizukoshi Y, Kobayashi T. Effects of lidocaine administration on hemodynamics and cytokine responses to endotoxemia in rabbits. *Crit Care Med.* 2000;28(3):755–759. doi:10.1097/00003246-200003000-00025.
54. Gudin J, Nalamachu S. Utility of lidocaine as a topical analgesic and improvements in patch delivery systems. *Postgrad Med.* 2020;132(1):28–36. doi:10.1080/00325481.2019.1702296.
55. El-Boghdadly K, Pawa A, Chin KJ. Local anesthetic systemic toxicity: Current perspectives. *Local Reg Anesth.* 2018;11:35–44. doi:10.2147/LRA.S154512.
56. E. Brookes M, Eldabe S, Batterham A. Ziconotide monotherapy: A systematic review of randomised controlled trials. *Curr Neuropharmacol.* 2016;15(2):217–231. doi:10.2174/1570159x14666160210142056.
57. McDowell GC, Pope JE. Intrathecal ziconotide: Dosing and administration strategies in patients with refractory chronic pain. *Neuromodulation.* 2016;19(5):522–532. doi:10.1111/ner.12392.
58. Pope JE, Deer TR. Ziconotide: A clinical update and pharmacologic review. *Expert Opin Pharmacother.* 2013;14(7):957–966. doi:10.1517/14656566.2013.784269.
59. Deer TR, Pope JE, Hanes MC, McDowell GC. Intrathecal therapy for chronic pain: A review of morphine and ziconotide as firstline options. *Pain Med (United States).* 2019;20(4):784–798. doi:10.1093/pm/pny132.
60. Finnerup NB, Sindrup SH, Jensen TS. The evidence for pharmacological treatment of neuropathic pain. *Pain.* 2010;150(3):573–581. doi:10.1016/j.pain.2010.06.019.
61. Uchitel OD, Di Guilmi MN, Urbano FJ, Inchauspe CG. Acute modulation of calcium currents and synaptic transmission by gabapentinoids. *Channels.* 2010;4(6). doi:10.4161/chan.4.6.12864.
62. Patel R, Bauer CS, Nieto-Rostro M, Margas W, Ferron L, Chaggar K, et al. α2δ-1 gene deletion affects somatosensory neuron function and delays mechanical hypersensitivity in response to peripheral nerve damage. *J Neurosci.* 2013;33(42):16412–16426. doi:10.1523/JNEUROSCI.1026–13.2013.
63. Chincholkar M. Analgesic mechanisms of gabapentinoids and effects in experimental pain models: A narrative review. *Br J Anaesth.* 2018;120(6):1315–1334. doi:10.1016/j.bja.2018.02.066.

64. Kukkar A, Bali A, Singh N, Jaggi AS. Implications and mechanism of action of gabapentin in neuropathic pain. *Arch Pharm Res*. 2013;36(3):237–251. doi:10.1007/s12272-013-0057-y.
65. Zanos P, Moaddel R, Morris PJ, Riggs LM, Highland JN, Georgiou P, et al. Ketamine and ketamine metabolite pharmacology: Insights into therapeutic mechanisms. *Pharmacol Rev*. 2018;70(3):621–660. doi:10.1124/pr.117.015198.
66. Zhou HY, Chen SR, Pan HL. Targeting N-methyl-D-aspartate receptors for treatment of neuropathic pain. *Expert Rev Clin Pharmacol*. 2011;4(3):379–388. doi:10.1586/ecp.11.17.
67. Kamp J, Van Velzen M, Olofsen E, Boon M, Dahan A, Niesters M. Pharmacokinetic and pharmacodynamic considerations for NMDA-receptor antagonist ketamine in the treatment of chronic neuropathic pain: an update of the most recent literature. *Expert Opin Drug Metab Toxicol*. 2019;15(12):1033–1041. doi:10.1080/17425255.2019.1689958.
68. Sharma SK, Vij AS, Sharma M. Mechanisms and clinical uses of capsaicin. *Eur J Pharmacol*. 2013;720(1–3):55–62. doi:10.1016/j.ejphar.2013.10.053.

19 Pathophysiology of Migraine

Leon S. Moskatel and Nathaniel M. Schuster

Permissions for figures obtained.

19.1 INTRODUCTION

19.1.1 What Is a Migraine?

Primary headache disorders are readily characterized in the International Classification of Headache Disorders, 3rd edition (ICHD-3), into one of four classifications: migraine, tension-type headaches, trigeminal autonomic cephalalgias (TAC), and the other primary headache disorders. The definition of *migraine* has evolved with time, with the most recent criteria being those of the ICHD-3 (Box 1):

BOX 1.1: MIGRAINE WITHOUT AURA

Previously used terms:
Common migraine; hemicrania simplex.
Description:

Recurrent headache disorder manifesting in attacks lasting 4–72 hours. Typical characteristics of the headache are unilateral location, pulsating quality, moderate or severe intensity, aggravation by routine physical activity and association with nausea and/or photophobia and phonophobia.

Diagnostic criteria:

A. At least five attacks[1] fulfilling criteria B-D
B. Headache attacks lasting 4–72 hr (untreated or unsuccessfully treated)[2;3]
C. Headache has at least two of the following four characteristics:
   1. unilateral location
   2. pulsating quality
   3. moderate or severe pain intensity
   4. aggravation by or causing avoidance of routine physical activity (e.g., walking or climbing stairs)

DOI: 10.1201/9781003094302-19

D. During headache at least one of the following:
1. nausea and/or vomiting
2. photophobia and phonophobia
E. Not better accounted for by another ICHD-3 diagnosis.

Source: ICHD-3.

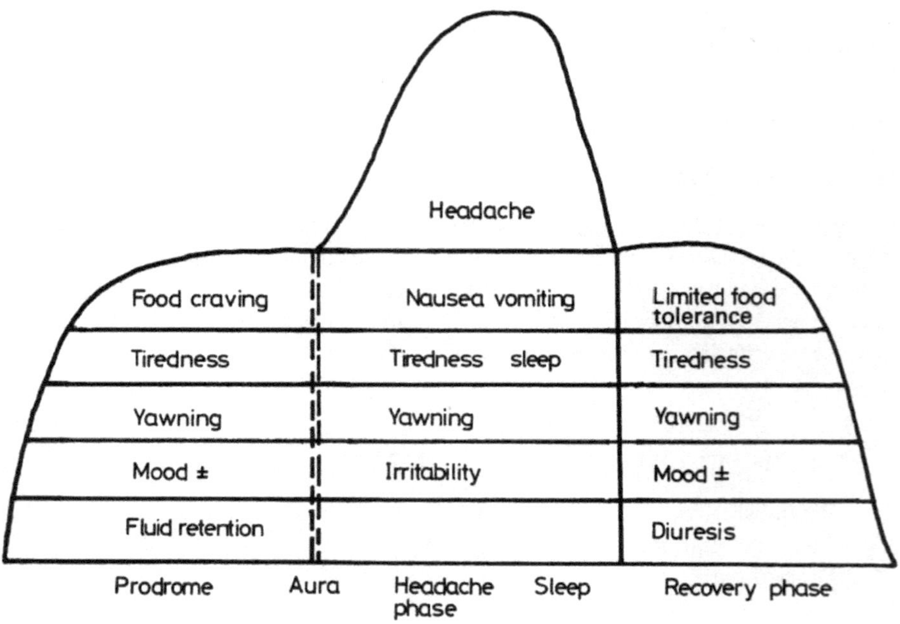

FIGURE 19.1 Migraine phases.

Source: From Blau, J. N., et al., JNNP (1984) (https://jnnp.bmj.com/content/jnnp/47/5/437.full.pdf).

Alternatively, tension-type headaches can have a wide variety of phenotypes but are characterized by their absence of migrainous features (such as nausea, photophobia, and phonophobia), the absence of autonomic features (such as lacrimation, eyelid edema, and facial sweating), and the lack of interference with one's daily activities. TACs, a family of primary headache disorders which includes cluster headache, present as side-locked head pain with associated ipsilateral autonomic features.

Beyond this, migraine attacks are defined by a trio of phases: (1) the prodromal phase (previously called premonitory phase), (2) the headache pain phase, and (3) the postdrome. The prodromal phase presents hours to days prior to the headache itself and encompasses a variety of disparate symptoms, including mood changes, urinary frequency, photophobia, and phonophobia.

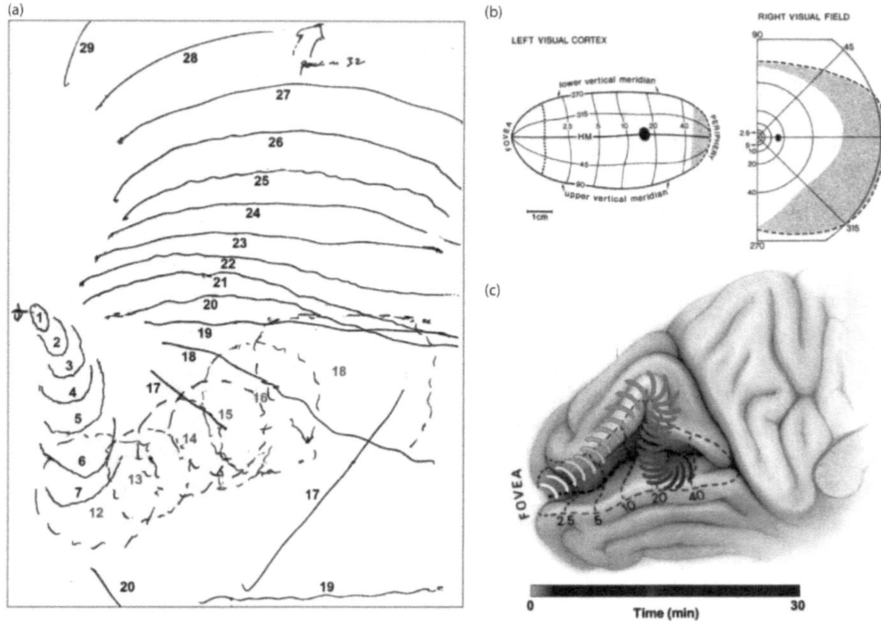

FIGURE 19.2 Drawings of migraine aura.

Source: From Hansen, J. M., et al., "Distinctive anatomical and physiological features of migraine aura revealed by 18 years of recording," ***Brain*** **(2013).**

The final minutes to hours of the prodromal phase and/or the onset of the headache phase may also include aura symptoms, such as the fortification spectra or scintillating scotoma (Figure 19.2), as well as possible sensory or motor symptoms. The headache phase itself lasts between 4 and 72 hours and includes the pain component as well as associated nausea, photophobia, and phonophobia. This is then followed by a postdrome phase, characterized by symptoms including tiredness and difficulty concentrating. The postdrome can last up to 48 hours. Most patients with migraine will then experience an interictal period prior to the next attack, during which they will be symptom-free. Patients with chronic migraine (CM, defined as at least 15 headache days and at least 8 migraine days per month) may continue to experience a wide variety of these symptoms as their high frequency of attacks results in little to no interictal period.

19.2 MIGRAINE EPIDEMIOLOGY

Migraine is a common neurological disorder with a 1-year prevalence of 14.4%. Indeed, when broken down by sex, this translates to up to 18.9% of women and 9.8% of men, with the prevalence peaking at 35–39 years (Stovner et al., 2018). Around puberty, this gap in migraine prevalence by sex is minimal but rapidly increases in the 18–29 demographic, and the difference remains throughout the rest of the ages. As a result of its broad prevalence, it is the world's seventh leading cause of disability as of 2015, and the first cause of disability in people under 50 as of 2018 (Steiner et al., 2018). At least 31% of patients with migraine have reported missing at least one day of work or school within the past 3 months, with at least 4.5% performing suboptimally for at least 3 days. In addition to the primary condition, patients with migraine, particularly chronic migraine, have worse socioeconomic status, higher rates of comorbid medical and psychiatric conditions, and higher health-care utilization and costs (Bigal et al., 2008; Buse et al., 2010; Stewart et al., 2010). About 6.8% to 8.8% of people with migraine have chronic migraine (Lipton et al., 2019). Patients with CM had twice as many primary care visits, three times as many neurology visits, and 1.5 times the number of emergency department visits than those experiencing fewer than 15 headache days per month (Burch et al., 2019). In terms of comorbid conditions, analysis of a Scottish database of 1.5 million primary care patients found a higher rate of 25 of 31 comorbidities in patients with CM, including anxiety and depression at rates of at least three times higher than the overall population (McLean and Mercer, 2017).

Beyond the high prevalence, there is also a heritable component of migraine that is continuing to be elucidated. Genetic epidemiologic studies have shown that the first-degree relatives of a patient with migraine without aura have a 1.9 times risk of migraine without aura and 1.4 times the risk of migraine with aura. Conversely, first-degree relatives of migraine with aura have almost 4 times the risk of migraine with aura and no increased risk of migraine without aura (Russell et al., 1996). Twin studies have also shown an increased concordance rate for migraine, particularly among monozygotic twins (Ulrich et al., 1993; Russell et al., 2002). Familial hemiplegic migraine (FHM) is a subset of migraine where genetic defects prompting the illness have been identified. One of these genes is CACNA1A (FHM1), which encodes the α_1 subunit of a voltage-dependent P/Q Ca^{2+} channel that is widely expressed throughout the central nervous system (Ophoff et al., 1996; Joutel et al., 1993). As these channels are involved in glutamate release and, consequently, cortical spreading depression (further discussed later), mutations in this gene may result in significantly higher susceptibility and facilitated subcortical propagation of cortical spreading depression (Ferrari et al., 2001; Eikermann-Haerter et al., 2009).

Beyond familial hemiplegic migraine, large genome-wide association studies (GWAS) have started to identify genes that may predispose to migraine with and without aura (Gormley et al., 2016). These include genes that add a variety of steps in the migraine transduction pathway; some genes regulate glutamate neurotransmission (MTDH, LRP1, and MEF2D) (Chasman et al., 2011), others affect ion channels (KCNK5 and TRPM8) and ion homeostasis (SLC24A3), and a couple target synaptic development and spasticity (Gormley et al., 2016).

19.3 THE HISTORICAL VASCULAR THEORY OF MIGRAINE

The first written description of migraine appeared 3,500 years ago as a case report in the Ebers Papyrus, where a courtesan in the court of the pharaoh was found to have "sickness of half the head" as well as vomiting and malaise (Aretaeus of Cappadocia, 1856). In Ancient Greece, Hippocrates first described the visual aura as well as it manifesting as an antecedent to headache. By the first century, migraine had been well-described, though with faulty underlying pathology; the unilateral nature was attributed to the falx cerebri preventing the bilateral spread of the headache, and the migraine itself was attributed to excess yellow bile (Didsbury, 1936).

Over the intervening centuries, migraine was believed to be a "vascular headache," with dilatation of the vessels triggering the episodes. Elements of this emerged as early as 1664 and continued to be refined throughout the 1800s until being fully described by Harold Wolff in 1948 (Goadsby, 2009; Wolff, 1948). Research supporting this theory includes trials in which infusion of vasodilatory molecules such as pituitary adenylate cyclase–activating peptide induced migraine in headache patients, but not controls (Schytz et al., 2009). Furthermore, ergotamine, a stalwart in the treatment of headaches until its displacement in the 1990s by the triptans, was a noted vasoconstrictor (Tunis and Wolff, 1953). However, reassessment of these studies posits that it is less the vasodilatory effect of the molecules and, instead, their receptor site activation; vasoactive intestinal polypeptide (VIP) has been shown to trigger dilation, but not migraine, while nitroglycerin has been shown to cause migraine without downstream changes in intra- or extracranial vessels (Rahmann et al., 2007; Schoonman et al., 2008).

Mild vasodilation of intracranial and extracranial arteries was noted in calcitonin gene–related peptide (CGRP)–induced migraine headache, but the observed 9–12% effect was unlikely to be the culprit for the headaches (Asghar et al., 2011). In addition, from a purely translational standpoint, patients with prominent throbbing headaches have been studied, and the throbbing rate was found to be strongly dyssynchronous from the pulsating rate, further removing the headache from the vasoactivity of blood vessels (Ahn, 2010).

19.4 THE ROLE OF THE HYPOTHALAMUS, CORTICAL SPREADING DEPRESSION, AND THE TRIGEMINOCERVICAL COMPLEX IN MIGRAINE

Our understanding of migraine has then pivoted to focus away from this vascular notion and toward a comprehensive neurovascular theory. In this theory, the trio of migraine phases constitutes a cycle with distinct physiologic changes occurring throughout.

During initiation of the headache, the hypothalamus is now thought to play a critical role. In nitroglycerin-triggered migraine attacks, nitroglycerin has been shown to generate increased hypothalamic activity in the hours directly before the onset of the headache (Maniyar et al., 2014). Daily functional magnetic resonance imaging of a single migraine patient over 30 days revealed that the hypothalamus is significantly more active in the 24 hours preceding migraine pain. In turn, this showed an altered functional coupling between the hypothalamus, the spinal trigeminal nuclei, and the region of the dorsal rostral pons (Schulte and May, 2016).

While it has been speculated that overactivation in the hypothalamus before the onset of the headache represented a decrease in the inhibitory effect on the trigeminocervical complex, this activation was not observed during the 30-day study, when preictal and baseline scans were compared (Maniyar et al., 2014; Schulte and May, 2016). Yet a strong and specific activation was noted in the dorsal rostral pons during the

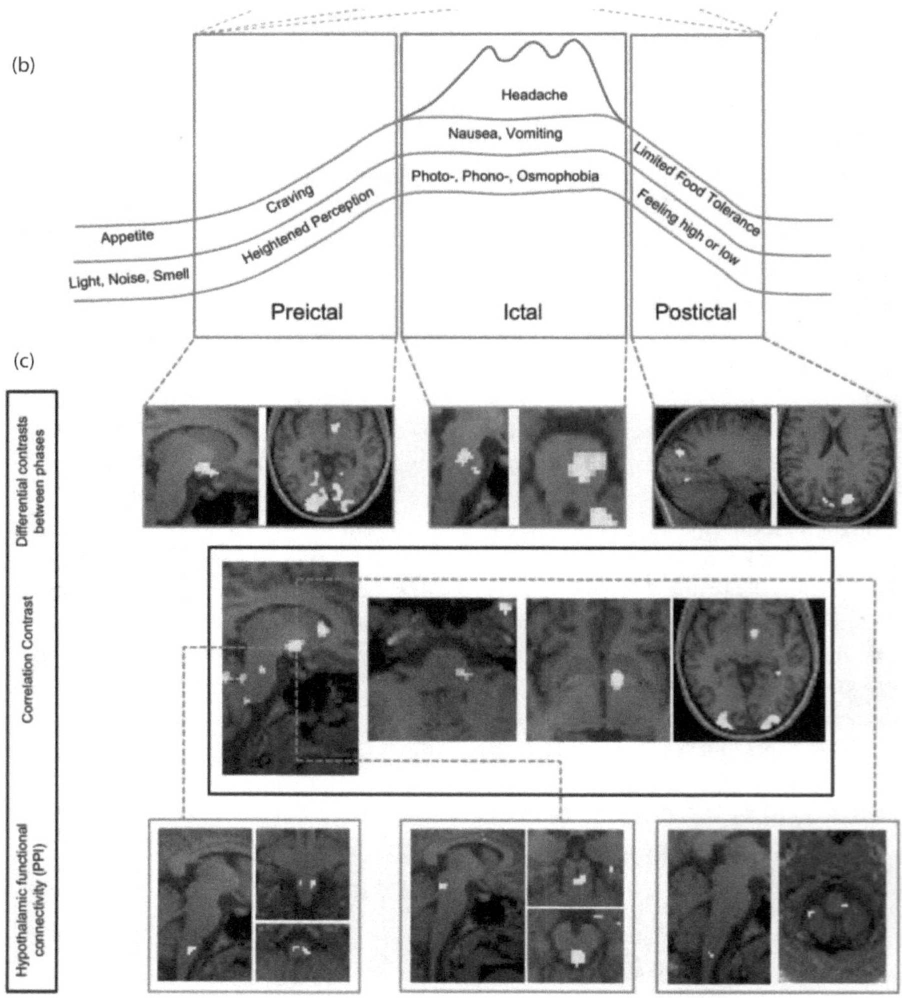

FIGURE 19.3 From Schulte 2016. Only need (B) and (C)—from the caption if we adapt for this article can remove (A) and relabel (B) and (C) as (A) and (B). Will require permission.

ictal phase; the dorsal rostral pons has been previously associated with migraine attack generation (Schulte and May, 2016; Weiller et al., 1995; Bahra et al., 2001; Stankewitz et al., 2011).

Cortical spreading depression is also thought to play an important role in the onset of migraine. This phenomenon was discovered in 1944 by the Brazilian physician Dr. Aristides de Azevedo Pacheco Leao and represents a slow (2–6 mm/min) spreading wave of neuronal and glial depolarization after electrical or chemical stimulation that is then followed by up to half an hour of inhibition of cortical activity, associated with the initiation and progression of aura symptoms (Pietrobon and Moskowitz, 2013). On a cellular level, a large ionic flux stems from a marked decrease in neuronal membrane resistance associated with an increase in extracellular potassium and neurotransmitters, as well as an increase in intracellular sodium and calcium (Ayata et al., 2006). Further evidence for CSD's role in migraine stems from studies showing that commonly used migraine preventive medications may inhibit CSD. In a mouse model study, potassium chloride–induced CSDs were roughly halved in the mice treated with the preventive medications topiramate, valproate, propranolol, amitriptyline, and methysergide as compared to controls (Ayata et al., 2006).

CSD then translates into pain through potentially activating the dural sensory afferents that are branches of the trigeminal nerve and feed into the trigeminocervical

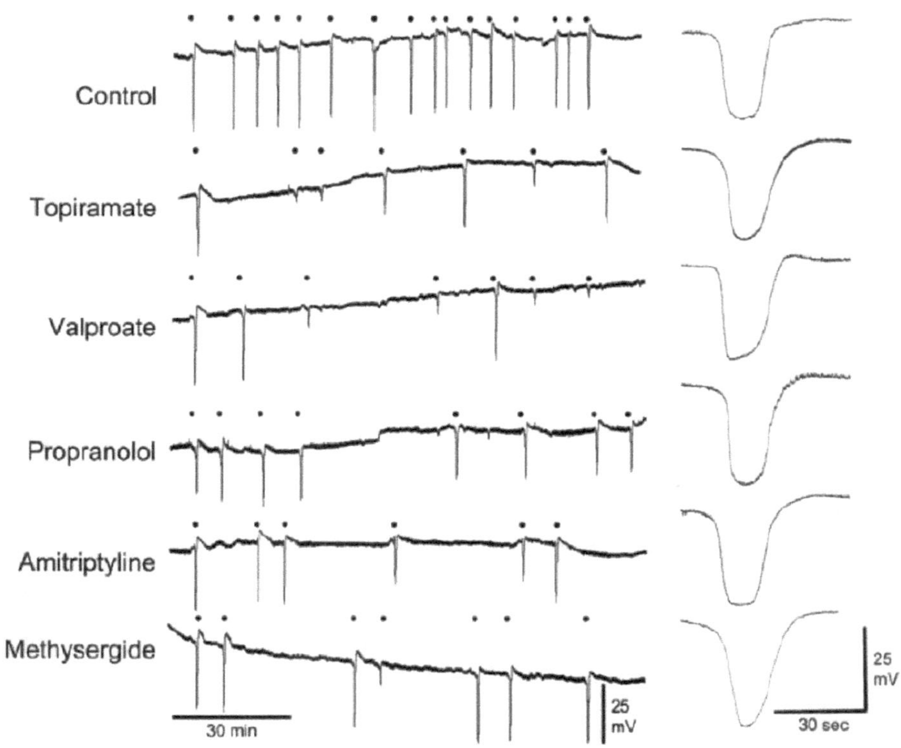

FIGURE 19.4 Inhibition of cortical spreading depression after chronic treatment with migraine prophylactic drugs. Representative electrophysiological tracings from frontoparietal cortex are shown from isoflurane-anesthetized animals after saline or drug treatment. After chronic treatment, significantly fewer cortical spreading depressions (CSD) were observed in response to topical KCl (1M) application. In the control animal, 16 were recorded over 2 hours, whereas 6 to 8 CSDs were present in the drug-treated animals. Black dots indicate individual CSDs. There was no statistically significant difference in DC shift amplitude, or duration and slope at half-maximal amplitude between control and drug-treated groups. Individual CSDs from representative experiments are shown on the right on an expanded time scale. Topiramate 80 mg/kg/day, valproate 100 mg/kg/day, DL-propranolol 20 mg/kg/day, amitriptyline 20 mg/kg/day, methysergide 1 mg/kg/day, for at least 4 weeks.

Source: Adapted from Ayata (2006).

complex. Nerve activation studies in mice have shown that stimulation of the greater occipital nerve induces central excitability of dural afferent inputs. In this study, the authors applied C fiber activator mustard oil to the cutaneous receptor field or the suboccipital muscles, innervated by the greater occipital nerve, and this resulted in increased excitability of dural responses in a large proportion of the neurons. This suggests a strong association between the trigeminal nucleus caudalis (also called the spinal trigeminal nucleus or trigeminocervical complex) and the upper cervical segments (Bartsch and Goadsby, 2002). Another study by the same authors demonstrated that second-order neurons were sensitized by stimulation of nociceptive afferent C fibers of the dura mater, which are trigeminal sensory afferents (Bartsch and Goadsby, 2003). These two studies together demonstrate how trigeminal and cervical sensory afferents can sensitize each other via the trigeminocervical complex.

The trigeminocervical complex also has ascending pathways that transmit to multiple nuclei throughout the brain stem, thalamus, hypothalamus, and basal ganglia (Malick et al., 2000). These nuclei further transmit to a plethora of cortical areas, including somatosensory, motor, auditory, visual, and olfactory zones, that are, in turn, related to the cognitive, emotional, and sensory processing aspects of the nociceptive signals. This signal interpretation then manifests as the non-pain symptoms of migraine, including photophobia, phonophobia, osmophobia, and cognitive dysfunction (Burstein et al., 2015; Noseda et al., 2011).

19.5 MECHANISM OF ACTION OF ONABOTULINUMTOXINA IN MIGRAINE

OnabotulinumtoxinA (onaA, Botox®, AbbVie, Dublin, Ireland) has become the standard of care for chronic migraine prevention. Based on the results of the PREEMPT 1 and 2 studies, it received US Food and Drug Administration approval for chronic migraine prevention in 2010 and has minimal side effects (Dodick et al., 2010). Yet its mechanisms of action are still being elucidated. The neurotoxin itself irreversibly blockades the pre-synaptic release of acetylcholine at the neuromuscular junction, causing muscle relaxation (Sugiyama, 1980). This action occurs by cleaving soluble N-ethylmaleimide-sensitive factor attachment protein receptor (SNARE) proteins, inhibiting the pre-synaptic release of these neurotransmitters, including acetylcholine. After initial reports of pain reduction in patients treated for its original indications, such as dystonia and blepharospasms, it was investigated for the treatment of chronic pain, with the assumption being that its effect was a result of muscle relaxation, causing decompression of blood vessels and sensory nerves (Binder et al., 2000).

Yet subsequent studies indicated onaA could be acting proximal to the neuromuscular junction as well. Indeed, retrograde and anterograde transport in axons has been observed, as well as transsynaptic transport from nerve terminals to adjacent neurons and glial cells (Maienschein et al., 1999). This is supported by animal studies, including a rat diabetic neuropathy model, which showed that peripheral onaA injections resulted in decreased mechanical and thermal hypersensitivity on both the ipsilateral and contralateral sides (Bach-Rojecky et al., 2010). In a separate rat model of formalin-induced inflammation, unilateral preventative onaA injections led to decreased rodent-specific central pain behavior. Taken together, these indicate the potential role of onaA as a modulator of decreased central sensitization as a result of decreased afferent firing (Do et al., 2018). In relation to human treatment of migraine with onaA, this may mean that injections, for example, in close proximity to the greater and lesser occipital nerves, or the supratrochlear nerves, may induce decreased meningeal nociception due to axonal transport to higher-order neurons.

A separate mechanism of onaA involves the decreased release of neurotransmitters and neuropeptides, including CGRP, substance P, serotonin, glutamate, gamma-aminobutyric acid, norepinephrine, dopamine, enkephalin, and glycine from trigeminal sensory afferents (Do et al., 2018). The primary mechanism for this involves onaA's cleavage of the SNARE proteins in trigeminal sensory afferents (separate from its effects on motor neurons at neuromuscular junctions), thus preventing vesicle fusion with the membrane, preventing its synaptic release (Montecucco and Molgó, 2005). This reduction in neurotransmitters results in decreased nociception. For example, one study showed that 10 and 14 days after onaA injections, there was decreased CGRP expression in the fourth and fifth lumbar spinal dorsal horn (Lee et al., 2011). Substance P has also been shown to be decreased in a similar matter, given a different mechanism for analgesia (Chien et al., 2012). Glutamate has also been shown in guinea pig models to be decreased as a result of onaA, which potentially translates into analgesia in some experimental models of pain and sensitization induced by capsaicin and mild heat (Bittencourt et al., 2014; McMahon et al., 1992).

Beyond neurotransmitters, onaA has also been shown to inhibit the surface expression of nociceptive receptors, including TRPV1, TRPA1, TRPM8, P2X3, and $GABA_A$ (Do et al., 2018). TRPV1 is a non-selective, ligand-gated cation channel that is activated by mechanical and chemical stimuli, leading to a prominent role in vascular tone and, consequently, pain and neurogenic inflammation (Jordt et al., 2000; Zhang and Gutterman, 2011). TRPA1 can function similarly, and indeed, some migraine triggers, such as cigarette smoke components, are TRPA1 agonists (Andrè et al., 2008). Similarly, the migraine-induction effect of nitric oxide (NO) has been found to be related, at least in part, to the nociceptive action on TRPV1 and TRPA1 (Miyamoto et al., 2009). Since surface expression of the TRP family is modulated by SNARE-dependent exocytosis, onaA cleavage of SNARE prevents this action (Camprubí-Robles et al., 2009). Supporting this includes two rodent models. In the first, pre-treatment with onaA inhibited the nociceptive response from capsaicin (a TRPV1 agonist) and mustard oil (a TRPA1 agonist) (Zhang et al., 2016). In the second, decreased nocifensive behaviors were seen when rodents were pre-treated with onaA before receiving capsaicin or allyl isothiocyanate (TRPA1 agonist) (Shimizu et al., 2012).

19.6 CALCITONIN GENE–RELATED PEPTIDE AND ITS ROLE IN MIGRAINE

Recent novel treatments for migraine have stemmed from a better understanding of the role of calcitonin gene–related peptide (CGRP) in migraine pathogenesis. CGRP is a 37-amino-acid-long neuropeptide with both alpha and beta variants. Alpha-CGRP is utilized by both the central and peripheral nervous systems and is preferentially expressed in sensory neurons. It is also the predominant isoform expressed in trigeminal ganglia neurons. Conversely, beta-CGRP is used by enteric nerves and the pituitary gland. The receptor for CGRP is present throughout the head and neck, including the cortex, thalamus, amygdala, external lateral and external medial parabrachial nuclei, the nucleus of the solitarius tract, small nuclei in the vagus, trigeminal, spinal lamina, dorsal root ganglia, and cerebral arteries (Villalón and Olesen, 2009).

In the context of migraine, CGRP is released from activated trigeminal sensory nerves and centrally modulates vascular nociception. It is abundant in perivascular trigeminal nerve fibers and in the spinal trigeminal nucleus (Villalón and Olesen, 2009). Infusions of exogenous CGRP into patients with a history of migraine have indeed induced migraine-like headaches, whereas a placebo did not (Lassen et al., 2002). Additionally, a similar experiment showed infusions of exogenous CGRP into patients without a history of migraine produced a feeling of head fullness, but not an actual headache (Howden et al., 1988; Shekhar et al., 1991). Subsequent studies showed that CGRP receptor activation increased the expression of inducible nitric oxide synthase and stimulated the release of nitric oxide from trigeminal ganglion cells. This release then facilitates the potent vasodilation of intracranial and extracranial vessels (Villalón and Olesen, 2009).

Given the role of CGRP in migraine, it has long been seen as a potential target for therapeutics. Several early small-molecule CGRP receptor antagonists (gepants), including olcegepant and telcagepant, were initially studied, and while they were found to be effective, their development was stopped due to hepatotoxicity and other reasons (Olesen et al., 2004; Ho et al., 2008, 2014). Research then shifted toward monoclonal antibodies targeting both CGRP and its receptor, including erenumab, galcanezumab, fremanezumab, and eptinezumab (Goadsby et al., 2017; Detke et al., 2018; Silberstein et al., 2017; Ashina et al., 2020). These medications were found to be safe and effective and have become an important tool in migraine prevention, with erenumab, galcanezumab, and fremanezumab arriving on the US market in 2018, and eptinezumab in 2020. The gepant class was then revisited, with rimegepant and ubrogepant demonstrating efficacy for acute treatment of migraine while avoiding the hepatotoxicity seen with earlier gepants and arriving on the US market in 2020 (Lipton et al., 2019; Voss et al., 2016). Two additional gepants, atogepant and zavegepant, are currently in clinical trials (Goadsby et al., 2019; Croop et al., 2021).

19.7 SEROTONIN RECEPTOR AGONISTS FOR ACUTE MIGRAINE TREATMENT

Advances in our understanding of the pathophysiology of migraine and CGRP have evolved our notions of the mechanism of action of the quintessential disease-specific acute medication class the triptans and its sister, the ditans. Previously, the mechanism of the triptan class, which are selective agonists of the 5-HT_{1B} and 5-HT_{1D} receptors, was thought to be a function of vasoconstricting overly dilatated vessels by direct action on vascular smooth muscles, inhibition of the release of vasoactive neuropeptides, and inhibition of the nociceptive neurotransmission pathway through the trigeminocervical complex in the upper spinal cord and brain stem (Goadsby, 1998). However, further work has yielded that this more specifically involves the stabilization of peripheral nerve endings, leading to decreased CGRP and substance P (Levy et al., 2004). The degree to which vasoconstriction plays in this is ongoing (Johnston and Rapoport, 2010). Yet it is exactly because of that worrisome vasoconstriction that the ditan class of selective 5-HT_{1F} agonists, including lasmiditan, was developed as the triptans are contraindicated in patients with uncontrolled hypertension, as well as in those with cardiovascular and cerebrovascular diseases (Xavier et al., 2017). Indeed, in vivo studies have not shown meaningful vasoconstriction at currently used doses (Rubio-Beltrán et al., 2019). That said, the mechanism of action is similar to triptans, as lasmiditan-induced activation of 5-HT_{1F} receptors inhibits the release of CGRP from trigeminal afferent nerves in the peripheral nervous system (Usman and Balaban, 2016).

19.8 SUMMARY

A comprehensive understanding of migraine pathophysiology continues to evolve as more elements of this complex disease process are elucidated. Additional work will be conducted to better trace the signal transduction pathways and nature of cortical spreading depression to map out the trajectory of a migraine. A better comprehension of migraine genetics could allow for more precise diagnoses and targeted treatments. Disease-specific treatments based on advancements in our understanding of migraine pathophysiology have improved care for the patient with migraine, as shown first by the development of triptans and more recently in the efforts to study the role of CGRP, and ultimately to translate this into two newest classes of medication for the treatment of migraine.

REFERENCES

Ahn, Andrew H. 2010. On the Temporal Relationship Between Throbbing Migraine Pain and Arterial Pulse. *Headache: The Journal of Head and Face Pain* 50: 1507–10. https://doi.org/10.1111/j.1526-4610.2010.01765.x.

Andrè, Eunice, Barbara Campi, Serena Materazzi, et al. 2008. Cigarette Smoke–Induced Neurogenic Inflammation Is Mediated by α, β-Unsaturated Aldehydes and the TRPA1 Receptor in Rodents. *The Journal of Clinical Investigation* 118: 2574–82. https://doi.org/10.1172/JCI34886.

Aretaeus of Cappadocia. 1856. *The Extant Works of Aretaeus, the Cappadocian.* Translated by Francis Adams. Sydenham Society, pp. 294–96.

Asghar, Mohammad S., Adam E. Hansen, Faisal M. Amin, et al. 2011. Evidence for a Vascular Factor in Migraine. *Annals of Neurology* 69: 635–45. https://doi.org/10.1002/ana.22292.

Ashina, Messoud, Joel Saper, Roger Cady. 2020. Eptinezumab in Episodic Migraine: A Randomized, Double-Blind, Placebo-Controlled Study (PROMISE-1). *Cephalalgia* 40: 241–54. https://doi.org/10.1177/0333102420905132.

Ayata, Cenk, Hongwei Jin, Chiho Kudo, Turgay Dalkara, and Michael A. Moskowitz. 2006. Suppression of Cortical Spreading Depression in Migraine Prophylaxis. *Annals of Neurology* 59: 652–61. https://doi.org/10.1002/ana.20778.

Bach-Rojecky, Lidija, Melita Šalković-Petrišić, and Zdravko Lacković. 2010. Botulinum Toxin Type A Reduces Pain Supersensitivity in Experimental Diabetic Neuropathy: Bilateral Effect after Unilateral Injection. *European Journal of Pharmacology* 633: 10–14. https://doi.org/10.1016/j.ejphar.2010.01.020.

Bahra, A, MS Matharu, C Buchel, RSJ Frackowiak, and PJ Goadsby. 2001. Brainstem Activation Specific to Migraine Headache. *The Lancet* 357: 1016–17. https://doi.org/10.1016/S0140–6736(00)04250–1.

Bartsch, T., and P. J. Goadsby. 2003. Increased Responses in Trigeminocervical Nociceptive Neurons to Cervical Input after Stimulation of the Dura Mater. *Brain* 126: 1801–13. https://doi.org/10.1093/brain/awg190.

Bartsch, Thorsten, and Peter J. Goadsby. 2002. Stimulation of the Greater Occipital Nerve Induces Increased Central Excitability of Dural Afferent Input. *Brain* 125: 1496–1509. https://doi.org/10.1093/brain/awf166.

Bigal, Marcelo E., Daniel Serrano, Michael Reed, and Richard B. Lipton. 2008. Chronic Migraine in the Population: Burden, Diagnosis, and Satisfaction with Treatment. *Neurology* 71: 559–66. https://doi.org/10.1212/01.wnl.0000323925.29520.e7.

Binder, William J., Mitchell F. Brin, Andrew Blitzer, Larry D. Schoenrock, and Janice M. Pogoda. 2000. Botulinum Toxin Type A (BOTOX) for Treatment of Migraine Headaches: An Open-Label Study. *Otolaryngology–Head and Neck Surgery* 123: 669–76. https://doi.org/10.1067/mhn.2000.110960.

Bittencourt da Silva, Larissa, Ali Karshenas, Flemming W. Bach, et al. 2014. Blockade of Glutamate Release by Botulinum Neurotoxin Type A in Humans: A Dermal Microdialysis Study. *Pain Research and Management* 19: 126–32. https://doi.org/10.1155/2014/410415.

Blau, J. N. 1984. Migraine Pathogenesis: The Neural Hypothesis Reexamined. *Journal of Neurology, Neurosurgery & Psychiatry* 47: 437–42. https://doi.org/10.1136/jnnp.47.5.437.

Burch, Rebecca C., Dawn C. Buse, and Richard B. Lipton. 2019. Migraine: Epidemiology, Burden, and Comorbidity. *Neurologic Clinics* 37: 631–49. https://doi.org/10.1016/j.ncl.2019.06.001.

Burstein, Rami, Rodrigo Noseda, and David Borsook. 2015. Migraine: Multiple Processes, Complex Pathophysiology. *Journal of Neuroscience* 35: 6619–29. https://doi.org/10.1523/JNEUROSCI.0373–15.2015.

Buse, D. C., A. Manack, D. Serrano, C. Turkel, and R. B. Lipton. 2010. Sociodemographic and Comorbidity Profiles of Chronic Migraine and Episodic Migraine Sufferers. *Journal of Neurology, Neurosurgery & Psychiatry* 81: 428–32. https://doi.org/10.1136/jnnp.2009.192492

Camprubí-Robles, M., R. Planells-Cases, and A. Ferrer-Montiel. 2009. Differential Contribution of SNARE-Dependent Exocytosis to Inflammatory Potentiation of TRPV1 in Nociceptors. *The FASEB Journal* 23: 3722–33. https://doi.org/10.1096/fj.09–134346.

Chasman, Daniel I., Markus Schürks, Verneri Anttila, et al. 2011. Genome-Wide Association Study Reveals Three Susceptibility Loci for Common Migraine in the General Population. *Nature Genetics* 43: 695–98. https://doi.org/10.1038/ng.856.

Chien, Chiang-Ting, Hsin-Min Lee, Chia-Ching (Josh) Wu, and Ping-Chia Li. 2012. Inhibitory Effect of Botulinum Toxin Type A on the NANC System in Rat Respiratory Models of Neurogenic Inflammation. *Archives of Biochemistry and Biophysics* 524: 106–13. https://doi.org/10.1016/j.abb.2012.05.016.

Croop, Robert, Jennifer Madonia, Charles Conway, et al. 2021. Intranasal Zavegepant Is Effective and Well Tolerated for the Acute Treatment of Migraine: A Phase 2/3 Dose-Ranging Clinical Trial (4976). *Neurology* 96 (15 Supplement). https://n.neurology.org/content/96/15_Supplement/4976.

Detke, Holland C., Peter J. Goadsby, Shufang Wang, et al. 2018. Galcanezumab in Chronic Migraine: The Randomized, Double-Blind, Placebo-Controlled REGAIN Study. *Neurology* 91: e2211–21. https://doi.org/10.1212/WNL.0000000000006640.

Didsbury, G. 1936. Considérations Sur La Migraine d'après Arétée de Cappadoce. *Bull Soc Franc d'Hist Med*, 260–67

Do, T. P., J. Hvedstrup, and H. W. Schytz. 2018. Botulinum Toxin: A Review of the Mode of Action in Migraine. *Acta Neurologica Scandinavica* 137: 442–51. https://doi.org/10.1111/ane.12906.

Dodick, David W., Catherine C. Turkel, Ronald E. DeGryse, Sheena K. Aurora, Stephen D. Silberstein, Richard B. Lipton, Hans-Christoph Diener, and Mitchell F. Brin. 2010. OnabotulinumtoxinA for Treatment of Chronic Migraine: Pooled Results from the Double-Blind, Randomized, Placebo-Controlled Phases of the PREEMPT Clinical Program. *Headache: The Journal of Head and Face Pain* 50: 921–36. https://doi.org/10.1111/j.1526-4610.2010.01678.x.

Eikermann-Haerter, Katharina, Ergin Dileköz, Chiho Kudo, 2009. Genetic and Hormonal Factors Modulate Spreading Depression and Transient Hemiparesis in Mouse Models of Familial Hemiplegic Migraine Type 1. American Society for Clinical Investigation. January 5, 2009. https://doi.org/10.1172/JCI36059.

Ferrari, Michel D., and Gisela M. Terwindt. 2001. "Familial Hemiplegic Migraine." *The Genetics of Neurological Disorders* (pp. 123–137). Oxford University Press.

Goadsby, Peter J. 2009. The Vascular Theory of Migraine—A Great Story Wrecked by the Facts. *Brain* 132: 6–7. https://doi.org/10.1093/brain/awn321.

Goadsby, Peter J. Serotonin receptors and the acute attack of migraine. 1998. Clinical neuroscience (New York, NY) 5, no. 1: 18–23.

Goadsby, Peter J., David W. Dodick, Joel M. Trugman, et al. 2019. Orally Administered Atogepant Was Efficacious, Safe, and Tolerable for the Prevention of Migraine: Results From a Phase 2b/3 Study (S17.001). *Neurology* 92 (15 Supplement). https://n.neurology.org/content/92/15_Supplement/S17.001.

Goadsby, Peter J., Uwe Reuter, Yngve Hallström, et al. 2017. A Controlled Trial of Erenumab for Episodic Migraine. *New England Journal of Medicine* 377: 2123–32. https://doi.org/10.1056/NEJMoa1705848.

Gormley, Padhraig, Verneri Anttila, Bendik S. Winsvold, et al. 2016. Meta-Analysis of 375,000 Individuals Identifies 38 Susceptibility Loci for Migraine. *Nature Genetics* 48: 856–66. https://doi.org/10.1038/ng.3598.

Hansen, Jakob Møller, Serapio Michael Baca, Paul VanValkenburgh, and Andrew Charles. 2013. Distinctive Anatomical and Physiological Features of Migraine Aura Revealed by 18 Years of Recording. *Brain* 136: 3589–95. https://doi.org/10.1093/brain/awt309.

Ho, Tony W, Michel D Ferrari, David W Dodick, et al. 2008. Efficacy and Tolerability of MK-0974 (Telcagepant), a New Oral Antagonist of Calcitonin Gene-Related Peptide Receptor, Compared with Zolmitriptan for Acute Migraine: A Randomised, Placebo-Controlled, Parallel-Treatment Trial. *The Lancet* 372: 2115–23. https://doi.org/10.1016/S0140-6736(08)61626-8.

Ho, Tony W., Kathryn M. Connor, Ying Zhang, et al. 2014. Randomized Controlled Trial of the CGRP Receptor Antagonist Telcagepant for Migraine Prevention. *Neurology* 83: 958–66. https://doi.org/10.1212/WNL.0000000000000771.

Howden, C. W., Catherine Logue, Karen Gavin, et al. 1988. Haemodynamic Effects of Intravenous Human Calcitonin-Gene-Related Peptide in Man. *Clinical Science* 74: 413–18. https://doi.org/10.1042/cs0740413.

Johnston, Mollie, and Alan Rapoport. 2010. Triptans for the Management of Migraine. Drugs 70: 1505–18. https://doi.org/10.2165/11537990-000000000-00000.

Jordt, Sven-Eric, Makoto Tominaga, and David Julius. 2000. Acid Potentiation of the Capsaicin Receptor Determined by a Key Extracellular Site. *Proceedings of the National Academy of Sciences* 97: 8134–39.

Joutel, Anne, Marie-Germaine Bousser, Valérie Biousse, et al. 1993. A Gene for Familial Hemiplegic Migraine Maps to Chromosome 19. *Nature Genetics* 5: 40–45. https://doi.org/10.1038/ng0993-40.

Lassen, LH, PA Haderslev, VB Jacobsen, et al. 2002. Cgrp May Play A Causative Role in Migraine. *Cephalalgia* 22: 54–61. https://doi.org/10.1046/j.1468–2982.2002.00310.x1.

Lee, Won-Ho, Teo Jeon Shin, Hyun Jeong Kim, Jin-Koo Lee, Hong-Won Suh, Sang Chul Lee, and Kyle Seo. 2011. Intrathecal Administration of Botulinum Neurotoxin Type A Attenuates Formalin-Induced Nociceptive Responses in Mice. *Anesthesia & Analgesia* 112: 228–35. https://doi.org/10.1213/ANE.0b013e3181ffa1d7.

Levy, Dan, Moshe Jakubowski, and Rami Burstein. 2004. Disruption of Communication between Peripheral and Central Trigeminovascular Neurons Mediates the Antimigraine Action of 5HT1B/1D Receptor Agonists. *Proceedings of the National Academy of Sciences* 101: 4274–79. https://doi.org/10.1073/pnas.0306147101.

Lipton, Richard B., Robert Croop, Elyse G. Stock. 2019. Rimegepant, an Oral Calcitonin Gene–Related Peptide Receptor Antagonist, for Migraine. *New England Journal of Medicine* 381: 142–49. https://doi.org/10.1056/NEJMoa1811090.

Maienschein, Vera, Markus Marxen, Walter Volknandt, and Herbert Zimmermann. 1999. A Plethora of Presynaptic Proteins Associated with ATP-Storing Organelles in Cultured Astrocytes. *Glia* 26: 233–44. https://doi.org/10.1002/(SICI)1098–1136(199905)26:3<233::AID-GLIA5>3.0.CO;2–2.

Malick, Amy, Rew M. Strassman, and Rami Burstein. 2000. Trigeminohypothalamic and Reticulohypothalamic Tract Neurons in the Upper Cervical Spinal Cord and Caudal Medulla of the Rat. *Journal of Neurophysiology* 84: 2078–2112. https://doi.org/10.1152/jn.2000.84.4.20782.

Maniyar, Farooq Husain, Till Sprenger, Teshamae Monteith, Christoph Schankin, and Peter James Goadsby. 2014. Brain Activations in the Premonitory Phase of Nitroglycerin-Triggered Migraine Attacks. *Brain* 137: 232–41. https://doi.org/10.1093/brain/awt3201.

McLean, Gary, and Stewart W. Mercer. 2017. Chronic Migraine, Comorbidity, and Socioeconomic Deprivation: Cross-Sectional Analysis of a Large Nationally Representative Primary Care Database. *Journal of Comorbidity* 7: 89–95. https://doi.org/10.15256/joc.2017.7.114.

McMahon, H.T., P Foran, J.O. Dolly, M Verhage, V.M. Wiegant, and D.G. Nicholls. 1992. Tetanus Toxin and Botulinum Toxins Type A and B Inhibit Glutamate, Gamma-Aminobutyric Acid, Aspartate, and Met-Enkephalin Release from Synaptosomes. Clues to the Locus of Action. *Journal of Biological Chemistry* 267: 21338–43. https://doi.org/10.1016/S0021–9258(19)36614–1.

Migraine without aura. ICHD-3 The International Classification of Headache Disorders 3rd edition. https://ichd–3.org/1-migraine/1–1-migraine-without-aura/ (accessed 16 Mar 2021)

Miyamoto, Takashi, Adrienne E. Dubin, Matt J. Petrus, and Ardem Patapoutian. 2009. TRPV1 and TRPA1 Mediate Peripheral Nitric Oxide-Induced Nociception in Mice. *PLOS ONE* 4: e7596. https://doi.org/10.1371/journal.pone.0007596.

Montecucco, Cesare, and Jordi Molgó. 2005. Botulinal Neurotoxins: Revival of An Old Killer. *Current Opinion in Pharmacology, Respiratory/Musculoskeletal* 5: 274–79. https://doi.org/10.1016/j.coph.2004.12.006.

Noseda, Rodrigo, Moshe Jakubowski, Vanessa Kainz, David Borsook, and Rami Burstein. 2011. Cortical Projections of Functionally Identified Thalamic Trigeminovascular Neurons: Implications for Migraine Headache and Its Associated Symptoms. *Journal of Neuroscience* 31: 14204–17. https://doi.org/10.1523/JNEUROSCI.3285–11.2011.

Olesen, Jes, Hans-Christoph Diener, Ingo W. Husstedt, et al. 2004. Calcitonin Gene–Related Peptide Receptor Antagonist BIBN 4096 BS for the Acute Treatment of Migraine. *New England Journal of Medicine* 350: 1104–10. https://doi.org/10.1056/NEJMoa030505.

Ophoff, Roel A, Gisela M Terwindt, Monique N Vergouwe, et al. 1996. Familial Hemiplegic Migraine and Episodic Ataxia Type-2 Are Caused by Mutations in the Ca2+ Channel Gene CACNL1A4. *Cell* 87: 543–52. https://doi.org/10.1016/S0092–8674(00)81373–2

Pietrobon, Daniela, and Michael A Moskowitz. 2013. Pathophysiology of Migraine. *Annual Review of Physiology* 75: 365–91.
Rahmann, A, T Wienecke, JM Hansen, J Fahrenkrug, J Olesen, and M Ashina. 2008. Vasoactive Intestinal Peptide Causes Marked Cephalic Vasodilation, but Does Not Induce Migraine. *Cephalalgia* 28: 226–36. https://doi.org/10.1111/j.1468–2982.2007.01497.x.
Rubio-Beltrán, Eloísa, Alejandro Labastida-Ramírez, Kristian A. Haanes, Antoon van den Bogaerdt, Ad J. J. C. Bogers, Eric Zanelli, Laurent Meeus, et al. 2019. Characterization of Binding, Functional Activity, and Contractile Responses of the Selective 5-HT1F Receptor Agonist Lasmiditan. British Journal of Pharmacology 176: 4681–95. https://doi.org/10.1111/bph.14832.
Russell, MB, L Iselius, and J Olesen. 1996. Migraine Without Aura and Migraine with Aura Are Inherited Disorders. *Cephalalgia* 16: 305–9. https://doi.org/10.1046/j.1468–2982.1996.1605305.x.
Russell, Michael Bjørn, Vibeke Ulrich, Morten Gervil, and Jes Olesen. 2002. Migraine Without Aura and Migraine with Aura Are Distinct Disorders. A Population-Based Twin Survey. *Headache: The Journal of Head and Face Pain* 42: 332–36. https://doi.org/10.1046/j.1526–4610.2002.02102.x.
Schoonman, G. G., J. van der Grond, C. Kortmann, R. J. van der Geest, G. M. Terwindt, and M. D. Ferrari. 2008. Migraine Headache Is Not Associated with Cerebral or Meningeal Vasodilatation—A 3T Magnetic Resonance Angiography Study. *Brain* 131: 2192–2200. https://doi.org/10.1093/brain/awn094.
Schulte, Laura H., and Arne May. 2016. The Migraine Generator Revisited: Continuous Scanning of the Migraine Cycle over 30 Days and Three Spontaneous Attacks. *Brain* 139: 1987–93. https://doi.org/10.1093/brain/aww097.
Schytz, Henrik Winther, Steffen Birk, Troels Wienecke, Christina Kruuse, Jes Olesen, and Messoud Ashina. 2009. PACAP38 Induces Migraine-like Attacks in Patients with Migraine without Aura. *Brain* 132: 16–25. https://doi.org/10.1093/brain/awn307.
Shekhar, Y. Chandra, Inder S. Anand, Raghav Sarma, et al. 1991. Effects of Prolonged Infusion of Human Alpha Calcitonin Gene-Related Peptide on Hemodynamics, Renal Blood Flow and Hormone Levels in Congestive Heart Failure. *The American Journal of Cardiology* 67: 732–36. https://doi.org/10.1016/0002–9149(91)90531-O.
Shimizu, Toshihiko, Mamoru Shibata, Haruki Toriumi, et al. 2012. Reduction of TRPV1 Expression in the Trigeminal System by Botulinum Neurotoxin Type-A. *Neurobiology of Disease* 48: 367–78. https://doi.org/10.1016/j.nbd.2012.07.010.
Silberstein, Stephen D., David W. Dodick, Marcelo E. Bigal, et al. 2017. Fremanezumab for the Preventive Treatment of Chronic Migraine. *New England Journal of Medicine* 377: 2113–22. https://doi.org/10.1056/NEJMoa1709038.
Stankewitz, A., H. L. Voit, U. Bingel, C. Peschke, and A. May. 2011. A New Trigemino-Nociceptive Stimulation Model for Event-Related FMRI. *Cephalalgia* n/a (n/a). Accessed April 26, 2021. https://doi.org/10.1111/j.1468–2982.2009.01968.x.
Steiner, Timothy J., Lars J. Stovner, Theo Vos, R. Jensen, and Z. Katsarava. 2018. Migraine Is First Cause of Disability in under 50s: Will Health Politicians Now Take Notice? *The Journal of Headache and Pain* 19: 17. https://doi.org/10.1186/s10194-018-0846-2
Stewart, Walter F., G. Craig Wood, Aubrey Manack, et al. 2010. Employment and Work Impact of Chronic Migraine and Episodic Migraine. *Journal of Occupational and Environmental Medicine* 52: 8–14. https://doi.org/10.1097/JOM.0b013e3181c1dc56
Stovner LJ, Nichols E, Steiner TJ, et al. 2018. Global, regional, and national burden of migraine and tension-type headache, 1990–2016: a systematic analysis for the Global Burden of Disease Study 2016. *The Lancet Neurology* 17(11): 954–76.
Sugiyama, H. 1980. Clostridium Botulinum Neurotoxin. *Microbiological Reviews* 44: 419.
Tunis, M Martin, and Harold G Wolff. 1953. STUDIES ON HEADACHE: Long-Term Observations of the Reactivity of the Cranial Arteries in Subjects with Vascular Headache of

the Migraine Type. *A.M.A. Archives of Neurology & Psychiatry* 70: 551–57. https://doi.org/10.1001/archneurpsyc.1953.02320350003001.

Ulrich, Vibeke, Morten Gervil, Kirsten O Kyvik, Jes Olesen, and Michael B Russell. 1993. The Inheritance of Migraine with Aura Estimated by Means of Structural Equation Modelling, *J Med Genet* 36: 225–7.

Usman, Habiba O., and Carey D. Balaban. 2016. Distribution of 5-HT1F Receptors in Monkey Vestibular and Trigeminal Ganglion Cells. Frontiers in Neurology 7. https://doi.org/10.3389/fneur.2016.00173.

Villalón, Carlos M, and Jes Olesen. 2009. The Role of CGRP in the Pathophysiology of Migraine and Efficacy of CGRP Receptor Antagonists as Acute Antimigraine Drugs, 15.

Voss, Tiffini, Richard B. Lipton, David W. Dodick. 2016. A Phase IIb Randomized, Double-Blind, Placebo-Controlled Trial of Ubrogepant for the Acute Treatment of Migraine. *Cephalalgia* 36: 887–98. https://doi.org/10.1177/0333102416653233.

Weiller, C., A. May, V. Limmroth, M. Jüptner, H. Kaube, R. V. Schayck, H. H. Coenen, and H. C. Dlener. 1995. Brain Stem Activation in Spontaneous Human Migraine Attacks. *Nature Medicine* 1: 658–60. https://doi.org/10.1038/nm0795–658.

Wolff, Harold G. 1948. Headache and Other Head Pain. In *Headache and Other Head Pain*, 648–648.

Xavier, Alphienes, Mageshwaran Lakshmanan, and Vikneswaran Gunaseelan. 2017. The journey of the non-vascular relief for migraine: from 'triptans' to 'ditans'. *Current Clinical Pharmacology* 12, no. 1: 36–40.

Zhang, David X., and David D. Gutterman. 2011. TRP Channel Activation and Endothelium-Dependent Dilation in the Systemic Circulation. *Journal of Cardiovascular Pharmacology* 57: 133–39. https://doi.org/10.1097/FJC.0b013e3181fd35d1.

Zhang, XiChun, Andrew M Strassman, Victor Novack, Mitchell F Brin, and Rami Burstein. 2016. Extracranial Injections of Botulinum Neurotoxin Type A Inhibit Intracranial Meningeal Nociceptors' Responses to Stimulation of TRPV1 and TRPA1 Channels: Are We Getting Closer to Solving This Puzzle? *Cephalalgia* 36: 875–86. https://doi.org/10.1177/0333102416636843.

20 Genetics of Pain

Sopyda Yin, Jacob Caylor, Eric Nelson, Christina Cui, Zabrina Reyes, and Imanuel Lerman

20.1 INTRODUCTION

20.1.1 Overview and Epidemiology

According to the IASP definition, *pain* is an unpleasant sensory and emotional experience associated with or resembling actual or potential tissue damage. Classically, *acute pain* is defined as a duration of less than 3 months, while *chronic pain* persists beyond this benchmark. Both the experience of acute pain and the conversion to chronic pain are largely variable in the general population. The estimated prevalence of chronic pain ranges from 11 to 40% in the United States.[1] Chronic pain patients are more likely to suffer anxiety and depressive disorders, restricted activity, and poor health acuity.[2] There is a clear need to further explore comorbidities that contribute to chronic pain which may translate into more accurate diagnosis and treatment.[3] More granular stratification of heterogeneous pain diagnoses could aid in the identification of pain etiologies and targeted treatments. One such example is the opioid crisis in the United States. The United States is one of the top consumers of opioids, and its prescribing culture has led to an opioid overdose epidemic.[4] Our limited understanding of individual pain response to analgesics can culminate in patient morbidity and mortality.

The prevalence and high societal costs associated with chronic pain have led to a growing health problem that contributes to increased morbidity and mortality.[3] The widely variable spectrum of pain response may be due to alterations in peripheral and central pain processing. Moreover, patients with a similar pain generator can *also* have variable responses to standard therapy. Currently, the management of chronic pain states is suboptimal due to several interfering factors.[5] The overarching challenges in treating these conditions stem largely from interindividual variability regarding the development of chronic pain conditions, severity of pain experienced, and response to analgesics, including opioids and NSAIDs.[6–9] However, emerging work is now uncovering genetic links that contribute to debilitating chronic pain—in addition to known environmental contributors, such as cultural, demographic, and biopsychosocial factors.[10]

20.2 GENETICS OF PAIN OVERVIEW

The era of modern genetics has revolutionized research within medicine. The initial foundations for the field were laid by Gregor Mendel and his pea plant experiments

DOI: 10.1201/9781003094302-20

in the 1860s, followed by the discovery of DNA structure by Franklin and Wilkins. While our understanding of genetics is constantly evolving, key concepts, such as genotypes, phenotypes, polymorphisms, and alleles, remain core in clinic evaluation. A *genotype* refers to an individual's unique genetic makeup and is the molecular basis for phenotype, an individual's observable characteristics. Genotypes are made of unique combinations of alleles, or one of two variations of a gene that an individual carries. Common variations of alleles in a population are known as *polymorphism*.

These core concepts pertain mostly to monogenic disorders with Mendelian inheritance patterns. In other words, our basic understanding of genetic inheritance focuses on one single gene inherited in a classical recessive/dominant fashion. In comparison, *non-Mendelian inheritance* refers to patterns that fall outside of this dichotomy. Some disease processes are triggered by a combination of both genetic factors and environmental contributions, which is the focus of the field of epigenetics. Twin studies are also commonly used to evaluate the relative importance of genetic versus environmental impact on phenotypes. Yet other disease processes involve polygenic inheritance, in which multiple genes contribute to one phenotype. This diversity in patterns of inheritance is further complicated by the sheer number of genes found within the human genome.

In 2003, the International Human Gene Sequencing Consortium successfully sequenced and published the complete sequence of the human genome, ushering in the era of genomics. The resources needed to sequence genomes have decreased significantly over time. The boom in sequencing capabilities reflects the growth in computing power described by Moore's law, which states that computing power doubles every two years. However, newer technologies have allowed for faster sequencing capabilities and the increased application of genome-wide association studies (GWAS). These studies cycle through hundreds of thousands of genes to find associations with a specified disease process. The most common genetic variation studied using GWAS is single base pair change, known as single nucleotide polymorphism (SNP). GWAS is one field in the development of large molecular database studies. The "omics" revolution has now evolved to include proteomics, metabolomics, and epigenomics. Within pain medicine, GWAS and other studies have been applied to understand the etiology of pain syndromes and differences in drug metabolism.

Numerous familial aggregation and twin studies showcase large heritability components with regard to chronic pain.[5] For example, monozygotic twins display an increased likelihood for similar experimental pain sensitivity, and cold and heat tolerance.[11] Additionally, monozygotic twins display similar occurrence rates of various pain-related conditions, such as musculoskeletal pain, migraine, low back pain, and menstrual pain.[12–17] From this, it's evident that heritable pain genes exist, and that they influence pain states. Moreover, further understanding the role these pain genes hold in the development and severity of chronic pain may improve targeted treatment modalities for patients.

The role of genetics in the acute and chronic pain experience is complicated and incompletely identified, to say the least. While Mendelian genetics and inheritance patterns may help us identify contributing factors to the development, maintenance, and therapeutic response of chronic pain, in reality, socioeconomic, environmental, and psychosocial factors contribute to this phenotype. This is evidenced by the wide result variability in clinical heritability studies (twin studies), though both clinical and preclinical models demonstrate a degree of pain heritability.[11, 18] With the advancement of genetic testing, it is now possible to more thoroughly catalog human genes and potentially identify polygenic contributions to the chronic pain phenotype. With the advent of lower-cost whole genome and exome sequencing, we expect that this research space will flourish in the years to come. Since 2005, publications regarding pain and gene association studies have exponentially increased.[5] In this chapter, we'll discuss various updates in pain genetics about ion channels, drug metabolism, opioid receptors, neurotransmitter release, and catabolism, as well as sexual differences in chronic pain.

20.3 GENETIC INFLUENCE ON PAIN DEVELOPMENT AND SEVERITY

While mendelian, single-gene mutation inheritance patterns of pain pathology are rare, they exist and help guide our evaluation of other complex polygenic pain phenotypes. These single-gene pain disorders have furthered our understanding of pain pathogenesis and potential drug targets. Here, we will examine two cases of monogenic polymorphisms which affect the pain experience.

Cox and colleagues (2006) reported on a 10-year-old Pakistani child street performer who would place knives through his forearms and walk over burning hot coals, all without feeling or expressing any form of pain.[19] Subsequently, their group identified six individuals from three consanguineous families who similarly were insensate to pain. Each individual presented similarly with evidence of extensive lip and tongue injuries, widespread bruising and cuts, numerous fractures, and osteomyelitis. Despite the extent of these injuries, these individuals were unequivocally insensate to all pain modalities. Of particular note, however, the pain-insensate cohort retained sensation to touch, temperature, proprioception, tickle, and pressure. Additionally, muscle strength, tone, reflexes, and joint appearance were normal.[19] Due to the familial nature of these conditions, the researchers suspected a strong genetic component.

Following genome sequence analysis, three various nonsense mutations were localized to chromosome 2q24.3, which contains the *SCN9A* gene locus, encoding the a-subunit of the voltage-gated sodium channel $Na_V1.7$.[20] This ion channel is strongly expressed in peripheral sensory neurons, particularly nociceptive small-diameter neurons in the dorsal root ganglia, nerves involved largely in afferent pain input.[21–23] Furthermore, $Na_V1.7$ is localized toward nerve terminals and is known to regulate action potential initiation.[22, 24] Subsequent laboratory studies analyzed wild-type versus mutant human $Na_V1.7$ in human embryonic kidney cells, which produced a loss of function (LoF) mutation in the channel, effectively preventing action potential propagation.[19] This surprising finding stunned researchers, as this single gene mutation in *SCN9A* resulted in multimodal peripheral pain insensitivity and was aptly termed channelopathy-associated congenital insensitivity to pain (CACIP).[19] Of particular note, diminished pain sensation due to LoF mutations in *SCN9A* was only caused by this particular channelopathy, leaving the neuron otherwise completely intact.[25–28] Before the discovery of the impacts of *SCN9A* LoF mutations in humans, preclinical animal studies exploring potential pain targets had experimented with defects in $Na_V1.7$ and displayed significantly decreased pain response to acid in mole rats and complete loss of acute mechanical and inflammatory pain in mice.[29, 30] Interestingly, congenital insensitivity to pain had been known to exist in other heritable chronic painless syndromes, such as hereditary and sensory autonomic neuropathies (HSAN) types I–V.[21] Similar to CACIP, these syndromes, also associated with single gene mutations that produce painless states, are due to (1) either neuronal cell destruction or (2) impaired neuronal propagation and migration, thus leading to additional adverse health effects.[31] Clearly, the $Na_V1.7$ channelopathy, although an exceedingly rare mutation, is known to produce severe and debilitating conditions.

In contrast to CACIP, a recent *SCN9A* mutation was discovered that promotes pain hypersensitivity, termed *primary erythromelalgia* (PE).[20] In PE, patients present with episodic erythema, swelling, and painful burning sensation in the hands, feet, ears, and face.[20] The episodes are triggered by heat and exercise, which can relegate these unfortunate patients to reside in frigid environs and avoid exercise. The bouts can become so severe that, often, pain relief is only provided by immersion in an ice bath. As the patients age, they experience more frequent and severe episodes, oftentimes daily bouts of burning, stinging, and throbbing pain ranging from minutes to hours. Although CACIP and PE range on different ends of the pain spectrum, both conditions are caused by *SCN9A* gene locus mutation.

In PE, various gain-of-function (GoF) mutations occur within *SCN9A*, causing missense variants in $Na_V1.7$.[32] These variants alter the electrophysiological state of DRG neurons by increasing the open-state probability of $Na_V1.7$. This facilitates activation and slows deactivation of these neurons, enhancing nociceptive signaling and producing continual cardinal symptoms of extreme pain and sensitivity.[31] Similar to patients with CACIP, patients with GoF mutations in $Na_V1.7$ do not experience any autonomic abnormalities, such as anhidrosis, orthostatic hypotension, or gastrointestinal dysfunction, causing fewer global health effects.[10]

The monogenic impact of *SCN9A* on pain experience is evident. Both LoF and GoF variants described produce distinct phenotypic pain states that exist on opposite ends of the spectrum, where CACIP leads to a life devoid of all pain, increasing the risk of injury and infection, and PE produces paroxysmal unbearable and debilitating bouts of pain. With its Mendelian genetic inheritance patterns, its primary localization to DRG neurons, and its minimal impact on neuronal development and integrity, $Na_V1.7$ has emerged as a prime target for both pain genetics research and analgesic drug development.[5] Various pharmaceutical companies, including Xenon Pharmaceuticals and Pfizer Inc., have developed experimental inhibitory medications targeting these channels, including XEN402 and PF-05089771, respectively.[33] These medications have shown promise in treating postherpetic trigeminal neuralgia and primary erythromelalgia,[34, 35] however, have not yet shown success in large randomized clinical trials. Most recently, Navega Therapeutics developed an epigenetic strategy using CRISPR-dCas9 and zinc fingers, called long-lasting analgesia via targeted in vivo epigenetic repression of $Na_V1.7$ (LATER), to repress $Na_V1.7$ expression. This CRISPR-dCas9 $Na_V1.7$ expression repression reduced preclinical hyperalgesia and chemotherapy-induced chronic pain that may translate to human therapy in the near future. It is hoped that such strategies that may target $Na_V1.7$ function could not only alleviate clinical pain from various peripheral neuropathies but also lessen the impact of the opioid crisis.[19]

20.4 GENETIC INFLUENCE ON THERAPEUTIC RESPONSE

In addition to affecting the development and maintenance of pain, genetic factors also affect the therapeutic efficacy of our treatments for these pain syndromes. Specifically, systemically administered analgesics demonstrate interindividual heterogeneity due to differences in pharmacokinetics and pharmacodynamics. *Pharmacokinetics* (PK) represents the process of drug metabolism, from first administration through elimination. This principle dictates the amount of active metabolite of the drug or effect site concentration available to exert its biochemical effect (i.e., turn on or turn off the target receptor). Physiologic processes, such as drug–protein or drug–lipid binding, metabolism enzymatic activation or deactivation, and active or passive elimination, change the amount of drug available to exert the drug effect. *Pharmacodynamics* (PD), on the other hand, represents the process whereby a drug exerts its biological effect. This may be through activation or inhibition of a receptor, by alteration of DNA/RNA/protein synthesis/translation/transcription, or through binding of other molecules. From this brief overview of PK and PD, it is clear that changes in genetic code that alter critical protein/epitope components result in differences in enzyme and/or receptor kinetics that change the biological response to an administered drug. This is the principle of pharmacogenomics, while in pain medicine, we refer to the pharmacogenomics of analgesics. In pain medicine pharmacogenomics, well-studied and prescribed analgesics are opioids and nonsteroidal anti-inflammatory drugs (NSAIDs). We will discuss some well-described genetic differences in these analgesic therapies.

As an example of PK, the cytochrome P450 (CYP) family of proteins is a catalytic enzyme class that is involved in drug metabolism, particularly phase I reactions.[36] Polymorphisms in these genes may result in different isoforms which affect drug metabolism and, thus, availability. Among the CYP family, CYP2C9 emerges as the principal enzyme accountable for the breakdown of NSAIDs, with the most salient genetic variants being CYP2C9*2 and CYP2C9*3, which are characterized by diverse SNPs and higher allele frequencies in the human population.[37, 38] Genetic differences within CYP2C9 can classify individuals as either normal or poor metabolizers of NSAIDs. Individuals lacking CYP2C9*2 or CYP2C9*3 are considered normal metabolizers, while those with the CYP2C9*2/3 genotype are classified as poor metabolizers of NSAIDs.[39] Poor metabolizers identified through CYP2C9 genotyping have an increased risk of developing NSAID-related gastrointestinal adverse events. Impaired NSAID metabolism due to these detrimental CYP2C9 mutations results in a prolonged half-life and increased drug exposure. Multiple studies have reported that individuals with detrimental CYP2C9 variant alleles in homozygosity have a significantly higher risk of NSAID-related gastrointestinal adverse events.[39]

Steroid medications like lidocaine, commonly used as a local anesthetic in pain intervention, are metabolized by specific alleles of cytochrome P450 enzymes, such as CYP3A4. As demonstrated in a study involving a patient with sepsis, reduced levels of lidocaine metabolites were observed by CYP3A4 activity.[40, 41] The altered metabolism mediated by CYP3A4 can impact pain management by potentially reducing the effectiveness of lidocaine in providing pain relief.

Responsible for the metabolism of the notable opioids tramadol, hydrocodone, and codeine, CYP2D6 accounts for 20% of all drug metabolism.[42] Depending on the number of CYP2D6 gene copies and other variations within the gene, a patient can be classified as a poor, intermediate, extensive, or ultrarapid metabolizer.[43] For example, a poor metabolizer may have only one copy of the CYP2D6 gene, while an ultrarapid metabolizer may have multiple copies on each chromosome. As CYP2D6 is responsible for the conversion of codeine and hydrocodone to the bioactive form, it is clear that differential metabolism of these drugs may lead to either (1) poor metabolizer-mediated inadequate pain relief due to less-active metabolite, that is, in the case of a poor metabolizer, or (2) ultrarapid metabolizer potential severe side effects, such as respiratory depression. Multiple case reports demonstrate the consequences of this variable metabolism with codeine due to unknown metabolizer status related to CYP2D6 copy number, including an ultrarapid metabolizer: morphine overdosed infant via a codeine-treated mother's breastmilk.[44, 45] Extensive and ultrarapid opioid metabolism is not the only problem with this genetic variance in CYP2D6—being a poor metabolizer is a risk factor for severe post-operative pain, as evidenced by a 250-patient cohort who received fentanyl analgesia.[46]

Genes that affect drug transport play a role in the PK of plasma drug concentration. For instance, the ABCB-1 gene encodes for a P glycoprotein that is an opioid efflux transporter, particularly in the kidney, intestines, and brain.[47, 48] As the gene is known to have several polymorphisms, certain SNPs are associated with decreased expression and activity of the P glycoprotein, and thus, opioids may accumulate to higher concentrations in the central nervous system for longer periods of time.[49] In multiple studies, poor exporter patients (low p glycoprotein) demonstrated improved post-operative pain scores and lower opioid use; however, in at least one study, there was an association with higher adverse events.[47, 48, 50]

Genetic variations also affect the PD of drugs, specifically in patients who have target receptor polymorphisms. Two such receptors include the mu-opioid receptor gene (OPRM1) and melanocortin 1 receptor (MC1R). Polymorphisms in these genes demonstrated increased sensitivity to opioid analgesia and improved pain control when given opioids.[51, 52] Although it remains unlikely that any single SNP or polymorphism is responsible for the differences in efficacy and pain relief amongst patients, identifying contributors to algesia and analgesia is critical to further our understanding of how these genes interact to create a phenotype.[53]

Figure 20.1 illustrates the interindividual variation of opioid effects. As medicine evolves toward individual, personalized patient treatment, pharmacogenomics will play an ever-greater role in evaluating and identifying therapies for disease syndromes—especially in pain medicine.[54] Understanding interindividual genetic variability specifically concerning genes that affect PK and PD will ultimately allow clinician-scientists to optimize efficacy and minimize side effects of drug therapy.[54] Even now, pharmacogenetics has made its way into the perioperative space, and widely available commercial products are likely to follow in the near future. This

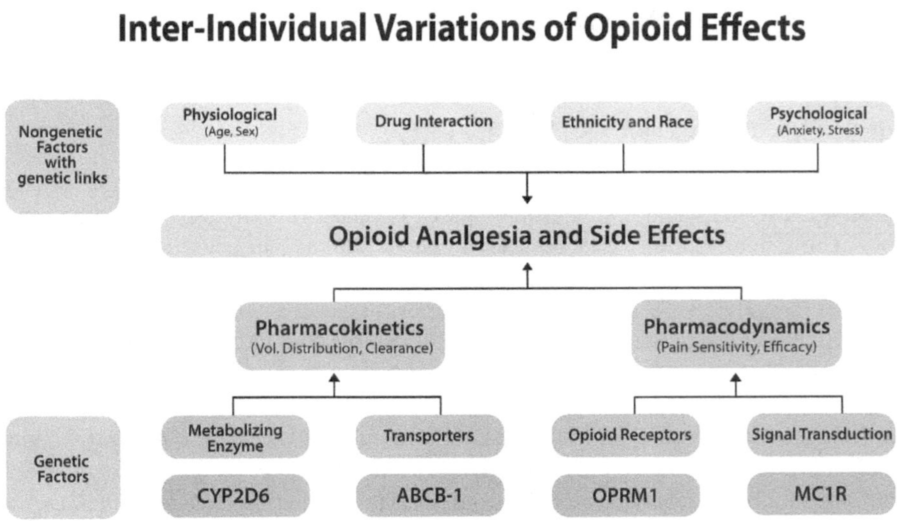

FIGURE 20.1 Interindividual variations of opioid effects. Many factors contribute to the patient's analgesic response to administered pharmacotherapy. These include patient, environment, physiologic, and drug factors that contribute to perceived analgesia.

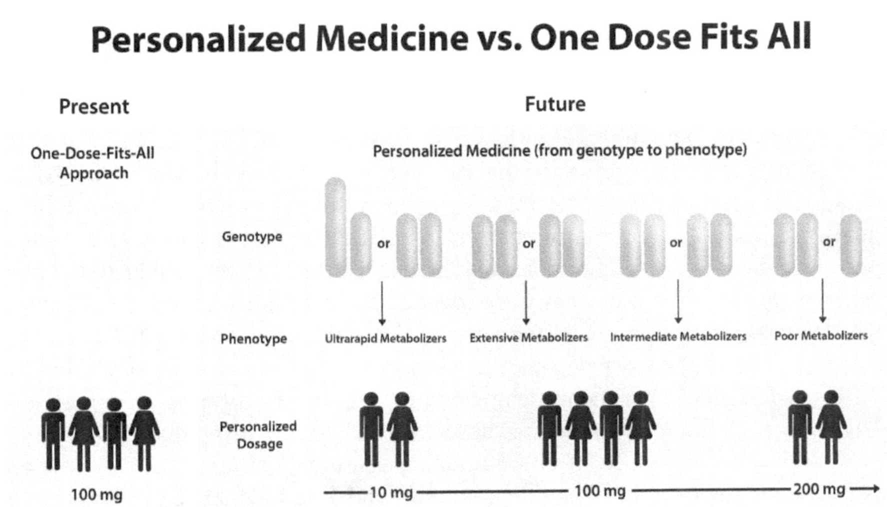

FIGURE 20.2 Personalized medicine vs. one-dose-fits-all. In current clinical practice, medications are started and dose-adjusted using readily available patient information. In the future, we expect that this information will be combined with patient-specific genetic factors to provide targeted therapies and interventions that may improve our therapy or preemptively dose-limit patients prone to side effects at higher dosages.

will better allow providers to choose not only the best drug for a patient but also the most optimal dosage.[49] Figure 20.2 illustrates the benefits of personalized medicine.

20.5 SEX DIFFERENCES IN PAIN PROCESSING

Our understanding of the interaction between genetics and pain is driven by poorly understood terms, including neurobiological, psychosocial, and environmental factors. These contributions may confound results obtained in acute or chronic pain studies and likely include heterogeneous chronic pain pathophysiology (e.g., osteoarthritis, spondylolysis, fractures, and/or deformities). It is known that sex-specific differences in chronic pain syndromes exist—the involved pathways and differential response to therapies have also begun to emerge.[55] Interestingly, in addition to lower pain tolerance and decreased thresholds in experimental models, females also exhibit an increased incidence of neuropathic pain, musculoskeletal pain, fibromyalgia, low back pain, and migraine.[55] This begs the question: What sex-specific mechanisms of chronic pain pathogenesis are at play, and what therapies have sex-dependent therapeutic benefit?

Historically, preclinical models used for pain research have been male animals, in an attempt to limit hormonal variation and standardize basic science research. This has been challenged, recently, as evidence has demonstrated that we have been neglecting female-specific pain pathways. Sorge et al. (2011) first showed the presence of a spinal toll-like receptor 4 (TLR4) pathway that was male-specific and testosterone-dependent in a mechanical allodynia mouse model.[56] Interestingly, they found that if they supplemented female animals with testosterone, they would switch to the male-specific TLR4 pathway instead of their default independent pathway.[56] This apparent sexual dimorphism was further characterized in 2015 when Sorge and Mogil noted both shared and exclusive pathways to developing allodynia between animal sexes.[57] In males, they noted that the development of allodynia was dependent on microglia upregulation of the P2X4 receptor pathway, which also involved the synthesis of brain-derived neurotrophic factor (BDNF).[57] Using carefully designed experiments involving sex hormones and knockouts, they further demonstrated that female mechanical hypersensitivity was dependent on adaptive immunity (likely T cells) rather than the microglia in the males.[57] When the female pain pathway is suppressed, they revert to the male-specific pathway. This work has been supported by carefully redesigned experiments demonstrating sex-specific differences in preclinical hyperalgesic pain models and the subsequent therapeutic response.[58, 59]

The increased incidence of autoimmune disease and chronic pain in women may be related through this adaptive immunity and T cell–dependent development of allodynia. Interestingly, an immune reaction to myelin basic protein (MBP), a component of the protective nerve sheath, can lead to allodynia via T cell recognition.[60] Confirming this work, Chernov et al. (2018) induced mechanical allodynia in female animals only when injecting MBP fragments into sciatic nerve.[61] Gene expression profiles confirmed this observed sexual dimorphism, and later work even demonstrated that female animals became seropositive for autoantibodies to this MBP.[62] Though it remains heavily disputed within the literature, sex differences have also been reported in opioid responsiveness and signaling.[63] Clinical studies and preclinical models do not universally agree regarding the purported increased efficacy of morphine in females.[64, 65] One working model explaining this difference is regarding microglia and TLR4 activation in females. Notably, Doyle et al. (2017) showed that microglia activation in the periaqueductal gray (PAG) in females had decreased analgesia compared to males. When naloxone was introduced and inhibited morphine's interaction with TLR4, females exhibited improved analgesia to male levels.[66] Further work is needed to clarify this relationship, but with advanced testing, such as transcriptomics and proteomics, in addition to other forms of genetic testing, we may finally clarify contributions to the development of chronic pain. In recent work, Ray et al. (2019) demonstrated sexual dimorphism in 149 genes associated with chronic pain, neuroimmunity, and inflammation.[67] We expect that these pathways will continue to be elucidated, which may lead to the identification of sex-based diagnostics and therapeutics for the treatment of pain.

20.6 CONCLUSIONS

Chronic pain is a widely heterogeneous condition with extreme patient-to-patient variation in analgesic response to administered medications and treatments. Moreover, the available medications and therapies we have for patients are limited in their efficacy or have significant risks. The implications of genomic medicine when applied to acute and chronic pain are potentially significantly advantageous. While the clinical application of genomic medicine to chronic pain treatment is currently limited, future investigations may open this field to offer novel drug targets or modify existing pharmacologic models to optimize sex-specific pain control.

REFERENCES

1. Dahlhamer J, Lucas J, Zelaya C, et al. Prevalence of chronic pain and high-impact chronic pain among adults—United States, 2016. *Morbidity and mortality weekly report*. 2018;67(36):1001.
2. Guerje O, Von Korff M, Simon G, Gater R. Persistent pain and well-being. *A World Health Organization study in primary care JAMA*. 1998;280:147–151.
3. Simon LS. Relieving pain in America: A blueprint for transforming prevention, care, education, and research. *Journal of pain & palliative care pharmacotherapy*. 2012;26(2):197–198.
4. Theisen K, Jacobs B, Macleod L, Davies B. The United States opioid epidemic: a review of the surgeon's contribution to it and health policy initiatives. 2018.
5. Mogil JS. Pain genetics: past, present and future. *Trends in genetics*. 2012;28(6):258–266.
6. Kehlet H, Jensen T, Woolf C. The mechanism of post-thoracotomy pain syndrome (PTPS). *Lancet*. 2006;367:1618–1625.
7. Bedson J, Croft PR. The discordance between clinical and radiographic knee osteoarthritis: a systematic search and summary of the literature. *BMC musculoskeletal disorders*. 2008;9(1):116.
8. Aubrun F, Langeron O, Quesnel C, Coriat P, Riou B. Relationships between measurement of pain using visual analog score and morphine requirements during postoperative intravenous morphine titration. *The Journal of the American Society of Anesthesiologists*. 2003;98(6):1415–1421.

9. Walker JS, Sheather-Reid RB, Carmody JJ, Day RO, Vial JH. Nonsteroidal anti-inflammatory drugs in rheumatoid arthritis and osteoarthritis. Support for the concept of "responders" and "nonresponders". *Arthritis & rheumatism: official journal of the american college of rheumatology*. 1997;40(11):1944–1954.
10. Belfer I. Nature and nurture of human pain. *Scientifica*. 2013;2013.
11. Norbury TA, MacGregor AJ, Urwin J, Spector TD, McMahon SB. Heritability of responses to painful stimuli in women: a classical twin study. *Brain*. 2007;130(11):3041–3049.
12. Do K-A, Treloar SA, Pandeya N, et al. Predictive factors of age at menopause in a large Australian twin study. *Human biology*. 1998:1073–1091.
13. Ferreira PH, Beckenkamp P, Maher CG, Hopper JL, Ferreira ML. Nature or nurture in low back pain? Results of a systematic review of studies based on twin samples. *European journal of pain*. 2013;17(7):957–971.
14. Honkasalo ML, Kaprio J, Winter T, Heikkilä K, Sillanpää M, Koskenvuo M. Migraine and concomitant symptoms among 8167 adult twin pairs. *Headache: the journal of head and face pain*. 1995;35(2):70–78.
15. Livshits G, Popham M, Malkin I, et al. Lumbar disc degeneration and genetic factors are the main risk factors for low back pain in women: the UK Twin Spine Study. *Annals of the rheumatic diseases*. 2011;70(10):1740–1745.
16. Svensson DA, Larsson B, Waldenlind E, Pedersen NL. Shared rearing environment in migraine: results from twins reared apart and twins reared together. *Headache: the journal of head and face pain*. 2003;43(3):235–244.
17. Ziegler DK, Hur YM, Bouchard Jr TJ, Hassanein RS, Barter R. Migraine in twins raised together and apart. *Headache: the journal of head and face pain*. 1998;38(6):417–422.
18. Nielsen CS, Stubhaug A, Price DD, Vassend O, Czajkowski N, Harris JR. Individual differences in pain sensitivity: genetic and environmental contributions. *Pain*. 2008;136(1–2):21–29.
19. Cox JJ, Reimann F, Nicholas AK, et al. An SCN9A channelopathy causes congenital inability to experience pain. *Nature*. 2006;444(7121):894–898.
20. Novella SP, Hisama FM, Dib-Hajj SD, Waxman SG. A case of inherited erythromelalgia. *Nature clinical practice neurology*. 2007;3(4):229–234.
21. Klugbauer N, Lacinova L, Flockerzi V, Hofmann F. Structure and functional expression of a new member of the tetrodotoxin-sensitive voltage-activated sodium channel family from human neuroendocrine cells. *The EMBO journal*. 1995;14(6):1084–1090.
22. Toledo-Aral JJ, Moss BL, He Z-J, et al. Identification of PN1, a predominant voltage-dependent sodium channel expressed principally in peripheral neurons. *Proceedings of the national academy of sciences*. 1997;94(4):1527–1532.
23. Sangameswaran L, Fish LM, Koch BD, et al. A novel tetrodotoxin-sensitive, voltage-gated sodium channel expressed in rat and human dorsal root ganglia. *Journal of biological chemistry*. 1997;272(23):14805–14809.
24. Cummins TR, Howe JR, Waxman SG. Slow closed-state inactivation: a novel mechanism underlying ramp currents in cells expressing the hNE/PN1 sodium channel. *Journal of neuroscience*. 1998;18(23):9607–9619.
25. Indo Y, Tsuruta M, Hayashida Y, et al. Mutations in the TRKA/NGF receptor gene in patients with congenital insensitivity to pain with anhidrosis. *Nature genetics*. 1996;13(4):485–488.
26. Bejaoui K, Wu C, Scheffler MD, et al. SPTLC1 is mutated in hereditary sensory neuropathy, type 1. *Nature genetics*. 2001;27(3):261–262.
27. Lafrenière RG, MacDonald ML, Dubé M-P, et al. Identification of a novel gene (HSN2) causing hereditary sensory and autonomic neuropathy type II through the Study of Canadian Genetic Isolates. *The American journal of human genetics*. 2004;74(5):1064–1073.
28. Slaugenhaupt SA, Blumenfeld A, Gill SP, et al. Tissue-specific expression of a splicing mutation in the IKBKAP gene causes familial dysautonomia. *The American journal of human genetics*. 2001;68(3):598–605.

29. Smith ESJ, Omerbašić D, Lechner SG, Anirudhan G, Lapatsina L, Lewin GR. The molecular basis of acid insensitivity in the African naked mole-rat. *Science*. 2011;334(6062):1557–1560.
30. Nassar MA, Stirling LC, Forlani G, et al. Nociceptor-specific gene deletion reveals a major role for Nav1. 7 (PN1) in acute and inflammatory pain. *Proceedings of the national academy of sciences*. 2004;101(34):12706–12711.
31. Zorina-Lichtenwalter K, Parisien M, Diatchenko L. Genetic studies of human neuropathic pain conditions: a review. *Pain*. 2018;159(3):583.
32. Dib-Hajj SD, Rush AM, Cummins T, et al. Gain-of-function mutation in Nav1. 7 in familial erythromelalgia induces the bursting of sensory neurons. *Brain*. 2005;128(8):1847–1854.
33. Bagal SK, Chapman ML, Marron BE, Prime R, Storer RI, Swain NA. Recent progress in sodium channel modulators for pain. *Bioorganic & medicinal chemistry letters*. 2014;24(16):3690–3699.
34. Price N, Namdari R, Neville J, et al. Safety and efficacy of a topical sodium channel inhibitor (TV-45070) in patients with postherpetic neuralgia (PHN): a randomized, controlled, proof-of-concept, crossover study, with a subgroup analysis of the Nav1. 7 R1150W genotype. *The clinical journal of pain*. 2017;33(4):310.
35. Cao L, McDonnell A, Nitzsche A, et al. Pharmacological reversal of a pain phenotype in iPSC-derived sensory neurons and patients with inherited erythromelalgia. *Science translational medicine*. 2016;8(335):335ra356–335ra356.
36. Rendic S, Carlo FJD. Human cytochrome P450 enzymes: a status report summarizing their reactions, substrates, inducers, and inhibitors. *Drug metabolism reviews*. 1997;29(1–2):413–580.
37. García-Martín E, Martínez C, Ladero JM, Agúndez JA. Interethnic and intraethnic variability of CYP2C8 and CYP2C9 polymorphisms in healthy individuals. *Molecular diagnosis & therapy*. 2006;10:29–40.
38. Zobdeh F, Eremenko II, Akan MA, et al. Pharmacogenetics and pain treatment with a focus on non-steroidal anti-inflammatory drugs (NSAIDs) and antidepressants: a systematic review. *Pharmaceutics*. 2022;14(6):1190.
39. Macias Y, Gómez Tabales J, Garcia-Martin E, Agundez JA. An update on the pharmacogenomics of NSAID metabolism and the risk of gastrointestinal bleeding. *Expert opinion on drug metabolism & toxicology*. 2020;16(4):319–332.
40. Darakjian L, Deodhar M, Turgeon J, Michaud V. Chronic inflammatory status observed in patients with type 2 diabetes induces modulation of cytochrome P450 expression and activity. *International journal of molecular sciences*. 2021;22(9):4967.
41. Jakob SM, Ruokonen E, Rosenberg PH, Takala J. Effect of dopamine-induced changes in splanchnic blood flow on MEGX production from lidocaine in septic and cardiac surgery patients. *Shock*. 2002;18(1):1–7.
42. Wang B, Yang L-P, Zhang X-Z, Huang S-Q, Bartlam M, Zhou S-F. New insights into the structural characteristics and functional relevance of the human cytochrome P450 2D6 enzyme. *Drug metabolism reviews*. 2009;41(4):573–643.
43. Robles CRF, Degnan M, Candiotti KA. Pain and genetics. *Current opinion in anesthesiology*. 2012;25(4):444–449.
44. Gasche Y, Daali Y, Fathi M, et al. Codeine intoxication associated with ultrarapid CYP2D6 metabolism. *New England journal of medicine*. 2004;351(27):2827–2831.
45. Koren G, Cairns J, Chitayat D, Gaedigk A, Leeder SJ. Pharmacogenetics of morphine poisoning in a breastfed neonate of a codeine-prescribed mother. *The Lancet*. 2006;368(9536):704.
46. Yang Z, Yang Z, Arheart KL, et al. CYP2D6 poor metabolizer genotype and smoking predict severe postoperative pain in female patients on arrival to the recovery room. *Pain medicine*. 2012;13(4):604–609.

47. Lötsch J, von Hentig N, Freynhagen R, et al. Cross-sectional analysis of the influence of currently known pharmacogenetic modulators on opioid therapy in outpatient pain centers. *Pharmacogenetics and genomics*. 2009;19(6):429–436.
48. Zwisler ST, Enggaard TP, Noehr-Jensen L, et al. The antinociceptive effect and adverse drug reactions of oxycodone in human experimental pain in relation to genetic variations in the OPRM1 and ABCB1 genes. *Fundamental & clinical pharmacology*. 2010;24(4):517–524.
49. Kapur BM, Lala PK, Shaw JL. Pharmacogenetics of chronic pain management. *Clinical biochemistry*. 2014;47(13–14):1169–1187.
50. Campa D, Gioia A, Tomei A, Poli P, Barale R. Association of ABCB1/MDR1 and OPRM1 gene polymorphisms with morphine pain relief. *Clinical pharmacology & therapeutics*. 2008;83(4):559–566.
51. Mogil J, Ritchie J, Smith S, et al. Melanocortin-1 receptor gene variants affect pain and μ-opioid analgesia in mice and humans. *Journal of medical genetics*. 2005;42(7):583–587.
52. Sia AT, Lim Y, Lim EC, et al. A118G single nucleotide polymorphism of human μ-opioid receptor gene influences pain perception and patient-controlled intravenous morphine consumption after intrathecal morphine for postcesarean analgesia. *The journal of the American society of anesthesiologists*. 2008;109(3):520–526.
53. Sadhasivam S, Chidambaran V. Pharmacogenomics of opioids and perioperative pain management. *Pharmacogenomics*. 2012;13(15):1719–1740.
54. Xie H-G, Frueh FW. Pharmacogenomics steps toward personalized medicine. 2005.
55. Fillingim RB, King CD, Ribeiro-Dasilva MC, Rahim-Williams B, Riley Iii JL. Sex, gender, and pain: a review of recent clinical and experimental findings. *The journal of pain*. 2009;10(5):447–485.
56. Sorge RE, LaCroix-Fralish ML, Tuttle AH, et al. Spinal cord Toll-like receptor 4 mediates inflammatory and neuropathic hypersensitivity in male but not female mice. *Journal of neuroscience*. 2011;31(43):15450–15454.
57. Sorge RE, Mapplebeck JCS, Rosen S, et al. Different immune cells mediate mechanical pain hypersensitivity in male and female mice. *Nature neuroscience*. 2015;18(8):1081.
58. Mapplebeck JCS, Dalgarno R, Tu Y, et al. Microglial P2X4R-evoked pain hypersensitivity is sexually dimorphic in rats. *Pain*. 2018;159(9):1752–1763.
59. Brings VE, Zylka MJ. Sex, drugs and pain control. *Nature neuroscience*. 2015;18(8):1059.
60. Liu H, Shiryaev SA, Chernov AV, et al. Immunodominant fragments of myelin basic protein initiate T cell-dependent pain. *Journal of neuroinflammation*. 2012;9(1):119.
61. chernov A, Hullugundi S, Eddinger K, et al. Transcriptomics analysis highlights the sexually dimorphic mechanical pain hypersensitivity mechanisms. Paper presented at: Society for Neuroscience 2018; San Diego, CA.
62. SK H, AV C, AG R, et al. The cryptic 68–104 region of myelin basic protein (MBP) causes pain from light touch exclusively in female rodents: autoimmune mechanisms of sexual dimorphism in mechanical allodynia. Paper presented at: Peripheral Nerve Society 2017; Barcelona, Spain.
63. Mogil JS. Sex differences in pain and pain inhibition: multiple explanations of a controversial phenomenon. *Nature reviews neuroscience*. 2012;13(12):859.
64. Mogil JS, Chesler EJ, Wilson SG, Juraska JM, Sternberg WF. Sex differences in thermal nociception and morphine antinociception in rodents depend on genotype. *Neuroscience & biobehavioral reviews*. 2000;24(3):375–389.
65. Niesters M, Dahan A, Kest B, et al. Do sex differences exist in opioid analgesia? A systematic review and meta-analysis of human experimental and clinical studies. *Pain*. 2010;151(1):61–68.
66. Doyle HH, Eidson LN, Sinkiewicz DM, Murphy AZ. Sex differences in microglia activity within the periaqueductal gray of the rat: a potential mechanism driving the dimorphic effects of morphine. *Journal of neuroscience*. 2017;37(12):3202–3214.
67. Ray P, Kahn J, Wangzhou A, et al. Transcriptome analysis of the human tibial nerve identifies sexually dimorphic expression of genes involved in pain, inflammation and neuro-immunity. *Frontiers in molecular neuroscience*. 2019;12:37.

21 Chronic Lower Back Pain
Etiology and Treatment

Christopher A. Woolley and Jeffrey L. Chen

21.1 INTRODUCTION

This chapter will address an important topic affecting many patients worldwide. The learning points include:

1. What are the demographics and etiology of chronic lower back pain?
2. What is the anatomy of the spine and pathophysiology behind chronic lower back pain?
3. What are some animal models used to study chronic lower back pain?
4. What are the main types of chronic lower back pain?
5. What is the presentation of chronic lower back pain?
6. What are the physical exam findings of chronic lower back pain?
7. What are some diagnostic tests to order in the evaluation of chronic lower back pain?
8. What are some common medical and interventional managements for chronic lower back pain?

21.2 DEMOGRAPHICS

Lower back pain is a very common disease that impacts individuals all over the world. It is estimated that the lifetime prevalence of lower back pain is over 70% in industrialized countries, and it has a 1-year prevalence of 15–45%. [1] Lower back pain can be classified as acute, subacute, or chronic. *Chronic lower back pain* (CLBP) is defined as low back pain persisting for longer than 12 weeks, or recurring pain after a period of healing. [2] According to the US Burden of Disease Collaborators, CLBP has accounted for the largest number of years lived with disability in the United States and is the sixth leading cause of disability-adjusted life years in *all* countries. [3, 4] Furthermore, health expenditures for patients with CLBP continue to increase, with a recent estimate of $88 billion spent in the United States annually for medical treatments for back pain, accounting for the third largest portion of total national health spending behind diabetes and ischemic heart disease. [3, 5]

Although CLBP can affect patients of any age, incidence rates peak between ages of 35 and 55 years. [6] Risk factors for CLBP are both physical and psychological.

DOI: 10.1201/9781003094302-21

Male gender, increased body height, and increased BMI are all independent risk factors for the incidence and prevalence of CLBP. People who work in professions with long-standing positions, or repetitive trunk movements, are also more likely to develop and to be affected by CLBP. Individuals with high levels of negative affectivity, anxiety, and depression, as well as low levels of social support, are also at an increased risk of developing CLBP. [2]

21.3 PATHOPHYSIOLOGY

21.3.1 The Spinal Cord

The human spinal cord is divided into four sections (from cephalad to caudal): cervical, thoracic, lumbar, and sacral. The spinal cord is protected by the vertebral column. There are 7 cervical, 12 thoracic, 5 lumbar, and 5 sacral vertebrae. Spinal nerves exit the cervical spinal cord above their corresponding vertebral body (e.g., the sixth cervical nerve roots [C6] exit above the C6 vertebral body). As there are 8 cervical nerves and 7 cervical vertebral bodies, the C8 nerve roots exit below the C7 vertebral body. In the thoracic, lumbar, and sacral spine, spinal nerves exit below their corresponding vertebral body. [7] The cervical and lumbar spine has a natural lordosis (anterior curvature), and the thoracic spine has a natural kyphosis (posterior curvature.)

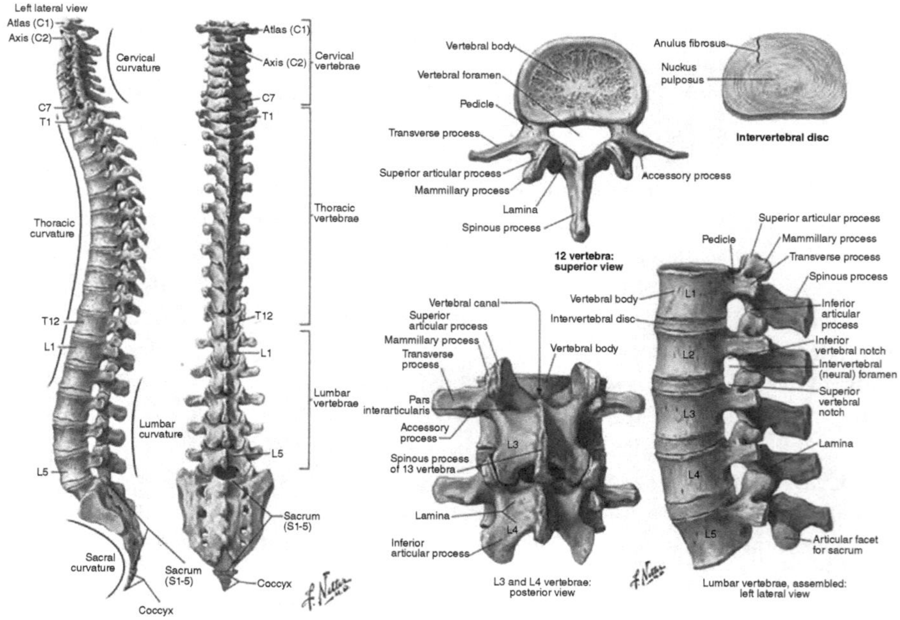

FIGURE 21.1 Bony anatomy of the spine.

Source: [8].

21.3.2 The Spinal Column

The spinal column provides support and protection for the spinal cord. It consists of two segments, the anterior segment and the posterior segment. The anterior segment is considered to be the weight-bearing segment and consists of the intervertebral bodies, vertebral discs, the anterior longitudinal ligaments (ALL), and the posterior longitudinal ligament (PLL.) The posterior segment provides protection to the vertebral bodies and intervertebral discs. [9] See Figure 21.2 for a cross-sectional illustration of the spinal column. [9]

21.3.2.1 Intervertebral Bodies and Discs

Intervertebral bodies make up the central structure of the anterior segment of the spinal column. In between these bodies lie symphysial joints containing intervertebral discs which contribute to spine stability and torsion. [10] The intervertebral discs are largely avascular, compressible structures that are able to distribute compressive loads. The intervertebral disc is comprised of the annulus fibrosis and the nucleus pulposus. The *annulus fibrosis* is a tough peripheral fibroelastic ring which contains the nucleus pulposus, a gel-like mucopolysaccharide filling. The nucleus pulposus may cause pain by irritating nerve roots if it spills out of the disc due to compression or injury. [9] The outer one-third of the intervertebral disc is well innervated, but there is controversy regarding whether this is a pain-producing structure. [11–14]

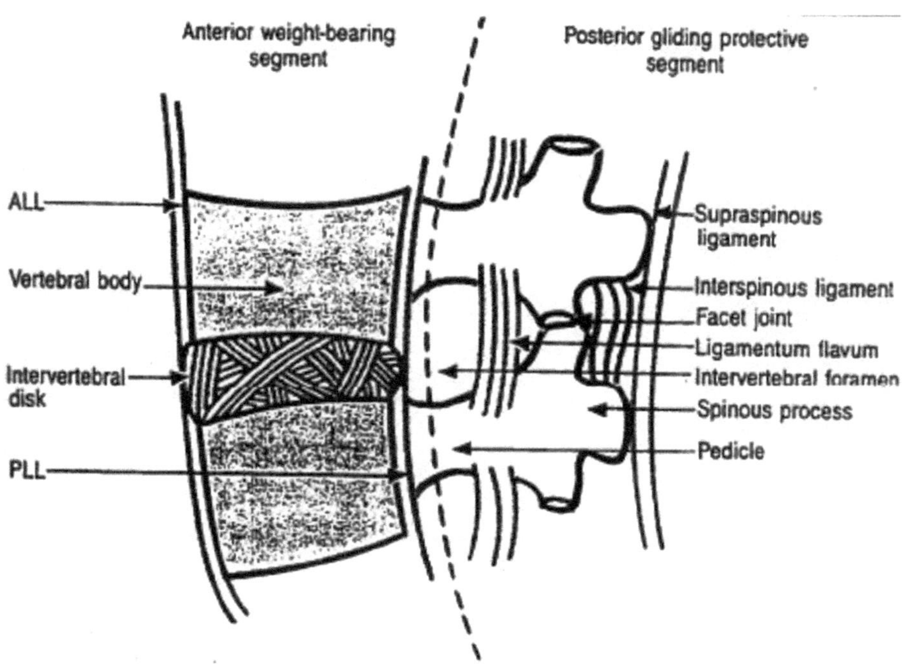

FIGURE 21.2 Cross section of two vertebrae and intervertebral disc.

Source: [9].

21.3.2.2 The Anterior Longitudinal Ligament (ALL) and Posterior Longitudinal Ligament (PLL)

The ALL and PLL extend the entire length of the spine. These two ligaments bind the anterior segment of the spinal column on either side and provide structural support to the intervertebral discs as well as prevent hyperextension and hyperflexion. [10] The PLL normally narrows at the L5–S1 region, which creates an area of weakness where herniation of intervertebral discs can occur. [9] The PLL appears to be the most heavily innervated spinal ligament, and the ligamentum flavum the least innervated. [15–17] Degenerative changes within these ligaments may result in chronic pain.

21.3.2.3 Facet Joints

The facet joints, also known as zygapophysial joints, z-joints, or apophyseal joints, are joints between the posterior articular processes of two neighboring vertebrae. [10] The facet joints are true diarthrodial joints, that is, consisting of cartilage lining bony surfaces and containing synovial fluid within a cavity. These joints have a rich nerve supply, including contributions from the afferent medial branches of the dorsal (posterior) rami. [18] The facet joints of the cervical spine are innervated by the medial nerve branches from the same spinal level and the level below the joint (i.e., the C4–C5 facet joint is innervated by C4 and C5 medial nerve branches). The facet joints of the thoracic and lumbar spine are innervated by the medial nerve branches from the same level and the level above the joint (i.e., the L3–L4 facet joint obtains somatic innervation from the medial branches of L2 and L3 spinal nerve roots). [19] Because the facet joints are deep structures and there is a higher ratio of C to A delta fibers, referral patterns of pain may be poorly localized.

21.3.2.4 Sacroiliac Joints (SIJ)

The sacroiliac joints are bilateral, synovial joints located between the sacrum and the ilium. They consist of synovial fluid bound by a ligamentous compartment posteriorly and an articular compartment anteriorly. The borders of the sacroiliac joint are the anterior sacroiliac ligament and posterior sacroiliac ligament. [9] Like the facet joint, the SI joints are highly innervated by free nerve endings. SI joint pain often refers down to the buttocks or posterior thighs but is unlikely to extend below the knee. [20]

21.3.3 Neural Pathways

Spine innervation is complex, with both sensory and sympathetic nervous systems contributing to pain pathways. At the lumbar level of the spinal cord, the spinal nerve roots are formed by dorsal and ventral segments. The dorsal (posterior) segments are somatic sensory nerves and carry sensory information from the periphery. The ventral (anterior) segments are somatic motor nerves and carry motor signals to the periphery. The cell bodies for sensory nerve fibers are located in the dorsal root ganglion (DRG), and the cell bodies for motor nerve fibers are located in the ventral horn of the spinal cord. [10] Laterally, the somatic sensory and somatic motor segments fuse and form the spinal nerve roots which exit through the intervertebral foramen.

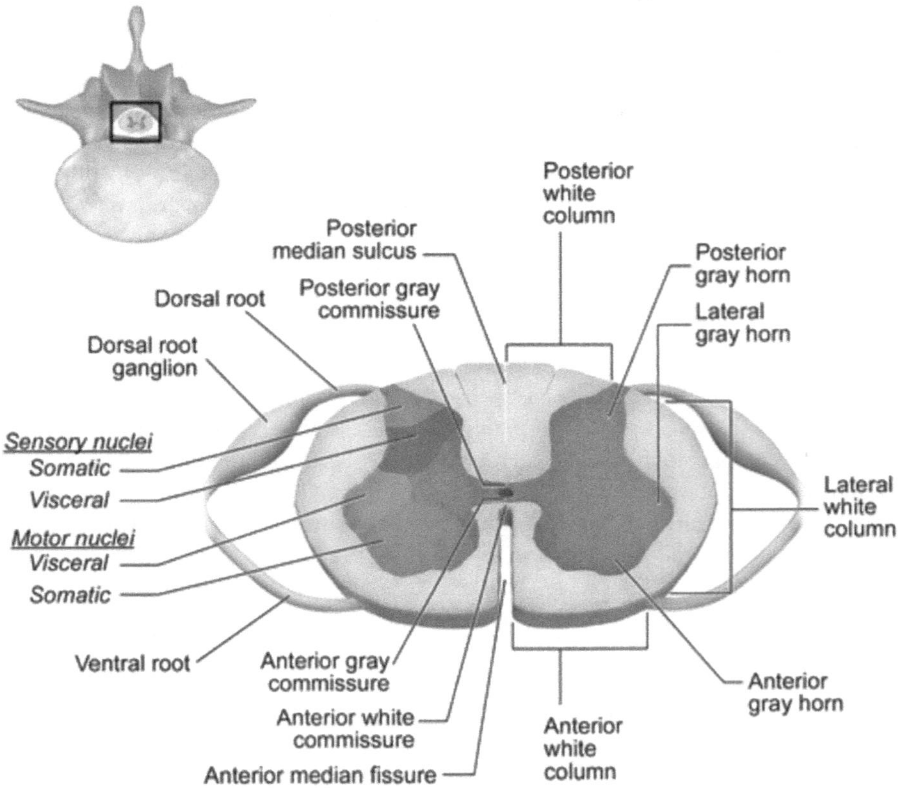

FIGURE 21.3 Lumbar spinal cord anatomy.

Source: [27].

[10] The end of the spinal cord, known as the conus medullaris, is located at the L1 or L2 vertebrae in adults. Below the conus medullaris, the nerve roots of L2–L5, S1–S5, and coccygeal nerve converge to form the cauda equina. The cauda equina, a bundle-like structure that extends caudally, exits the subarachnoid space through the lumbar cistern, typically located at the S1 vertebral level.

21.4 ANIMAL MODELS

Many animal models have been used to study the pathophysiologic events leading to CLBP. The induction of specific spinal pathologies in animal models is a beneficial tool in the study of pathology in humans. Neurogenic and inflammatory pain has been extensively studied in the rat model and has contributed to the breadth of information on the pathology of CLBP and current therapies. Up until the late 1990s, sciatica, a condition characterized as radiating pain from the thigh down the leg, was thought to be caused solely from vertebral disc herniation on surrounding L4 and L5 nerve roots. However, rat models were used to show that the pathophysiology of sciatic pain was more complex than previously thought. Several studies used porcine and rat models to demonstrate that the nucleus pulposus contains cytokines involved with neuroinflammatory changes when exposed to the epidural space and induces edema and reduced blood flow to adjacent nerve roots. [21, 22] What was once thought to be purely a mechanical source of pain was found to also be biochemical in nature. Further studies showed that in rat models, nerve root compression and disc herniation together produce pain behavior by altering cutaneous mechanosensitivity and thermosensitivity. [23] These studies also provided evidence for therapies such as corticosteroids, NSAIDs, and other anti-inflammatories in the treatment of sciatic pain.

The study of the conversion of acute post-operative to chronic pain has also benefited from animal model studies. Low back pain after lumbar surgery is a condition that persists or reoccurs in 40% of patients who undergo surgery on the lumbosacral spine. [23] Laminectomies, a surgical procedure where the lamina is removed from the vertebrae to relieve pressure on the dura of the spinal cord at particular levels, are performed to alleviate mechanical impingement of the dura and spinal cord. In 2008, Saxler et. al performed laminectomies in rat models and discovered that 6 weeks after surgery, levels of nociceptive CGRP and SP-immunopositive primary afferents were upregulated in the dura mater, and new and rearranged afferent sensory neurons had sprouted when compared to sham surgical rat models. [23] This evidence directly supported the hypothesis of plasticity of peripheral neuron terminals in mammals as a response to stimuli and the wound healing process and is suggestive that increased density of nociceptive afferent neurons is a cause of low back pain observed after lumbar surgery. [23]

21.5 CLASSIFICATIONS OF CHRONIC LOWER BACK PAIN (CLBP)

21.5.1 Myofascial Pain

Myofascial pain syndrome (MPS) is defined as pain originating from musculoskeletal trigger points or fascial planes. [24] It is a chronic pain syndrome that affects a focal or regional part of the body, and the dysfunction is located in, or referable to, the muscles or connective tissue. Trigger points are hypersensitive nodules located within taut bands of skeletal muscle and are often tender upon physical exam. It is characteristic on compression (digital palpation should be performed with an approximate force of 4 kg/cm^2) or can give rise to referred pain, tenderness, and autonomic phenomena. The pathophysiology of MPS is believed to be a result of early recruitment and late de-recruitment of small type I muscle fibers during submaximal levels of exertion. This results in fibers which are continuously activated and overloaded and often seen in cervical or postural muscles involved in low-intensity activities. [25, 26] MPS can present alone or alongside other types of back pain and must be properly identified in order to be treated appropriately. Myofascial pain is commonly associated with facet joint dysfunctions, disc herniation, osteoarthritis, migraine, tension-type headache, fibromyalgia, or visceral disorders.

21.5.2 Musculoskeletal (Facet Joint, Intervertebral Disc, and Sacroiliac Joint) Pain

21.5.2.1 Facet Joint Pain

Facet joint arthropathy is often a result of osteoarthritis of the lumbar spine but can affect the thoracic and cervical spine as well. Lumbar facet arthropathy can be classified as nociceptive pain and presents as lower back pain which occurs lateral to the spine and is commonly bilateral. The most common levels for facet joint arthropathy are L4/L5 and L5/S1. [19] The pain may radiate to the legs but will terminate at the knee and be mild in comparison to the back discomfort. [19] Pain is exacerbated with lumbar extension, prolonged standing, lying prone, and spinal rotation. Additionally, pain is typically worse in the morning and will temporarily improve with activity. Pain can be reproduced on physical exam via forward flexion, ipsilateral side bending, and ipsilateral rotation (lumbar quadrant/Kemp's test). [27]

21.5.2.2 Vertebral Disc Pain

The vertebral bodies may produce pain if they are invaded by metabolic or metastatic disease [9]. The source of pain in the intervertebral discs is typically the outer layer of the annulus fibrosus. *Discogenic pain* is caused by vertebral disc degeneration and is often a diagnosis of exclusion. Patients may present with nonspecific, axial lumbar back pain without radicular pain and may exhibit no spinal deformities on MRI. Intervertebral discs consist of three components: two vertebral end plates, a peripheral annulus fibrosus, and a central nucleus pulposus. One potential pain generator from this area is actually from the vertebral end plates. The basivertebral nerve, an extension of the sinuvertebral nerve, enters the vertebral body posteriorly via the central vascular foramen and at the end plates. There are often fibrovascular changes, or Modic type 1 or 2 changes, seen at the vertebral end plates at these levels on MRI. [28,29]

Disc degeneration, leading to inflammation and nerve irritation, may occur in the annulus fibrosis or the softer nucleus pulposus. The nucleus pulposus is largely composed of water and collagen and has been found to be highly pro-inflammatory. [10] Risk factors for disc degeneration include diabetes, advanced age, and obesity.

21.5.2.3 Sacroiliac Joint Pain

The sacroiliac (SI) joints are innervated by the dorsal primary rami and/or the ventral lumbopelvic rami. [10] Patients with SI joint pain have focal pain lateral and inferior to the lumbar spine, in the buttock, or posterolateral thigh. Pain is exacerbated with prolonged sitting or with the transitional movement from sitting to standing and can be reproduced with supine hip flexion, abduction, and external rotation (FABER test) or prone hip extension with knee extension (Yeoman's test.) [27], as well as with several other physical exam maneuvers.

21.5.3 Neuropathic Pain

Oftentimes, the source of CLBP will be a combination of both nociceptive and neuropathic pain. *Neuropathic pain* refers to pain caused by inherent conditions, such as injury, dysfunction, or disease of the spinal cord or nerve roots themselves. It has been suggested that neuropathic pain is often unrecognized, and thus underdiagnosed and undertreated. [4] Neuropathic pain is most commonly caused by a lesion to sprouting C fibers within damaged intervertebral discs, mechanical compression of a nerve (such as spinal stenosis), or irritation from inflammatory mediators released from a degenerating vertebral disc. [4]

While there is no gold standard test for the diagnosis of neuropathic CLBP, its differentiation from nociceptive pain is important as the treatment options differ. [30] Some of the most common signs and symptoms of neuropathic pain are pain that arises without stimulation, allodynia (an abnormal response to a non-painful stimuli), or hyperalgesia (an exaggerated response to a painful stimulus). [4] Pain is often characterized as "shooting," "stabbing," or feeling like "burning" or "pins and needles." Neuropathic pain is often associated with an area of numbness or decreased sensation in the similar dermatomal distribution.

Although the physical exam for neuropathic pain can be helpful, oftentimes it is nonspecific, varying from patient to patient, or evolving throughout the course of an illness within the same patient. In instances like this, more detailed radiological or neurological testing may be helpful. Electrodiagnostic studies, such as electromyography (EMG) with nerve conduction studies (NCS), or autonomic studies, such as quantitative sensory testing (QST), or in rare cases, intra-epidermal nerve fiber (IENF) biopsies, may be needed for accurate diagnosis.

21.6 PRESENTATION OF CHRONIC LOWER BACK PAIN

When evaluating a patient with chronic lower back pain, the provider should identify relevant aspects in the patient's medical history and perform a thorough physical exam.

CLBP should be differentiated from acute lower back pain, as these two conditions are treated differently. CLBP persists for longer than 12 weeks, or back pain that reoccurs after a period of healing and intermittently affects an individual. [2] Evaluation of pain typically begins by inquiring about any injury the patient may have sustained, any previous injuries, related symptoms, any treatments to date, and the efficacy of these treatments. To obtain information on the psychosocial impact of this CLBP, the provider may inquire about any effect the pain has had on function or impact on aspects of the patient's life. [10] Many providers find "pain drawings," or blank diagrams indicating the location and distribution of the patient's pain, a useful tool to elucidate specific regions of pain. [9] If the patient will be considered for interventional treatment at any point, a psychosocial evaluation is helpful in declaring suitable candidates for implantable devices. Every evaluation must address the presence of any "red flag" signs/symptoms, that is, any aspects that may warrant further diagnostic workup and/or immediate treatment. Red flag signs and symptoms can be found in Table 21.1.

21.6.1 Cauda Equina Syndrome

Cauda equina syndrome (CES) is an acute process that is defined as a dysfunction of the sacral and lumbar nerve roots as a result of compression, trauma, or infection.

TABLE 21.1
Physical Examination of Chronic Lower Back Pain

Position	Test	Area of Interest	Instructions	Normal Exam	Abnormal Exam
Standing	Toe raise	S1	Instruct patient to walk on toes.	No pain or weakness noted.	Foot unable to lift heel off the ground suggests S1 weakness.
	Heel walk	L5	Instruct patient to walk on heels.	No pain or weakness noted.	Foot unable to lift toes off the ground suggests L5 weakness.
	Gillet's test	SI joint	Flex hip and raise one foot off the ground.	Ipsilateral posterior superior iliac spine (PSIS) moves **inferior** relative to sacrum.	Ipsilateral PSIS moves **superiorly** relative to sacrum as patient compensates for pain by tilting pelvis.
Sitting	Hip flexion	L2, L3	Hip is passively and actively flexed.	No pain in ipsilateral L2, L3 distribution.	Pain along L2, L3 distribution.
	Ankle dorsiflexion	L4	Ankle is passively and actively dorsiflexed.	No pain in ipsilateral L4 distribution.	Pain along L4 distribution.
	Toe extension	L4–**L5**	Passive and active extension of the metatarsophalangeal joint.	No pain in ipsilateral L4, L5 distribution.	Pain along L4, L5 distribution.
	Patellar reflex	L3, **L4**	Gentle tap w/reflex hammer distal to meniscus.	Brisk knee=jerk reflex.	Diminished, hyperactive reflex, or clonus.
	Achilles reflex	L5, **S1**, S2	Gentle tap w/reflex hammer superior and posterior to calcaneus.	Brisk plantarflexion in response to stimulation.	Diminished, hyperactive reflex, or clonus.
Supine	Lasegue test	L5–S1	Flex hip and dorsiflex ankle, with ipsilateral knee in extension.	No pain in ipsilateral L5–S1 distribution.	Pain along L5–S1 distribution.

(*Continued*)

TABLE 21.1 (*Continued*)
Physical Examination of Chronic Lower Back Pain

Position	Test	Area of Interest	Instructions	Normal Exam	Abnormal Exam
	Patrick FABER test	SI joint	**F**lex hip, flex knee to 90°; **ab**duct and **e**xternally **r**otate thigh (**FABER**).	No pain in contralateral SI joint or ipsilateral groin.	Pain over the contralateral SI joint indicates SI joint pathology (FABER); ipsilateral groin pain indicates hip pathology (Patrick).
	Gaenslen's test	SI joint	Flex hip to patient's chest while allowing contralateral leg to drop off table. Apply opposing forces to anterior knee of flexed leg, and downward against contralateral leg.	No pain in the contralateral (lower leg) SI joint.	Pain over the contralateral (lower leg) SI joint.
Prone	Yeoman's test	SI joint	Flex knee to 90° and extend ipsilateral hip.	No pain in the ipsilateral SI joint.	Pain over the ipsilateral SI joint.

Source: [9, 27, 35–39].

[31, 32] CES is characterized by the red flag symptoms listed in **Table 21.1** and considered to be a medical emergency requiring immediate MRI and surgical evaluation for decompression of the impacted levels. The most common causes of CES are large lumbar disc herniation/prolapse, epidural hematoma, CNS infections, metastatic neoplasms, and trauma.

21.6.1.1 Red Flag Signs/Symptoms [10]

- History of cancer
- Unexpected weight loss
- Immunosuppression
- Prolonged steroid use
- IV drug use
- Urinary tract infection
- Increased pain at rest
- Fever

- Recent trauma
- Bladder/bowel incontinence
- Urinary retention
- Saddle anesthesia
- Sudden weakness

21.7 PHYSICAL EXAM FINDINGS OF CLBP

A proper physical exam can provide key diagnostic information on the etiology of the CLBP. We suggest a comprehensive stepwise approach discussed in detail in what follows:

21.7.1 Observation and Inspection

Observation of how a patient stands and walks is a simple starting point to an exam. A patient's natural stance can indicate anatomical variations, such as spinal lordosis, kyphosis, scoliosis, pelvic rotation, or leg shortening. Ambulation patterns can provide information about the presence of guarding, motor weakness, or asymmetrical weight-bearing. [9, 33] The provider should also note any pain the patient is experiencing with passive movements of the upper torso, including flexion, extension, lateral flexion, and lateral rotation. Any point tenderness to palpation over the spine should be noted, as this can indicate fracture or infection of the spine. Point tenderness over paraspinal muscles may indicate muscular pain or spasm. [33]

21.7.2 Physical Exam

The key portions of the physical exam to evaluate CLBP take place with the patient in the standing, sitting, supine, and prone positions. Passive movements stress non-contractile tissue, including joints, ligaments, bursa, fascia, nerve roots, and dura. Active movements stress both contractile tissue (muscles and tendons) and non-contractile tissues. See **Table 21.2** for important portions of the physical exam. It can be difficult to diagnose specific pathology based on a physical exam, as findings may suggest multiple areas of concern. However, CLBP is often due to a culmination of multiple causes.

While performing an exam, the provider must be aware of psychogenic manifestations of CLBP, or Waddell's signs. Waddell's signs, found in **Table 21.3**, indicate that a patient's pain is not due solely to structural pathology within the spine or surrounding musculature; three or more positive signs show clinical significance. Incorrectly used by some providers as a test to detect malingering, Waddell's signs should instead emphasize that CLBP must be viewed within a psychosocial context, and positive signs may represent fear and/or anxiety developed from the pain or an injury. These patients often do not respond well to solely physical treatment or surgery and benefit instead from a combination of physical treatment and therapy for psychosocial and behavioral aspects to their illness. [34]

TABLE 21.2
Physical examination of chronic lower back pain [9, 27, 35, 36, 37, 38, 39]

Position	Test	Area of Interest	Instructions	Normal Exam	Abnormal Exam
Standing	Toe Raise	S1	Instruct patient to walk on toes	No pain or weakness noted	Foot unable to lift heel off the ground suggests S1 weakness
	Heel Walk	L5	Instruct patient to walk on heels	No pain or weakness noted	Foot unable to lift toes off the ground suggests L5 weakness
	Gillet's test	SI joint	Flex hip and raise one foot off the ground	Ipsilateral posterior superior iliac spine (PSIS) moves **inferior** relative to sacrum	Ipsilateral PSIS moves **superiorly** relative to sacrum as patient compensates for pain by tilting pelvis
Sitting	Hip flexion	L2, L3	Hip is passively and actively flexed	No pain in ipsilateral L2, L3 distribution	Pain along L2, L3 distribution
	Ankle dorsiflexion	L4	Ankle is passively and actively dorsiflexed	No pain in ipsilateral L4 distribution	Pain along L4 distribution
	Toe extension	L4-**L5**	Passive and active extension of the metatarsophalangeal joint	No pain in ipsilateral L4, L5 distribution	Pain along L4, L5 distribution
	Patellar Reflex	L3, **L4**	Gentle tap w/ reflex hammer distal to meniscus	Brisk knee jerk reflex	Diminished, hyperactive reflex, or clonus
	Achilles Reflex	L5, **S1**, S2	Gentle tap w/ reflex hammer superior and posterior to calcaneus	Brisk plantarflexion in response to stimulation	Diminished, hyperactive reflex, or clonus
Supine	Laseague test	L5-S1	Flex hip and dorsiflex ankle, with ipsilateral knee in extension	No pain in ipsilateral L5-S1 distribution	Pain along L5-S1 distribution
	Patrick-FABER Test	SI joint	**F**lex hip, flex knee to 90*, **ab**duct and **e**xternally **r**otate thigh **FABER**	No pain in contralateral SI joint or ipsilateral groin	Pain over the contralateral SI joint indicates SI joint pathology (FABER) ipsilateral groin pain indicates hip pathology (Patrick)
	Gaenslen's Test	SI joint	Flex hip to patient's chest while allowing contralateral leg to drop off table. Apply opposing forces to anterior knee of flexed leg, and downward against contralateral leg	No pain in the contralateral (lower leg) SI joint	Pain over the contralateral (lower leg) SI joint
Prone	Yeoman's Test	SI joint	Flex knee to 90* and extends ipsilateral hip	No pain in the ipsilateral SI joint	Pain over the ipsilateral SI joint

TABLE 21.3
Waddell's Signs

Observation	Description
Superficial tenderness	Pain with gentle skin touch or rolling
Non-anatomical tenderness	Deep pain not localized to one structure or crossing over non-anatomical boundaries
Axial loading	Lumbar pain with downward pressure on top of patient's head
Acetabular rotation	Lumbar pain during the first 30 of passive/active external rotation of shoulder and pelvis in same plane in the standing position
Distracted straight leg raise discrepancy	Pain during supine straight leg test, but not when distracted and provider extends patient's knee in the seated position
Regional sensory disturbance	Non-physiologic regional disturbances of sensation or distribution of pain
Regional weakness	Weakness, cogwheeling, or a "giving way" of numerous muscle groups that are not explained by anatomical basis
Overreaction	Excessive verbalization, facial grimacing, or other pain behaviors out of proportion to test stimulus

Source: [9, 34].

21.8 DIAGNOSTIC TESTS

Clinical evaluation and physical exam can be supplemented by diagnostic tests. Generally, diagnostic imaging is recommended after a patient has had 6 weeks or more of medical management and physical therapy and has not seen improvement in their CLBP. [32, 40] Additionally, diagnostic imaging is considered when the provider is concerned for acute processes, such as cauda equina syndrome, fractures, or underlying conditions, like infection or malignancy. [32, 40]

While access to diagnostic tests is abundant, the provider must use discretion and clinical judgment on when diagnostic imaging is warranted in the diagnosis of CLBP. Unnecessary imaging can lead to additional unnecessary imaging, tests, referrals, or procedures. [40] The World Health Organization (WHO) endorses ordering diagnostic tests only for patients over the age of 50, or those with systemic disease or history of trauma. They suggest that adults who do not meet these criteria do not see benefit after diagnostic testing. [30] If the CLBP is nonspecific, it is recommended that imaging be delayed for 6 weeks while conservative treatments are utilized. [40] Diagnostic tests typically include conventional radiography (x-ray), computed tomography (CT), magnetic resonance imaging (MRI), electromyography, and quantitative sensory testing (QST).

21.8.1 Conventional Radiography, CT, and MRI

Conventional radiography, or plain film x-ray, is often the initial imaging study of choice as it quickly evaluates the overall integrity of the spine and pelvis; however, it does not provide any information about soft tissues. CT has the ability to evaluate bony structures as well as surrounding structures, however, is limited in its ability to diagnose extradural soft tissue disease, such as disc disease, though this can be improved with myelogram. CT does involve radiation exposure. MRI is used most frequently to establish a diagnosis for CLBP as it provides greater tissue contrast, shows superior soft tissue delineation, and involves no radiation exposure. [40]

21.8.2 Electromyography (EMG)

For patients who may have difficult-to-diagnose radicular pain, an MRI is not the optimal test for distinguishing between peripheral neuropathy, plexopathy, or radiculopathy. For this type of scenario, electromyography (EMG) may be utilized as an extension to physical exam. EMG is composed of a needle EMG and a nerve conduction study (NCS) that can assist in differentiating peripheral neuropathy from neuropathic CLBP. [4] While EMG has been shown to have good specificity (88%) for detecting radicular disease, it has a low sensitivity (46%). [41] EMG is primarily performed on upper and lower extremities and can provide information on sensory responses (delays or abnormal patterns of sensation) and motor amplitudes of specific nerves. Furthermore, EMG can provide evidence of denervation of certain muscle groups, which would indicate a proximal process and not a single peripheral neuropathy. [41]

21.8.3 Quantitative Sensory Testing (QST)

Quantitative sensory testing, or QST, is a form of testing where noxious nociceptive stimuli is applied to areas of the body distal to a centralized injury. QST can be helpful in revealing the pathological signs of neuropathic pain, particular small-fiber. [4] It is believed that in the setting of central irritation, such as spinal nerve impingement causing radicular pain, prolonged afferent nociceptive input causes a hypersensitivity of peripheral sensory neurons. [42, 43] As such, patients with CLBP due to a centralized source would have increased pain on QST. A variety of painful stimuli are used, including pressure stimulation, heat/cold stimulation, and electrical stimulation. Of the numerous stimuli, pressure and electrical stimuli have been determined to have high discriminative ability to distinguish CLBP and asymptomatic controls and may be the most reliable QSTs. [42]

21.9 MEDICAL AND INTERVENTIONAL MANAGEMENT OF CLBP

While acute lower back pain can be treated by rest and passive sensory modulating techniques, such as heat or massage, these techniques are not as effective at treating CLBP. For chronic pain, an active multimodal approach is indicated—including physical therapy, counseling, medical treatments, and interventional diagnostics and treatments.

21.9.1 Counseling and Physical Therapy

Chronic pain makes an impact on many aspects of a patient's life. Patients may experience loss of employment and wages, a decrease in independence, and a strain on their personal relationships. As a result of their CLBP, patients often experience low self-esteem, depression, and anxiety—all of which can exacerbate their pain and add to pain catastrophizing. An important step in treating a patient's CLBP is psychological counseling. Through counseling, patients can develop coping skills, practice relaxation techniques, or learn mindfulness meditation. [9]

Physical therapy and active movement are indicated in the treatment of CLBP. Aerobic exercises, resistance or light-weight training, stretching, and yoga are all validated components of treatment and are often recommended before any other treatment options are discussed.

21.9.2 Medical Treatments

21.9.2.1 NSAIDS, COX-2 Inhibitors, and Acetaminophen

Nonsteroidal anti-inflammatories (NSAIDS) are medications with anti-inflammatory, antipyretic, and analgesic effects. Normally, arachidonic acid is broken down by cyclooxygenase enzymes (COX-1 and COX-2) to produce pro-inflammatory prostaglandins. These prostaglandins cause direct sensitization of the terminals of C fibers, the main peripheral pain receptors in the body. Through inhibition of cyclooxygenase enzymes, NSAIDS prevent the production of prostaglandins and reduce this sensitization of C fibers. NSAIDS are mainly effective at providing pain relief from inflammatory components of pain. [9] NSAIDS are available in oral (ibuprofen), intravenous/intramuscular (ketorolac), and topical forms (diclofenac gel.)

Unfortunately, due to systemic side effects, NSAIDS are not recommended for long-term use and are mainly indicated for acute lower back pain or quelling exacerbations of CLBP. These side effects include GI irritation, an increased risk of bleeding, and nephrotoxicity, though these concerns are minimized with topical medications.

Celecoxib is an example of a specific COX-2 inhibitor. COX-2 inhibitors have a similar mechanism of action to NSAIDS; however, they only inhibit half of the cyclooxygenase pathway. As the COX-2 enzyme is only constitutively expressed in the brain and renal tissue, COX-2 inhibitors have less GI side effects yet still may cause renal dysfunction if used on a chronic basis. Additionally, COX-2 inhibitors have been found to increase the risk of thromboembolic events in patients with pre-existing cardiovascular disease and therefore should be avoided in these patients. Celecoxib is available in oral form only.

Acetaminophen is one of the most widely prescribed non-opioid analgesics for CLBP and considered to be a main first-line medical treatment in many types of chronic pain. [44] While the mechanism of action of acetaminophen is unknown, it has been theorized to inhibit nitric oxide synthase at the level of the spinal cord and reduce the activation of post-synaptic spinothalamic tract neurons as well as inhibit cyclooxygenase in the brain. [9] While acetaminophen does not have the GI, hematological, or nephrotoxic side effects as NSAIDS, it causes hepatotoxicity when consumed in large doses. Acetaminophen is available in oral and intravenous forms.

21.9.2.2 Anticonvulsants

While many anticonvulsants exist, lamotrigine, carbamazepine, and gabapentinoids are the most common anticonvulsants used to treat CLBP. All anticonvulsants, aside from the gabapentinoids, are limited in their chronic use due to hepatotoxicity and the frequent need for liver enzyme testing; thus, they will not be discussed further. Gabapentinoids are a class of medications that have been shown to be efficacious in the treatment of neuropathic CLBP, post-laminectomy pain, and post-amputation pain. [9] The two main gabapentinoids are gabapentin and pregabalin, both of which act by inhibiting the alpha-2 delta-2 ($\alpha 2\delta 2$) subunit of pre-synaptic voltage-gated calcium channels. [45] It is believed that through this inhibition, pathologically enhanced neurotransmission in primary afferent neurons is decreased. [45] While sometimes used acutely in the perioperative setting, gabapentinoids are typically initiated and titrated slowly over several weeks in order to avoid intolerance due to side effects. The most common side effects of these medications include sedation, dizziness, peripheral edema, dry mouth, fatigue, nausea, and weight gain. [45] While there is mixed evidence on the overall effectiveness of gabapentinoids on CLBP, until larger trials provide more evidence against their use, they remain a standard in a multimodal medicinal approach to patients with neuropathic pain.

21.9.2.3 Anti-Neuroleptics and Antiarrhythmics

21.9.2.3.1 Anti-Neuroleptics

Anti-neuroleptics, sometimes referred to as antidepressants, are used as adjuvants in the treatments of many types of chronic pain. Evidence on the effectiveness of anti-neuroleptics in the treatment of CLBP is controversial. Some studies indicate that these medications provide benefit to patients with CLBP associated with radiculopathy, while others claim they are not more helpful than placebo in treating pain and related symptoms. [45] Despite this lack of consensus, these medications are commonly used in the treatment of neuropathic CLBP. [9] Their efficacy is likely due to a combination of pain relief, sleep improvement, and antidepressant effects. While serotonin-specific reuptake inhibitors (SSRI's) may be used in the treatment of CLBP, tricyclic antidepressants (TCAs), such as amitriptyline and nortriptyline, are more commonly used. The doses used to treat CLBP are typically much lower than doses used for antidepressant effects.

The anti-neuroleptics assist in the activation of descending inhibitory neurons. In the brain stem, serotonergic and noradrenergic neurons inhibit C fiber input into the spinal cord. By inhibiting the reuptake of serotonin and norepinephrine, anti-neuroleptics potentiate the action of these neurotransmitters to further inhibit painful sensory information. Furthermore, anti-neuroleptics are NMDA and alpha-1 receptor antagonists, both of which provide additional neuropathic pain relief.

Anti-neuroleptics should be prescribed with caution due to their extensive side effect profile. TCAs, the most common anti-neuroleptic used in the treatment of CLBP, cause anticholinergic, antihistaminic, and antidopaminergic side effects.

Anticholinergic effects can range from dry mouth and constipation to urinary retention or sedation. Antihistaminic side effects also cause sedation. Due to their sedative nature, TCAs are often prescribed to be taken once nightly before bed and are not typically prescribed for daytime use.

Providers should be monitoring patients taking TCAs for signs of antidopaminergic effects. Antidopaminergic side effects, also known as extrapyramidal symptoms (EPS), include dystonia, dyskinesia, and akathisia. [46] As anti-neuroleptics are also alpha-1 inhibitors, patients should also be monitored for signs of orthostatic hypotension.

21.9.2.3.2 Antiarrhythmics

Antiarrhythmic medications are not commonly used in the treatment of CLBP in any form outside of topical uses. While antiarrhythmics have been shown to be effective at treating intractable radicular symptoms and allodynic components of CLBP, most of the data is mixed and comes from small trials. [47] Mexiletine (oral) and lidocaine (intravenous, topical) are both local anesthetics that block sodium channels and suppress activity of peripheral nerves. They are thought to provide analgesia by reducing firing of damaged nerves.

Nausea is the most common side effect of these antiarrhythmics. Tinnitus and perioral numbness/tingling are concerning symptoms that may also occur if dosing is titrated too quickly or if local anesthetics are given in large quantities. These symptoms are early indications of local anesthetic toxicity (LAST), and the medication dosage must be decreased, or discontinued, right away. LAST, the most devastating side effect of local anesthetics occurs with very high serum levels of local anesthetics and can result in seizures, coma, and cardiopulmonary collapse. [48]

21.9.2.4 Opioids

Once a cornerstone of chronic pain treatment, opioids became overprescribed, leading to an epidemic of dependence, addiction, and opioid-related deaths in the United States. In 2017, opioid abuse claimed more lives each year than motor vehicle accidents and homicides combined. [49] Opioids are no longer indicated for the treatment of CLBP; however, minimal doses are sometimes considered when all other conservative measures have failed. The American Pain Society (APS) and the American Academy of Pain Medicine (AAPM) created the first evidence-based guidelines for chronic opioid therapy for adults with chronic non-cancer pain in 2009, and since then, the Center for Disease Control (CDC) has issued an updated guideline in 2016 for physicians who may be prescribing opioids. [50] These principles should be applied to the treatment of CLBP. The main points from these recommendations are:

- Optimize all non-opioid therapies before prescribing the shortest-acting opioids at their lowest doses.
- Check prescription drug monitoring programs (PDMPs) and a urine drug screen at the time of initial prescription of an opioid and at each subsequent office visit/refill.
- Attempt to taper opioid usage at each return visit and offer prescriptions for self-administered naloxone to patients taking high levels of opioids.

Numerous studies have found little evidence to support the benefits of long-term opioid therapy for chronic pain, with some suggesting that chronic opioid use can lead to a worsened pain state and potential abuse. [50–52] For these reasons, the judicious prescription and management of opioids is essential in the treatment of CLBP.

The two main mechanisms of action of opioids occur in the brain and spinal cord. In the brain, opioid receptors are located in the periaqueductal gray matter. When these receptors are activated, descending fibers release norepinephrine and serotonin, which modulate the input of C fibers. At the level of the spinal cord, opioid receptors are located in the substantia gelatinosa in the dorsal horn (lamina II.) Activation of these opioid receptors inhibits the pre-synaptic release of substance P and slows neuronal firing by increasing the potassium conductance in the post-synaptic terminals. [9]

The side effects of opioids are well-known and dose-dependent. Common side effects include nausea, vomiting, constipation, pruritus, and somnolence. Respiratory depression is more likely to occur in opioid-naive patients or with very high doses. Titration of opioids should occur very slowly over the course of several weeks. If prescribing opioids, it is also recommended that the provider prescribe naloxone, an opioid antagonist which competes with opioids for mu receptors, resulting in opioid reversal.

21.9.3 Interventional Treatments

21.9.3.1 Trigger Point Injections

Trigger point injections can be performed for the treatment of myofascial pain or lumbosacral radiculopathy. [53] Injections of steroids, local anesthetics, or botulinum toxin can provide effective short-term and long-term pain relief. In addition, dry needling (no medication injection) has been shown to be as effective at pain relief as lidocaine, but with increased post-injection pain. Analgesia is believed to be due to mechanical disruption by the needle and the termination of the dysfunctional activity of involved motor end plates. [54]

21.9.3.2 Sacroiliac Joint Injections

Intra-articular injection of the sacroiliac (SI) joint is a targeted approach to relieve SI joint pain which has varied long-term success in the current literature. [55] Using fluoroscopic guidance, this procedure can be utilized for short-term pain relief or as a diagnostic procedure. A rare major complication associated with SI joint injections is incidental extra-articular injection of local anesthetic, which may contact the nearby sciatic nerve and result in transient, ipsilateral leg weakness or numbness which resolves on its own after the metabolism of local anesthetic.

21.9.3.3 Epidural Steroid Injections

Epidural steroid injections (ESI) are typically performed in the setting of CLBP with a radicular component or discogenic pain. These injections can be performed via an interlaminar, caudal, or transforaminal approach. The transforaminal technique allows for a more specific and targeted delivery of medication near the exiting nerve root. It is typically utilized when one or two particular nerve roots can be identified, via physical exam and/or imaging, as the cause of the patient's pain. An interlaminar technique can be utilized to target multiple nerve roots, or if a clear dermatomal pattern of pain is not identifiable. [19] While the interlaminar technique is historically the more common technique utilized, disadvantages include a decreased distribution of ventral spread of the epidural steroid and a higher risk for dural puncture than the transforaminal approach. A caudal epidural can be performed with the needle placed through the sacral hiatus and more commonly done in post-laminectomy cases. All approaches should be performed under fluoroscopic guidance and are well tolerated by most patients. Intrathecal injections or intravascular injections occur rarely with the use of fluoroscopic guidance. If intravascular injections do occur, they are often immediately identified under live fluoroscopy.

21.9.3.4 Medial Branch Blocks/Radiofrequency Ablations

The medial branch nerves of the spinal dorsal rami innervate the facet joints of the vertebral column. Facet joints and adjacent tissues contain many nociceptive receptors, which cause pain when irritated by mechanical stimulation or inflammation. [56] Medial branch blocks (MBB) are performed for centralized back pain, often due to facet joint arthropathy. MBBs are often used as a diagnostic blockade, performed with fluoroscopic guidance in an attempt to determine an individual's candidacy for radiofrequency ablation therapy (RFA). A positive diagnostic block is defined as greater than or equal to 50% pain reduction occurring using a local anesthetic (often 2% lidocaine) lasting for the duration of the anesthetic. [19] If a positive diagnostic block is achieved, the patient may be a candidate for RFA of the targeted medial branches.

RFA is a form of targeted thermal neural ablation of the medial branch nerve. Using fluoroscopy guidance, high-frequency electrical current is used in a pulsed or non-pulsed fashion to target the destruction of nerve fibers. RFA of the medial branch nerve can provide sustained pain relief in a patient who achieved a positive diagnostic MBB. After short-acting local anesthetic is administered at the target medial branch nerve, an electrode catheter is heated to 60–85°C for 60–90 seconds per location. [19] A rare, yet serious, complication that may occur with RFA is damage to the motor nerve component due to an incorrectly positioned electrode catheter. A catheter positioned too far anteriorly may inadvertently cause damage to the ventral ramus of the adjacent spinal nerve. A sign that the catheter is positioned too far anteriorly is the patient complaining of burning pain radiating down their ipsilateral leg immediately after ablation has begun. [19, 57] Patients often experience an increase in pain for the first few days following an RFA; however, after this period subsides, pain relief can last 8–12 months.

21.9.3.5 Intrathecal Drug Therapy

Intrathecal (IT) drug therapy consists of a permanent intrathecal catheter and an implanted subcutaneous pump that continuously infuses medications into the intrathecal space. There are three main benefits of intrathecal therapy when compared to traditional medication administration:

- IT therapy allows for the administration of pain medications in a selective fashion. By delivering smaller quantities of these medications in close proximity to spinal pain receptors in the substantia gelatinosa, many of the systemic side effects of the medications are experienced less frequently. [58]
- IT therapy allows for the continuous infusion of multiple types of medications, allowing these agents to target multiple pain receptors. Currently, only bupivacaine, morphine, ziconotide (which is only available in an intrathecal form), and baclofen are FDA-approved for intrathecal administration; however, several other medications are used, and their use is supported in the literature.
- IT pumps can continue to infuse in an outpatient setting, which allows patients to live a routine life, albeit with close medical follow-up.

IT pumps are implanted in the operating room, typically under monitored anesthetic care (MAC). Before an IT pump can be implanted, the patient proceeds through a trial injection of intrathecal medication or a trial catheter placement to estimate doses of medications required for pain relief, confirm position of the catheter, and assess overall efficacy of treatment. In the past, a trial for these devices involved placing the intrathecal catheter under fluoroscopic guidance in an inpatient setting and infusing medications for 7–14 days. More commonly at this time, patients can undergo a single intrathecal injection of the desired medication rather than trial an infusion for an extended period of time. If the patient achieves a 50% decrease in his/her pain level with functional improvement, then they are considered candidates for the placement of a permanent device. [58]

21.9.3.6 Neuromodulation: SCS, DRG, PNS

Neuromodulation is a category of interventional treatments aimed at targeting neuropathic pain via electrical stimulation.

21.9.3.6.1 Transcutaneous Electrical Nerve Stimulation (TENS)

Transcutaneous electrical nerve stimulation (TENS) is a low-cost, low-risk therapy that patients may utilize in their homes. TENS uses external electrical stimulation of the skin, which activates large-diameter sensory fibers at either a low-frequency/high-intensity "acupuncture-like" setting to induce muscular contraction or a high-frequency/low-intensity setting that creates a mild "tingling" sensation. [9, 59] It is proposed that TENS units utilize the gate control theory of pain, which states that activating large A-beta afferent nerve fibers will inhibit transmission in afferent A delta and C fibers in the dorsal horn of the spinal cord. [60]

21.9.3.6.2 Spinal Cord Stimulation (SCS)

Spinal cord stimulation (SCS) is an interventional therapy that is typically utilized for refractory chronic pain. The goal is to reduce pain by 50% or more and to improve the patient's quality of life. While the initial placement of a device is costly, SCS has also been found to reduce health-care resources in the treatment of the patient's pain over time. [60, 61] SCS has been approved for the treatment of complex regional pain syndromes (CRPS), failed back surgery syndrome, limb ischemia, and refractory angina pectoris. SCS has also been shown to be beneficial in the treatment of radicular pain following spine surgery, or for peripheral neuropathic pain. [59–61] SCS involves the implantation of leads into the epidural space, the insertion of an implantable pulse generator (IPG), and the application of electrical stimulation to these leads. This stimulation causes paresthesia overlapping the region of pain (tonic stimulation) or, in other modalities, causes pain relief without paresthesia (high-frequency—HF). Adequate stimulation depends on precise lead placement in order to isolate the dorsal column, lateral funicular tract, and dorsal root fibers. Paresthesia in these regions results in the inhibition of pain transmission via ascending nociceptive fibers as well as descending antinociceptive fibers without causing motor effects [60] and, in HF cases, more central modulation.

Prior to the placement of an SCS, several criteria must be met. The patient selection process for SCS should include [59, 60]:

- Clear diagnosis of neuropathic pain.
- Patient has pain that is resistant to conservative medicinal and interventional therapy.
- Patient has no significant psychological history or evidence of secondary gain.
- Successful trial and adequate response to trial stimulation.
- No surgical contraindications to implantation (coagulopathy, active infection, etc.).

21.9.3.6.3 Dorsal Root Ganglion (DRG) Stimulation

Dorsal root ganglion (DRG) stimulation is a newer form of neuromodulation used in the treatment for neuropathic pain. Whereas traditional SCS provides analgesia in patients with neuropathic pain conditions, studies indicate that DRG stimulation may provide improved analgesia amongst patients with mixed pain syndromes. [62, 63] DRG stimulation differs from traditional SCS by stimulating only the DRG, the region which holds the primary sensory neurons transmitting afferent nociception. Due to innervation patterns of afferent fibers, it has been hypothesized that the T12 area is the optimal target for lead placement for chronic axial low back pain. [62] Alternative levels are used for different targets, such as knee (L3, L4) or ankle (L4, L5). Like traditional SCS, DRG stimulation has been associated with increased pain relief, improvement of disability, and improved quality of life in patients with CLBP when compared to conservative therapies. [62] While most positive outcomes have been demonstrated in small sample sizes with relatively short follow-up durations, larger studies are likely to come in this developing field.

21.9.3.6.4 Peripheral Nerve Stimulation (PNS)

The concept of neuromodulation can be performed at the peripheral level as well, through peripheral nerve stimulation (PNS.) Via ultrasound (preferred), or fluoroscopy guidance, a stimulation lead can be implanted near the targeted peripheral nerve. By applying an electrical stimulus to a single nerve, or group of small nerve fibers, pain relief has been provided to patients with neuropathic CLBP. [59] Some evidence suggests that blockade of the nerve in question using local anesthetics can be predictive of benefit from PNS, though this is not always the case. Some commonly targeted peripheral nerves in the lower body include the ilioinguinal nerve, iliohypogastric nerve, genitofemoral nerve, lateral femoral cutaneous nerve, saphenous nerve, and sciatic nerve. While this is a novel therapy, results on long-term (2-year) efficacy are promising—with small trials showing significant reduction in pain and level of disability in patients with refractory low back and lower extremity pain. [64] There are temporary devices that can be left in place for up to 60 days, and others that are permanently implanted and have an external receiver.

21.9.3.7 Minimally Invasive Interventions

Minimally invasive lumbar interventions have increased in popularity since the 1970s as treatment options for patients with CLBP unresponsive to conservative care. While more invasive than SCS lead placement or intrathecal pump placement, these interventions are less invasive than traditional spine surgery and can be performed under monitored anesthetic care (MAC). Furthermore, by fixing anatomical abnormalities that may be the cause of a patient's pain, these procedures theoretically spare ongoing pain management and health-care resources. These interventions carry perioperative risks, including wound infections, implant infections, and bleeding, although given their minimally invasive nature, these risks are assumed to be less than that of traditional surgery.

21.9.3.7.1 Interspinous Spacers

Interspinous spacers are designed to help alleviate symptoms related to compression of spinal nerve roots, central stenosis, or other conditions causing neurogenic claudication. Current studies suggest that interspinous spacers may be efficacious in the treatment of spinal stenosis and degenerative disease of the lumbar spine unresponsive to conservative care. [65, 66] The Superion spacer is a titanium implant that is inserted between the spinous processes percutaneously and deployed to provide support and rigidity between the processes (**Figure 21.4**). [66] Once in place, the spacer will limit extension of the spine at the targeted level but preserve all other aspects of mobility. While interspinous spacers are a relatively novel treatment option, results suggest that patients experience an improvement of symptoms of CLBP due to spinal stenosis. [66]

21.9.3.7.2 Minimally Invasive Sacroiliac Joint Fusion (SIJF)

Sacroiliac joint fusion is a minimally invasive procedure for chronic sacroiliac joint dysfunction unresponsive to conservative treatment. [67] Most published evidence on the efficacy of SIJF focuses on the use of either triangular or cylindrical implants that bridge the ilium to the sacrum. [68] SIJF offers a therapy that has been shown to be superior to non-surgical management in refractory cases [69] though decreases mobility of the segment. Other devices with posterior placement can also be performed to distract and stabilize the joint.

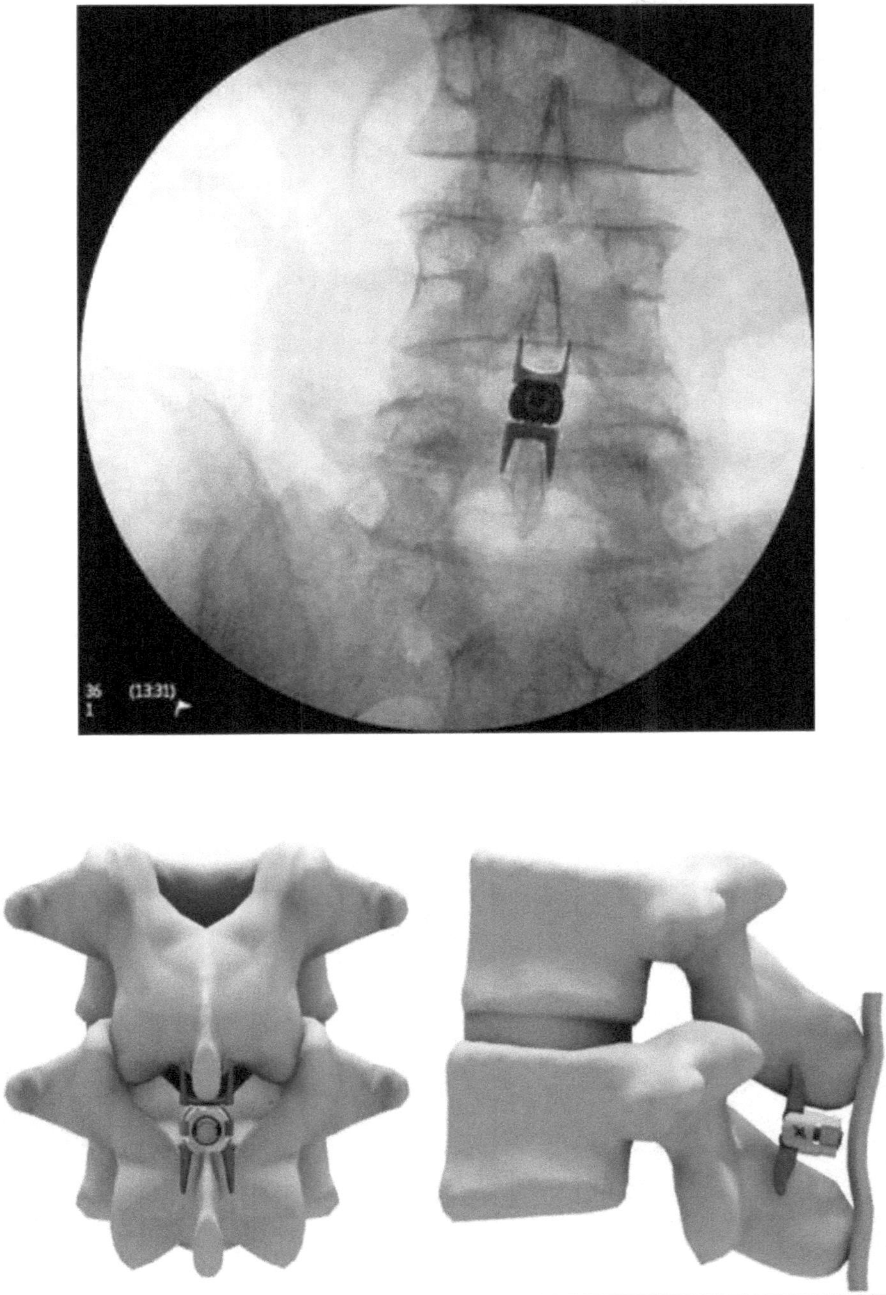

FIGURE 21.4 Superion spacer: (a) A/P view. (b) Lateral view. (c) Radiographic A/P view of properly placed spacer.

Source: [66].

21.9.3.7.3 Percutaneous Image-Guided Lumbar Decompression (PILD)

Percutaneous image-guided lumbar decompression (PILD) is a therapy used in the treatment of refractory pain caused by symptomatic central lumbar canal stenosis. PILD involves a percutaneous laminotomy and removal of small areas of ligamentum flavum in order to enlarge the diameter of a stenosed spinal segment to help relieve nerve compression in the targeted area. [70] Although PILD does carry a risk of dural puncture and epidural bleeding/hematoma, these events are reported to be very rare. [70] PILD has also been shown to be more cost-effective and have a decreased healing time than traditional laminectomy. [70]

21.9.3.7.4 Kyphoplasty/Vertebroplasty

Balloon kyphoplasty is a minimally invasive technique that has been used to stabilize and reduce pain from vertebral body compression fractures. [71] Through a percutaneous

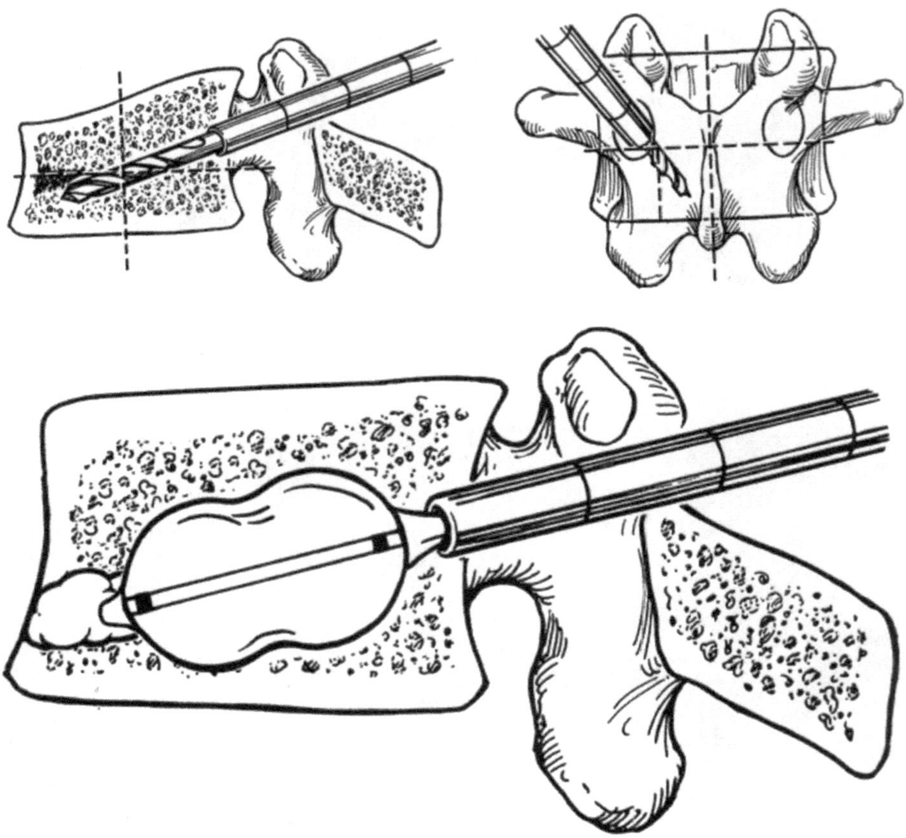

FIGURE 21.5 Balloon kyphoplasty. Drill inserted through cannula to create larger channel in bone: (a) Lateral view. (b) A/P view. (c) A balloon is deployed through the cannula and creates a cavity while compacting bone and elevating fractured areas. (d) Balloon has been removed, and cement is injected into the void.

Source: [71].

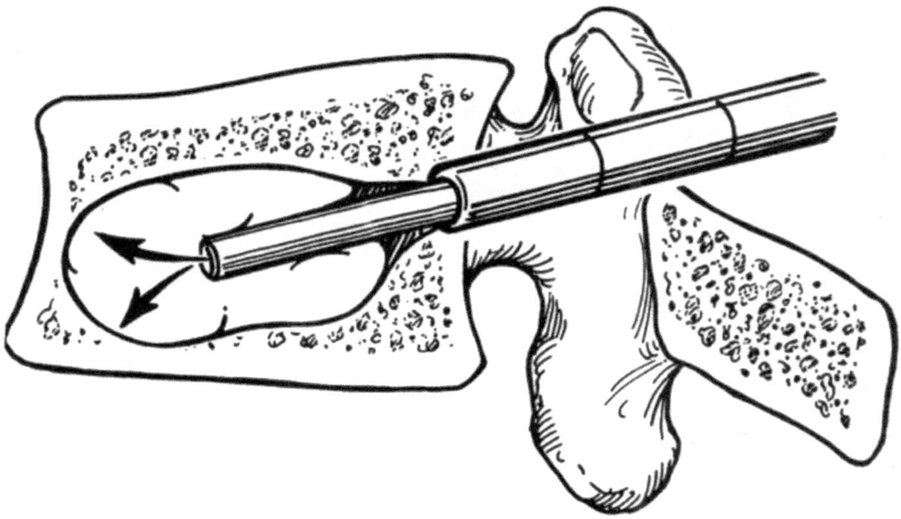

FIGURE 21.5 (Continued)

cannula, a channel is drilled through the pedicle into the fractured vertebra, and a balloon is inserted into the body. Once in place, the balloon is inflated, creating a cavity in the middle of the vertebral body and compressing bone particle. This compression can elevate the end plates of the vertebral body without expanding laterally or posteriorly, thus correcting kyphotic deformity. [71] Once the balloon is deflated and removed, a vertebroplasty can be performed to give the body increased strength and stability. [71]

21.9.3.8 Intraosseous Basivertebral Nerve Ablation

Intraosseous basivertebral nerve (BVN) ablation is a minimally invasive technique aimed at decreasing CLBP due to vertebral end plate dysfunction. Vertebral end plates, through trauma, degeneration, or malignancy, can release inflammatory mediators which modulate nociception via the BVN. Through a transpedicular approach, a thermal probe is inserted into the targeted vertebral body, and a radiofrequency ablation of the BVN is performed. Multiple lumbar vertebral levels can be percutaneously targeted, and it has been approved for targeting levels L3–S1 at the time of publication. [72] Although BVN ablation is a novel technique, there is evidence that it is superior to conservative non-surgical management in refractory CLBP due to vertebral body pathology. [73]

21.9.3.9 When Surgery Is Indicated

Urgent/emergent surgery is indicated when a patient has identifiable pathology on diagnostic imaging that is causing red flag symptoms. Elective surgery is typically reserved for patients with identifiable pathology demonstrated on diagnostic imaging and who were refractory to all other conservative treatments, who are having progressing neurologic decline, or who have an uncertain diagnosis.

21.10 CONCLUSION

This chapter provides a comprehensive summary of approaching chronic lower back pain, a common medical condition with a lifetime prevalence of 70% in industrialized countries. It outlines how to use a history and physical exam to determine a differential diagnosis for back pain, consisting of whether the pain is nociceptive, neuropathic, inflammatory, or myofascial in nature. It also outlines treatment algorithms based on subjective and objective findings in the patient. We provide a comprehensive summary of both pharmacological as well as interventional techniques for treatment of persistent back pain, giving the reader a guide as to how physicians approach this complex pain condition.

REFERENCES

1. Kaplan W, Wirtz VJ, Mantel-Teeuwisse A, *et al.* Priority medicines for Europe and the World: 2013 update. World Health Organization; Geneva, Switzerland; 2013.
2. Duthey B. Update on 2004 Background Paper, BP 6.24 Low back pain. Geneva: World Health Organization; 2013.
3. Shmagel A, Foley R, Ibrahim H. Epidemiology of chronic low back pain in US Adults: data from the 2009–2010 national health and nutrition examination survey. *Arthritis Care Res (Hoboken).* 2016;68(11):1688–1694. doi:10.1002/acr.22890
4. Baron R, Binder A, Attal N, Casale R, Dickenson AH, Treede RD. Neuropathic low back pain in clinical practice. *Eur J Pain.* 2016;20(6):861–873. doi:10.1002/ejp.838
5. Kim LH, Vail D, Azad TD, *et al.* Expenditures and health care utilization among adults with newly diagnosed low back and lower extremity pain. *JAMA Netw Open.* 2019;2(5):e193676. Published 2019 May 3. doi:10.1001/jamanetworkopen.2019.3676
6. Meucci RD, Fassa AG, Faria NM. Prevalence of chronic low back pain: systematic review. *Rev Saude Publica.* 2015;49:1. doi:10.1590/S0034–8910.2015049005874
7. Gray H. *Anatomy, Descriptive and Surgical: Gray's Anatomy*, Philadelphia: Courage Books/Running Press; 1974.
8. Netter FH. https://www.netterimages.com/lumbar-vertebrae-and-intervertebral-discspine-osteology-unlabeled-orthopaedics-frank-h-netter–1438.html Illustration of Lumbar Vertebrae and Intervertebral Disc. Spine: Osteology from the Netter Collection. C. Elsevier Inc. All rights reserved.
9. Wallace, M. University of California San Diego Dept. of Anesthesiology Center for Pain Medicine Core curriculum syllabus; 2012.
10. Allegri M, Montella S, Salici F, *et al.* Mechanisms of low back pain: a guide for diagnosis and therapy. *F1000Res.* 2016;5:F1000 Faculty Rev–1530. Published 2016 Jun 28. doi:10.12688/f1000research.8105.2
11. Bogduk, N. Diskography. *APS J.* 1994;3(3):149–154.
12. García-Cosamalón J, del Valle ME, Calavia MG, *et al.* Intervertebral disc, sensory nerves and neurotrophins: who is who in discogenic pain? *J Anat.* 2010;217(1):1–15. doi:10.1111/j.1469–7580.2010. 01227.x
13. Aprill C, Bogduk N. High-intensity zone: a diagnostic sign of painful lumbar disc on magnetic resonance imaging. *Br J Radiol.* 1992;65(773):361–369. doi:10.1259/0007-1285-65-773-361
14. Guyer RD, Ohnmeiss DD. Lumbar discography. Position statement from the North American Spine Society Diagnostic and Therapeutic Committee. *Spine (Phila Pa 1976).* 1995;20(18):2048–2059.

15. Grönblad M, Weinstein JN, Santavirta S. Immunohistochemical observations on spinal tissue innervation. A review of hypothetical mechanisms of back pain. *Acta Orthop Scand.* 1991;62(6):614–622. doi:10.3109/17453679108994512
16. Pionchon H, Tommasi M, Pialat J, *et al.* Etude de l'innervation des ligaments rachidiens à l'étage lombaire [Study of the innervation of the spinal ligaments at the lumbar level]. *Bull Assoc Anat (Nancy).* 1986;70(210):63–67.
17. Rhalmi S, Yahia LH, Newman N, Isler M. Immunohistochemical study of nerves in lumbar spine ligaments. *Spine (Phila Pa 1976).* 1993;18(2):264–267. doi:10.1097/00007632-199302000-00015
18. Inoue N, Orías AAE, Segami K. Biomechanics of the Lumbar Facet Joint. *Spine Surg Relat Res.* 2019;4(1):1–7. doi:10.22603/ssrr.2019–0017
19. Iannuccilli JD, Prince EA, Soares GM. Interventional spine procedures for management of chronic low back pain-a primer. *Semin Intervent Radiol.* 2013;30(3):307–317. doi:10.1055/s-0033–1353484
20. Fortin JD, Dwyer AP, West S, Pier J. Sacroiliac joint: pain referral maps upon applying a new injection/arthrography technique. Part I: Asymptomatic volunteers. *Spine (Phila Pa 1976).* 1994;19(13):1475–1482.
21. Omarker K, Myers RR. Pathogenesis of sciatic pain: role of herniated nucleus pulposus and deformation of spinal nerve root and dorsal root ganglion. *Pain.* 1998;78(2):99–105. doi:10.1016/s0304-3959(98)00119-5
22. Olmarker K, Rydevik B, Nordborg C. Autologous nucleus pulposus induces neurophysiologic and histologic changes in porcine cauda equina nerve roots. *Spine (Phila Pa 1976).* 1993;18(11):1425–1432.
23. Saxler G, Brankamp J, von Knoch M, Löer F, Hilken G, Hanesch U. The density of nociceptive SP- and CGRP-immunopositive nerve fibers in the dura mater lumbalis of rats is enhanced after laminectomy, even after application of autologous fat grafts. *Eur Spine J.* 2008;17(10):1362–1372. doi:10.1007/s00586-008-0741-7
24. Desai MJ, Saini V, Saini S. Myofascial pain syndrome: a treatment review. *Pain Ther.* 2013;2(1):21-36. doi:10.1007/s40122-013-0006-y
25. Hagg, G. M. Static work load and occupational myalgia: a new explanation model, *Electromyographical Kinesiology,* 1991;141–144.
26. Kaergaard A, Andersen JH. Musculoskeletal disorders of the neck and shoulders in female sewing machine operators: prevalence, incidence, and prognosis. *Occup Environ Med.* 2000;57(8):528–534. doi:10.1136/oem.57.8.528
27. Yeoman's test, Kemp's test. (2018, August 30). *Physiopedia.* Retrieved 21:30, June 28, 2020 from https://www.physio-pedia.com/index.php?title=Yeoman%27s_Test&oldid=197126.
28. Brown MF, Hukkanen MV, McCarthy ID, *et al.* Sensory and sympathetic innervation of the vertebral endplate in patients with degenerative disc disease. *J Bone Joint Surg Br.* 1997;79(1):147–153. doi:10.1302/0301–620x.79b1.6814
29. Antonacci MD, Mody DR, Heggeness MH. Innervation of the human vertebral body: a histologic study. *J Spinal Disord.* 1998;11(6):526–531.
30. Freynhagen R, Baron R. The evaluation of neuropathic components in low back pain. *Curr Pain Headache Rep.* 2009;13(3):185-190. doi:10.1007/s11916-009-0032-y
31. Gardner A, Gardner E, Morley T. Cauda equina syndrome: a review of the current clinical and medico-legal position. *Eur Spine J.* 2011;20(5):690-697. doi:10.1007/s00586-010-1668-3
32. Rao D, Scuderi G, Scuderi C, Grewal R, Sandhu SJ. The Use of Imaging in Management of Patients with Low Back Pain. *J Clin Imaging Sci.* 2018;8:30. doi: 10.4103/jcis.JCIS_16_18
33. Bratton RL. Assessment and management of acute low back pain. *Am Fam Physician.* 1999;60(8):2299–2308.

34. D'Souza RS, Dowling TJ, Law L. Waddell Sign. In: *StatPearls*. Treasure Island (FL): StatPearls Publishing; 2020.
35. Camino Willhuber GO, Piuzzi NS. Straight Leg Raise Test. In: *StatPearls*. Treasure Island (FL): StatPearls Publishing; 2020.
36. Raj MA, Varacallo M. Sacroiliac (SI) Joint Pain. In: *StatPearls*. Treasure Island (FL): StatPearls Publishing; 2020.
37. Visser LH, Woudenberg NP, de Bont J, *et al*. Treatment of the sacroiliac joint in patients with leg pain: a randomized-controlled trial. *Eur Spine J*. 2013;22(10):2310-2317. doi:10.1007/s00586-013-2833-2
38. Figliuzzi A, Alvarez R, Al-Dhahir MA. Achilles Reflex. In: *StatPearls*. Treasure Island (FL): StatPearls Publishing; 2020.
39. Ginanneschi F, Mondelli M, Piu P, Rossi A. Pathophysiology of knee jerk reflex abnormalities in L5 root injury. *Funct Neurol*. 2015;30(3):187–191. doi:10.11138/fneur/2015.30.3.187
40. Wáng YXJ, Wu AM, Ruiz Santiago F, Nogueira-Barbosa MH. Informed appropriate imaging for low back pain management: A narrative review. *J Orthop Translat*. 2018;15:21–34. doi: 10.1016/j.jot.2018.07.009
41. Callaghan BC, Burke JF, Feldman EL. Electrodiagnostic Tests in Polyneuropathy and Radiculopathy. *JAMA*. 2016;315(3):297–298. doi:10.1001/jama.2015.16832
42. Müller M, Curatolo M, Limacher A, *et al*. Predicting transition from acute to chronic low back pain with quantitative sensory tests-A prospective cohort study in the primary care setting. *Eur J Pain*. 2019;23(5):894–907. doi:10.1002/ejp.1356
43. O'Neill S, Manniche C, Graven-Nielsen T, Arendt-Nielsen L. Generalized deep-tissue hyperalgesia in patients with chronic low-back pain. *Eur J Pain*. 2007;11(4):415–420. doi: 10.1016/j.ejpain.2006.05.009
44. Chou R. Pharmacological management of low back pain. *Drugs*. 2010;70(4):387–402. doi:10.2165/11318690-000000000-00000
45. Shanthanna H, Gilron I, Thabane L, *et al*. Gabapentinoids for chronic low back pain: a protocol for systematic review and meta-analysis of randomised controlled trials. *BMJ Open*. 2016;6(11):e013200. doi:10.1136/bmjopen-2016–013200
46. D'Souza RS, Hooten WM. Extrapyramidal Symptoms (EPS). In: *StatPearls*. Treasure Island (FL): StatPearls Publishing; 2020.
47. Nicol AL, Hurley RW, Benzon HT. Alternatives to opioids in the pharmacologic management of chronic pain syndromes: a narrative review of randomized, controlled, and blinded clinical trials. *Anesth Analg*. 2017;125(5):1682–1703. doi:10.1213/ANE.0000000000002426
48. Barreveld A, Witte J, Chahal H, Durieux ME, Strichartz G. Preventive analgesia by local anesthetics: the reduction of postoperative pain by peripheral nerve blocks and intravenous drugs. *Anesth Analg*. 2013;116(5):1141–1161. doi:10.1213/ANE.0b013e318277a270
49. Christie GC. The President's Commission on Combating Drug Addiction and the Opioid Crisis Interim Report, 2017. Retrieved June 28th 2020 from https://www.whitehouse.gov/sites/whitehouse.gov/files/images/Final_Report_Draft_11-1-2017.pdf.
50. Dowell D, Haegerich TM, Chou R. CDC guideline for prescribing opioids for chronic pain—United States, 2016 [published correction appears in MMWR Recomm Rep. 2016;65(11):295]. *MMWR Recomm Rep*. 2016;65(1):1–49. doi:10.15585/mmwr. rr6501e1
51. Chou R, Fanciullo GJ, Fine PG, *et al*. Clinical guidelines for the use of chronic opioid therapy in chronic noncancer pain, *J Pain*, 2014;10(2):113–130.
52. Blendon RJ, Benson JM. The public and the opioid-abuse epidemic. *N Engl J Med*. 2018;378(5):407–411. doi:10.1056/NEJMp1714529
53. Saeidian SR, Pipelzadeh MR, Rasras S, Zeinali M. Effect of trigger point injection on lumbosacral radiculopathy source. *Anesth Pain Med*. 2014;4(4):e15500. doi:10.5812/aapm.15500

54. Borg-Stein J. Treatment of fibromyalgia, myofascial pain, and related disorders. *Phys Med Rehabil Clin N Am.* 2006;17(2):491–viii. doi:10.1016/j.pmr.2005.12.003
55. Cohen SP, Chen Y, Neufeld NJ. Sacroiliac joint pain: a comprehensive review of epidemiology, diagnosis and treatment. *Expert Rev Neurother.* 2013;13(1):99–116. doi:10.1586/ern.12.148
56. Shuang F, Hou SX, Zhu JL, *et al.* Clinical anatomy and measurement of the medial branch of the spinal dorsal ramus. *Medicine (Baltimore).* 2015;94(52):e2367. doi:10.1097/MD.0000000000002367
57. Van Zundert J, Vanelderen P, Kessels A, van Kleef M. Radiofrequency treatment of facet-related pain: evidence and controversies. *Curr Pain Headache Rep.* 2012;16(1):19–25. doi:10.1007/s11916-011-0237-8
58. De Leon-Casasola O. Intrathecal Therapy for the Management of Cancer and Noncancer Pain, Anesthesiology News, 2009;74–86.
59. Wallace M, Staats P. *Pain Medicine & Management: Just the Facts.* 2nd Edition New York, McGraw-Hill, 2005;398–402.
60. Atkinson L, Sundaraj SR, Brooker C, *et al.* Recommendations for patient selection in spinal cord stimulation. *J Clin Neurosci.* 2011;18(10):1295–1302. doi: 10.1016/j.jocn.2011.02.025
61. Barolat G, Oakley JC, Law JD, North RB, Ketcik B, Sharan A. Epidural spinal cord stimulation with a multiple electrode paddle lead is effective in treating intractable low back pain. *Neuromodulation.* 2001;4(2):59–66. doi:10.1046/j.1525–1403.2001. 00059.x
62. Chapman KB, Groenen PS, Patel KV, Vissers KC, van Helmond N. T12 dorsal root ganglion stimulation to treat chronic low back pain: a case series. *Neuromodulation.* 2020;23(2):203–212. doi:10.1111/ner.13047
63. Grider JS, Manchikanti L, Carayannopoulos A, *et al.* Effectiveness of spinal cord stimulation in chronic spinal pain: a systematic review. *Pain Physician.* 2016;19(1): E33–E54.
64. Ishak B, Campos B, Brunn H, Unterberg AW, Ahmadi R. Feasibility, safety, and efficacy of subcutaneous peripheral nerve field stimulation for the treatment of refractory low back pain: a two-year single-center study. *Neuroscience.* 2018;387:38–47. doi: 10.1016/j.neuroscience.2017.12.011
65. Kabir SM, Gupta SR, Casey AT. Lumbar interspinous spacers: a systematic review of clinical and biomechanical evidence. *Spine (Phila Pa 1976).* 2010;35(25):E1499–E1506. doi:10.1097/BRS.0b013e3181e9af93
66. Bini W, Miller LE, Block JE. Minimally invasive treatment of moderate lumbar spinal stenosis with the superion interspinous spacer. *Open Orthop J.* 2011;5:361–367. doi:10.2174/1874325001105010361
67. Darr E, Meyer SC, Whang PG, *et al.* Long-term prospective outcomes after minimally invasive trans-iliac sacroiliac joint fusion using triangular titanium implants. *Med Devices (Auckl).* 2018;11:113–121. doi:10.2147/MDER.S160989
68. Claus CF, Lytle E, Kaufmann A, *et al.* Minimally invasive sacroiliac joint fusion using triangular titanium versus cylindrical threaded implants: a comparison of patient-reported outcomes. *World Neurosurg.* 2020;133:e745–e750. doi: 10.1016/j.wneu.2019.09.150
69. Polly DW, Swofford J, Whang PG, *et al.* Two-year outcomes from a randomized controlled trial of minimally invasive sacroiliac joint fusion vs. non-surgical management for sacroiliac joint dysfunction. *Int J Spine Surg.* 2016;10:28. doi:10.14444/3028
70. Deer TR, Kapural L. New image-guided ultra-minimally invasive lumbar decompression method: the mild procedure. *Pain Physician.* 2010;13(1):35–41.
71. Garfin SR, Yuan HA, Reiley MA. New technologies in spine: kyphoplasty and vertebroplasty for the treatment of painful osteoporotic compression fractures. *Spine (Phila Pa 1976).* 2001;26(14):1511–1515. doi:10.1097/00007632-200107150-00002

72. Khalil JG, Smuck M, Koreckij T, *et al.* A prospective, randomized, multicenter study of intraosseous basivertebral nerve ablation for the treatment of chronic low back pain. *Spine J.* 2019;19(10):1620–1632. doi: 10.1016/j.spinee.2019.05.598
73. Fischgrund JS, Rhyne A, Franke J, *et al.* Intraosseous basivertebral nerve ablation for the treatment of chronic low back pain: 2-year results from a prospective randomized double-blind sham-controlled multicenter study. *Int J Spine Surg.* 2019;13(2):110–119. doi:10.14444/6015

Index

Note: Page numbers in *italics* indicate a figure and page numbers in **bold** indicate a table on the corresponding page.

D

I

K

L

M

Q

R

S

T

FSC
www.fsc.org
MIX
Papier | Fördert gute Waldnutzung
FSC® C083411

Kolibri 360 GmbH
Ferdinand-Jühlke-Straße 7
99095 Erfurt, Deutschland
produktsicherheit@kolibri360.de